Amyotrophic Lateral Sclerosis

A synthesis of research and clinical practic

Amyotrophic lateral sclerosis (ALS), otherwise known as Lou Gehrig's disease or motoneuron disease, is one of several degenerative diseases of the ageing nervous system. Commonly affecting those in their mid-50s and beyond, it is a progressive illness resulting in death within a few years. The decade of the brain has seen an explosion in research into this particular condition, which this text neatly synthesizes to construct a detailed and comprehensive overview. From its epidemiology, molecular biology and pathophysiology right through to clinical assessment and care, Professor Eisen and Doctor Krieger use their research expertise and extensive clinical experience to provide this practical and thought-provoking account.

> The range of subjects covered is astonishing ... their reviews are comprehensive and sophisticated. Their writing is clear and the several controversies are given balanced reviews. The ample illustrations have been selected thoughtfully ... This book ought to appeal to practising neurologists, medical students and residents and other health care workers involved with people who have ALS. Anyone interested in ALS will find material for thought and for practice.

From the Foreword by Professor L. P. Rowland.

Andrew Eisen is Professor of Neurology at the University of British Columbia and Head of the Neuromuscular Diseases Unit, Vancouver General Hospital, Canada. He has a particular interest in electromyography, spinal cord disease and ALS. Past President of both the Canadian Society of Clinical Neurophysiologists and the American Association of Electrodiagnostic Medicine, he has published 120 articles in prestigious medical journals, including 29 papers devoted to ALS. In addition to authorship of this book, he is an editor of two earlier publications on spinal cord disease: *Diseases of the Spinal Cord* (1992) and *Spinal Cord Disease: Basic Science, Diagnosis and Management* (1997).

Charles Krieger is Associate Professor of Neurology at the University of British Columbia, Vancouver, Canada, and has been involved in the care of ALS patients for more than 15 years. During this time his extensive research studies into the cause of ALS have resulted in the publication of more than 35 important original articles.

AMYOTROPHIC LATERAL SCLEROSIS

A synthesis of research and clinical practice

ANDREW EISEN

and

CHARLES KRIEGER

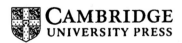

CAMBRIDGE
UNIVERSITY PRESS

CAMBRIDGE UNIVERSITY PRESS
Cambridge, New York, Melbourne, Madrid, Cape Town, Singapore, São Paulo

Cambridge University Press
The Edinburgh Building, Cambridge CB2 2RU, UK

Published in the United States of America by Cambridge University Press, New York

www.cambridge.org
Information on this title: www.cambridge.org/9780521581035

First published 1998
This digitally printed first paperback version 2006

A catalogue record for this publication is available from the British Library

Library of Congress Cataloguing in Publication data
Eisen, Andrew, 1936–
   Amyotrophic lateral sclerosis: synthesis of research and clinical
   practice/by Andrew Eisen and Charles Krieger.
      p. cm.
   ISBN 0 521 58103 6 (hb)
   1. Amyotrophic lateral sclerosis.   I. Krieger, Charles, 1954–.
   II. Title.
   [DNLM: 1. Amyotrophic Lateral Sclerosis.]
   RC406.A24E37   1998
   616.8'3–dc21   97-42597 CIP

ISBN-13 978-0-521-58103-5 hardback
ISBN-10 0-521-58103-6 hardback

ISBN-13 978-0-521-03426-5 paperback
ISBN-10 0-521-03426-4 paperback

To our wives, Kathleen and Alisa, and to the 700 patients with ALS who we have seen and whose plight has given us continual inspiration

Contents

Foreword

The past five years have seen the publication of several books on amyotrophic lateral sclerosis (ALS). Why another one now? Several answers are evident. Some of the previous books were focused on clinical management, or diagnosis, or pathology. None has been as comprehensive as this volume of Professor Eisen and his colleague Dr Krieger. The writing here is seamless, in contrast to multi-authored books. The range of subjects covered is astonishing, especially for a veteran like me. I can remember when there was almost no research on ALS, because there was not much to do except for clinico-pathological correlations. This book, however, considers the whole range in depth from epidemiology to clinical features. Why the predominance in men? How does age at onset or family history affect prognosis? What accounts for clusters? What is the current interpretation of the high incidence on Guam? The differential diagnosis is discussed in detail, including a judicious presentation of motoneuropathy. The authors also provide a full description of cellular pathology and theories of pathogenesis, including inherited human and mouse diseases, and transgenic murine models. Questions are raised and answered about the significance of ubiquitination, Bunina bodies, Lewy bodies, and neurofilaments. Apoptosis is explained. In a detailed discussion of pathogenesis, the authors consider the excitotoxic theory of pathogenesis, which they favour, and the autoimmune theory, which they find wanting. Naturally, electrophysiology gets full treatment, including the authors' theory that the disease begins in the upper motoneuron rather than in both upper and lower motoneurons simultaneously. In addition to the details of electromyography and nerve conduction studies, they also explain the use of transcranial magnetic stimulation. Modern imaging is advancing even in ALS, and includes magnetic resonance spectroscopy, which is also presented clearly. The authors are judicious in describing symptomatic therapy and they are optimistic about prospects for truly effective therapy in the near future.

In all of this, their reviews are comprehensive and sophisticated. Their writing is clear and the several controversies are given balanced reviews. The ample illustrations have been selected thoughtfully; the references are complete and up-to-date. This book ought to appeal to practising neurologists, medical students and residents and other health care workers involved with people who have ALS. Anyone interested in ALS will find material for thought and for practice.

Lewis P. Rowland, MD

Preface

In my dreams I climb the mountains high,
In my dreams I face the samurai.
In my dreams I stroke my lover's hair,
In my dreams I travel everywhere.
In my dreams I kiss and never tell,
In my dreams I'm not a languid shell.
In my dreams I never convalesce,
In my dreams I don't have ALS.

Laugh, I Thought I'd Die – My Life With ALS

Dennis Kay, 1993

Amyotrophic lateral sclerosis (ALS) research has escalated considerably during this, 'the decade of the brain'. Frequently read neurological–neuroscience journals contain at least one article related to ALS in virtually each issue. A current Medline search reveals more than 1000 titles relevant to ALS or motoneuron disease (MND). The latter term is still commonly used synonymously with ALS in much of Europe. The Internet too has a growing number of WEB sites devoted to ALS, but one in particular (http://http1.brunel.ac.ukö8080/ ~ hssrsdn/alsig/alsig.htm) has a weekly digest that maintains much current information of interest to patients, their care-givers and professionals. The subcommittee on ALS and Motoneuron Diseases of the World Federation on Neuromuscular Diseases, a standing committee of the World Federation of Neurology, has substantially expanded its activities. In the last four years, the committee has developed the first formal classification of ALS, criteria and valid end-points for therapeutic trials and a worldwide consortium directed towards the collaborative performance of therapeutic trials. An annual meeting, devoted to ALS research, which originated in England just a few years ago, has become international and sizeable, with several countries bidding each year to host subsequent meetings. The associated International Alliances of ALS/MND now represent almost every country in the world.

Several excellent, edited, multi-author texts on ALS have been published within the last five years, but books written by a single or, as in this case, two authors are uncommon. Their slant is different, more focused and obviously biased by personal perspective. This monograph is derived from our examination of 664 patients with ALS seen since 1982. We have tried to review those aspects of ALS that presently occupy the forefront. Many people have made major contributions to these topics. Some we know personally and some are good friends. We have enjoyed reviewing their work, but the references at the end of the book aim to be current rather than complete. The experience of studying many patients with a single disease gives one the opportunity to think about the particular disorder in depth. This provokes speculation and commentary that is not always shared by conventional dictum. For this we make no apology and hope that our thoughts will encourage debate and further research.

The book has eight chapters, each emphasizing a particular aspect of the disease. The chapters have a summarizing paragraph or two and are written so that each is largely 'stand-alone' which has necessitated some replication. The eight chapters deal with epidemiology, clinical aspects, pathology, aetiopathogenesis, physiology, imaging, overlap syndromes and therapy. New information in ALS is surfacing so rapidly that even as we were preparing the manuscript, aspects that were current when we started have become outdated. For example, the hope for brain-derived neurotrophic factor (BDNF) as a therapy for ALS was not to be, and the first attempts at using intracranial delivery of another trophic factor glial cell-derived neurotrophic factor (GDNF) are underway.

Andrew Eisen
Charles Krieger

Acknowledgements

Professor Lewis P. Rowland has reviewed the manuscript. We appreciate his most thoughtful comments and his generous Foreword.

Our sincere thanks to Heather Stewart and Ellen Higgins for their editorial expertise and support, and thanks to the neurologists of British Columbia who over many years have entrusted their patients with ALS to us.

We are very grateful for the material supplied to us by Drs Samuel Chou, San Francisco; Stirling Carpenter, Toronto; Jean-Pierre Julien and Heather Durham, Montreal; Shoichi Sasaki, Tokyo; and Drs Kenneth Berry, Gillian Gibson and Tom Beach in Vancouver.

Abbreviations

AA	amino acid
AALS	Appel rating scale for amyotrophic lateral sclerosis
AD	Alzheimer's disease
ALS	amyotrophic lateral sclerosis
AMPA	α-amino-3-hydroxy-5-methyl-1,4-isoxazole-proprionic acid
ASP	[^{3}H]-D-aspartate
BCAA	branched chain amino acid
BDNF	brain-derived neurotrophic factor
BIPAP	bimodal passive airway pressure
BMAA	β-N-methylamino-L-alanine
BOAA	β-N-oxalylamino-L-alanine
CaBP	calbindin-D$_{28K}$
CAG	repeating trinucleotide sequence
CaMKII	Ca^{2+} calmodulin-dependent kinase II
CB	calbindin
CDF	cholinergic differentiation factor
CGRP	calcitonin gene-related peptide
Cho	choline
CIDP	chronic idiopathic demyelinating polyneuropathy
CJD	Creutzfeldt–Jakob (Jakob–Creutzfeldt) disease
C–M	corticomotoneuronal
CMAP	compound muscle action potential
CNS	central nervous system
CNTF	ciliary neurotrophic factor
COPD	chronic obstructive pulmonary disease
Cr	creatine
CR	calretinin
CSF	cerebrospinal fluid
CT	computerized tomography
Cu	copper
Cu/Zn–SOD	copper/zinc–superoxide dismutase
CUSM	cumulative sum analysis
DAP	3,4-diaminopyridine
DDPAC	disinhibition–dementia–Parkinson–amyotrophy complex

DHEA	dehydroepiandrosterone
DHEAS	dehydroepiandrosterone sulphate
DNA	deoxyribonucleic acid
DOPAC	3,4-dihydroxyphenylacetic acid
DRG	dorsal root ganglion
DTR	deep tendon reflex
EAA	excitatory amino acid
EAAC1	glutamate transporter
EDC	extensor digitorum communis
EEG	electroencephalogram
EMG	electromyography
EPSP	excitatory postsynaptic potential
FALS	familial amyotrophic lateral sclerosis
FGF	fibroblast growth factor
FD	fluorodopa
FDA	Food and Drug Administration
FDG	$[^{18}F]$-2-fluoro-2-deoxy-D-glucose
FDI	first dorsal interosseus
F^1 H-MRS	functional H-magnetic resonance spectroscopy
FMRI	functional magnetic resonance imaging
FTD	frontotemporal dementia
FVC	forced vital capacity
GABA	γ-aminobutyric acid
G-ALS	Guamanian amyotrophic lateral sclerosis
GD1b	ganglioside GD1b
GDH	glutamate dehydrogenase
GDNF	glial cell-derived neurotrophic factor
GFAP	glial fibrillary acidic protein
GLAST	glial glutamate transporter
GLT-1	glutamate transporter-1
GLU	glutamate
GM1	ganglioside GM1
H_2O_2	hydrogen peroxide
HLA-DR	human leucocyte antigen-DR
^{1}H-MRS	proton magnetic resonance spectroscopy
IBM	inclusion body myositis
ICD	International Classification of Diseases
ICU	intensive care unit
IGF	insulin-like growth factor
IgG	immunoglobulin G
IL-6	interleukin-6
^{123}I-IMP	N-isopropyl-p-^{123}I-amphetamine
IVIg	intravenous immunoglobulin
KSP repeats	lysine–serine–proline repeats
LIF	leukaemia inhibitory factor
LMN	lower motoneuron
MAPK	mitogen-activated protein kinase
MEP	motor evoked potential
MHC	major histocompatibility complex
MMN	multifocal motor neuropathy
MMNCB	multifocal motor neuropathy with conduction block
mnd 1	motoneuron degeneration 1

MND	motoneuron disease
MOA-B	mono-oxidase-β inhibitor
MPTP	1-methyl-4-phenyl-1,2,3,6-tetrahydropyridine
MRC	Medical Research Council
MRI	magnetic resonance imaging
MRS	magnetic resonance spectroscopy
MS	multiple sclerosis
MSV	murine sarcoma virus
MUAP	motor unit action potential
MUP	motor unit potential
MUNE	motor unit numerical estimate
NA	N-acetyl acetate
NAA	N-acetyl aspartate
NAAG	N-acetyl aspartyl-glutamate
NAC	n-acetyl cysteine
NADH	nicotinamide adenine dinucleotide
NAIP	neuronal apoptosis inhibitory protein
NDA	new drug application
NGF	nerve growth factor
NF	neurofilament
NF-H	high molecular weight neurofilament
NF-L	low molecular weight neurofilament
NF-M	medium molecular weight neurofilament
NMDA	N-methyl-D-aspartate
NO	nitric oxide
NOS	nitric oxide synthase
NSAID	non-steroidal anti-inflammatory drug
NT-3	neurotrophin-3
NT-4	neurotrophin-4
O^{2-}	superoxide ion
$ONOO^-$	peroxynitrite anion
PCr	phosphocreatine
PD	Parkinson's disease
PEG	percutaneous endoscopically placed gastrostomy
PET	positron emission tomography
PKA	protein kinase A
PKC	protein kinase C
PKM	protein kinase M
PLS	primary lateral sclerosis
PMA	progressive muscular atrophy
PMP	peripheral myelin protein
PNS	peripheral nervous system
PP	protein phosphatase
PP1	protein phosphatase 1
PP2A	protein phosphatase 2A
PPMA	post-polio progressive muscular atrophy
PSMA	progressive spinal muscular atrophy
PSTH	peristimulus time histogram
PUMNS	possible upper motoneuron signs
PV	parvalbumin
rCBF	regional cerebral blood flow
rhCNTF	recombinant ciliary neurotrophic factor

rhIGF-1	myotrophin
SIP	sickness impact profile
SFEMG	single fibre electromyography
SMA	spinal muscular atrophy
SMN	survival motoneuron gene
SNAP	sensory nerve action potential
SOD1	superoxide dismutase
SPECT	single photon emission computed tomography
T	Tesla
99m Tc-Hm PAO	technetium-99m hexamethylpropylene amine
TGF-β	transforming growth factor-β
TMS	transcranial magnetic stimulation
TQNE	Tufts Quantitative Neuromuscular Exam
Trk	tyrosine kinase receptor
TrkC	receptor for NT-3
UMN	upper motoneuron
WFN	World Federation of Neurology

1
Epidemiological considerations

Demographics

The demographic, epidemiological and electrophysiological data described in this and subsequent chapters are based on 664 patients with definite or probable amyotrophic lateral sclerosis (ALS) as defined by the El Escorial criteria (Brooks, 1994). All of the patients were examined by one of the authors (AE) between 1984 and 1996 (Table 1.1). The data are representative of typical populations of ALS patients as reported previously (Brooks, 1996). It is well established that the age-adjusted incidence of the neurodegenerative disorders (Alzheimer's disease (AD), Parkinson's disease (PD) and ALS) rises sharply with ageing and, as shown in Figure 1.1, this is true for our own data.

Gender

The overall male:female ratio of our cohort was 1.33:1. Epidemiological studies of sporadic ALS unanimously agree that the disease is more frequent in men, although the male:female ratios quoted are variable. In older patients, particularly those over 65 years, the male:female ratio begins to approach 1:1 (Chancellor et al., 1993a). Based on our own data, there is a significant negative correlation between age and the male:female ratio of ALS. This is shown in Figure 1.2, and it probably reflects the greater longevity enjoyed by women. However, this benefit is limited because of an increased risk of developing ALS. In younger patients (those less than 40 years) there is a much higher frequency of ALS amongst young men (Christensen, Hojer-Pedersen and Jensen, 1990; Strong, Hudson and Alvord, 1991; Eisen et al., 1993c). But, as is shown in Figure 1.2, there is a significant correlation between age and the male:female ratio of ALS, and male predominance of ALS declines with each decade.

Table 1.1. *Demographics of patients seen in the British Columbia ALS Clinic between 1984 and 1996*

	All	Men	Women
Number	664	379	285
Mean age (years) ± SD	60.6 ± 13.65	59.5 ± 13.9	61.65 ± 12.9
Minimum age (years)	14	14	17
Maximum age (years)	89	89	89
Number with spinal onset (%)	445 (67)	283 (63.6)	162 (36.4)
Number with bulbar onset (%)	219 (33)	99 (45.2)	120 (54.8)
Mean duration (years)*	3.6 ± 3.1	4.0 ± 3.8	3.2 ± 2.5

* Based on 414 patients who were followed to time of death.

Total ALS Cohort N = 664

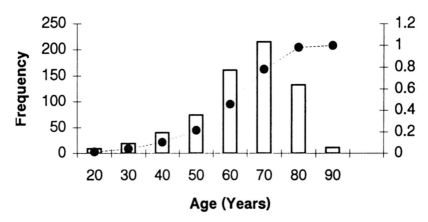

Figure 1.1. Frequency distribution by age of 664 patients with ALS. The raw data suggest that there is a decrease in frequency of ALS after about age 65 years. However, cumulative analysis, shown by the interrupted line, shows that amongst patients who do develop ALS, the frequency is highest in the elderly. Under 45 years, the chances of developing ALS are small but, as indicated, thereafter there is a steep rise in the frequency distribution curve. This might imply that the effects of neuronal ageing, which increases the risk of developing ALS, start in the fourth decade.

Others have made the same observation (Chancellor *et al.*, 1993a). Of our total patient population 46 (7 per cent) were aged 75 years or older when the diagnosis of ALS was made, and 28 of these were women, so that midway through the seventh decade of life the male:female ratio in favour

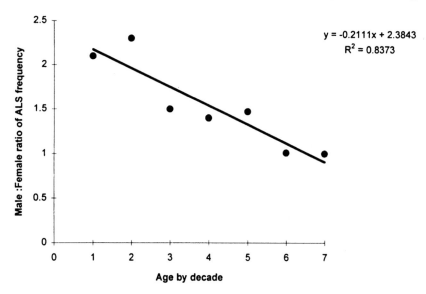

Figure 1.2. Relationship between age (x-axis) shown by decade and male:female ratio of ALS (y-axis). There is a linear decline in the ratio which in the young favours men, but by age 70 years there is an equal chance for men and women to develop ALS. In the old old (greater than 85 years) the frequency of ALS is higher in women.

of men had reversed (M:F = 0.6:1). The higher incidence of ALS in younger men is not readily explained. It may partly relate to the rate of decline in the serum concentrations of the neurosteroid dehydroepiandrosterone (DHEA). Serum concentrations of DHEAS, the sulphate of DHEA, normally declines with age. As shown in Figure 1.3, men with ALS have much lower age-predicted serum DHEAS concentrations than do women (Eisen, Pearmain and Stewart, 1995). Figure 1.3 shows the individual DHEAS concentrations expressed as a percentage of age-predicted normal values. We have measured serum DHEAS in 56 men and 35 women with ALS. In 63.2 per cent of men and 30.6 per cent of women, the DHEAS serum concentrations were below age-predicted values. This gives a male:female ratio of abnormal concentrations of about 2:1, which is similar to the usually quoted men:women ratio for ALS. The finding suggests that the greater frequency of lowered DHEAS concentrations in men plays a role in their greater risk of developing ALS. How this may happen is not known, but DHEA is discussed as a possible therapy for ALS in Chapter 7.

Men N = 56

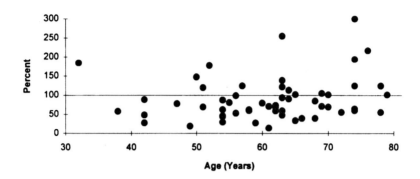

Women N = 35

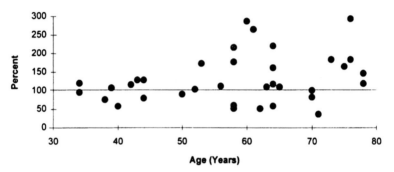

Figure 1.3. Scatterplot relating dehydroepiandrosterone sulphate (DHEAS) serum concentrations (ml/l) and patient's age. The values are expressed as a percentage of normal for the age. This is indicated by the solid line at 100 per cent. The serum DHEAS is frequently reduced in men (top scatterplot) but in only about a third of women.

Age

The frequency distribution of age of ALS onset for all patients is shown in Figure 1.4. The same figure also shows the frequency distribution for men and women separately. The peak incidence for men occurred over a 15-year period between 55 and 70 years but for women there was a more steadily increasing incidence starting at about 50 years of age and reaching a peak at about 70 years. The gender difference can be explained by the larger number of younger men with ALS and the greater mean life-span of women. There are very few firm data regarding ALS in the elderly (aged 75

Women N = 285

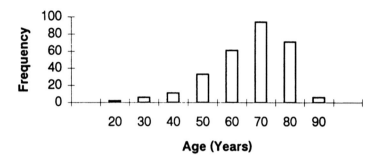

Men N = 379

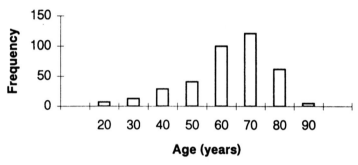

Figure 1.4. Histograms showing the frequency distribution by age for women and men with ALS. Overall, the peak age at which ALS developed in our cohort was 65–70 years. For women there is a steady rise in the frequency up to this age. For men the age range at which ALS develops is spread over the sixth and seventh decades.

years and over), but the apparent decrease in the incidence of ALS after age 70 years probably reflects a rapidly rising mortality rate after this age from other diseases that compete with the probability of developing ALS. Also, progressive loss of strength and difficulty in walking in elderly subjects who are frequently frail may be easily discarded as simply being due to 'old age' and the possibility of ALS is overlooked. This too would erroneously lower incidence of the disease in the elderly.

ALS commencing under the age of 40–45 years is well recognized but unusual. The incidence of young sporadic ALS may be increasing, but present data are insufficient to make a firm statement on this point. Eighty-three of our patients (52 men and 31 women) were aged 45 years

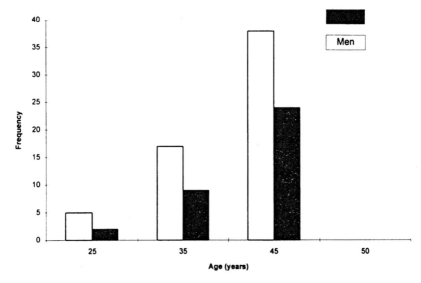

Figure 1.5. Young-onset ALS. This is defined as an onset at, or less than, 45 years of age. As shown in the bar chart, the frequency of young-onset disease in men is much greater than in women.

or younger (Fig. 1.5). Why young men develop ALS so much more frequently than young women is not known. Most young-onset disease turns out to be typical sporadic ALS, but lower motoneuron features often predominate for many months. During this period there are several disorders, mimicking ALS, which are commoner in younger patients. Progressive muscular atrophy (PMA), Kennedy's syndrome (X-linked progressive bulbar spinal muscular atrophy) and Ben Hamida syndrome, better known as juvenile ALS, need to be considered. Ben Hamida syndrome is inherited as an autosomal recessive trait and progresses very slowly. However, a specific genetic defect has not been identified and it is probably better to refer to these disorders as Ben Hamida variants (Ben Hamida, Hentati and Ben Hamida, 1990). They seem to be largely restricted to Tunisia, Turkey and possibly other mid-Eastern countries which border the Mediterranean Sea. Three clinical subgroups have been identified. Group 1 is characterized by upper limb amyotrophy and spastic paraplegia, combining upper and lower motoneuron deficits. There may also be bulbar involvement. This group most closely resembles classic sporadic ALS. Group 2 combines hereditary spastic paraplegia with peroneal atrophy. Group 3 is essentially primary lateral sclerosis with minimal lower motoneuron features involving the hand or peroneal musculature. These and other disorders that resemble ALS are discussed further in Chapter 2.

Increasing mortality

The incidence of a disease refers to the number of new cases in a population over a given time, which for ALS is usually expressed as the number of new cases per 100 000 population per year. Globally, the incidence of ALS varies from about 0.3 to over 2 per 100 000 population. Incidence rates are used to establish the prevalence of ALS, which is defined as the total number of patients per 100 000 population. The prevalence of ALS varies from about 2.5 to 4.5 times that of its incidence (a low of 0.75–9 per 100 000 population). Prevalance rates are more variable than incidence rates because they are dependent upon disease duration, which varies with the level of care and other factors. For example, survival is likely to be prolonged by early implementation of bimodal passive airway pressure (BIPAP) and percutaneous endoscopically placed gastrostomy (PEG) (Hopkins, Tatarian and Pianta, 1996; Kasarskis and Neville, 1996). Prevalence will be increased in the future as 'palliative' therapies such as riluzole are developed (Brooks, 1996). Mortality rates are defined as the number of deaths annually per 100 000 population, and these are increasing for ALS as the population ages (Lillienfeld *et al.*, 1989; Kurtzke, 1991; Chancellor and Warlow, 1992; Briani *et al.*, 1996; Brooks, 1996). There is a close association between increased life expectancy and increasing mortality from ALS (Neilson *et al.*, 1993; Brooks, 1996). Life expectancy has risen, and continues to rise. It has been estimated that by the year 2021, deaths from ALS will have increased by approximately 20 per cent (Neilson *et al.*, 1993). By the year 2000, the USA will have over 5 million people who are 85 years and older and more than 10 million people who are over the age of 65 years. Based upon available data from 18 different countries, between 1951 to 1958, the mean worldwide age-adjusted death rate from ALS was 0.76 ± 0.28 per 100 000 population. For the years 1966–1971, this had doubled to 1.37 ± 0.41 per 100 000 population ($p < 0.0001$). Between 1985 and 1992, the worldwide mortality from ALS exceeded 2 per 100 000 population and within the last five years is approaching 3 per 100 000 (Brooks, 1996).

Incidence rates have also shown similar significant increases. Before 1975, the incidence rate of ALS per 100 000 population was 0.99 ± 0.41, since when it has steadily risen to 1.3 ± 0.63 ($p < 0.01$). Mortality rates from ALS are a reasonable approximation of its incidence, and increasing mortality rates from ALS have been interpreted to indicate that there has been an increase in the incidence of ALS (Chancellor *et al.*, 1993b; Neilson *et al.*, 1993). The accuracy of mortality data is dependent on the vagaries of death certificates and definition of disease. As a group of disorders becomes better clarified so that they can be separated into definitive entities, the International Classification of Diseases (ICD) also changes. Prior to 1969, ALS was not separated from other sporadic or familial motoneuron diseases (MND). However, non-ALS MND patients comprise only a small fraction of the total number of MND cases so that their inclusion is unlikely to have significantly biased the results. If anything, the incidence would have been overestimated. Recent evidence, from the UK, indicates that the diagnostic accuracy of ALS based upon death certificates has a positive predictive value of 90 per cent, with a false-negative rate of 6 per cent (Chancellor *et al.*, 1993b). Similar studies regarding the diagnostic accurracy of ALS based on death certificates need to be done in North America to confirm the same high predictive value in that and other continents. On the other hand, coded hospital discharge data are inaccurate for ascertaining a diagnosis of ALS and in their present form cannot be used reliably to measure disease incidence. Possible explanations for the recent increase in the incidence of ALS are (1) better case ascertainment, (2) improved diagnosis, (3) increasing longevity, and (4) survival of a susceptible subpopulation who survived other potentially fatal diseases earlier in life, and who are now at risk for developing ALS.

It is unlikely that improved diagnosis or better case ascertainment can fully explain the increased incidence of ALS in the developed countries, but this may be a factor in underdeveloped countries. Although most non-neurologists may only see one or two cases of ALS during their careers, few patients with ALS in developed countries fail to reach the attention of a neurologist during the course of their disease. The diagnosis remains dependent upon a clinical constellation, and this has not substantially changed since Charcot's time. The El Escorial diagnostic criteria are detailed in Chapter 2 and should help exclude diseases mimicking ALS that could falsely increase the recorded disease incidence (Brooks, 1994).

Laboratory aids other than electromyography have not helped in the confirmation of ALS. Improved diagnostic imaging has been helpful in revealing structural lesions in patients who appear to have ALS. These diagnostic techniques would tend to decrease the apparent incidence of ALS.

Geographic distribution

The incidence rates of ALS vary in different places. Although these figures are confounded by non-standardized case ascertainment and diagnosis, they suggest a correlation between age-specific incidence of ALS and distance from the Equator (Chancellor and Warlow, 1992). If one excludes areas within the South Pacific in which there are high, albeit declining, incidences of ALS, it is widely believed that the incidence of ALS throughout the rest of the world is uniform and the reported variations are thought to reflect inaccuracies in ascertainment. However, Chancellor and Warlow (1992) reviewed the incidence rates for ALS from nine surveys which were judged to have nearly complete case ascertainment. The crude annual incidence rates ranged from a low of 0.6 per 100 000 to a high of 2.6 per 100 000. When the incidence rates were standardized to the Scottish population, the differences were statistically significant, suggesting a true geographic variation. Other studies have also shown there to be a relationship between the incidence of ALS and latitude (Eisen and Calne, 1992; McGuire *et al.*, 1996; Brooks, 1996). Like multiple sclerosis, there is a significant positive correlation between incidence of ALS and latitude degrees north ($p < 0.001$) (Fig. 1.6). These data might imply a transmittable agent which is more readily expressed in northern climates. It could also be that populations living in northern latitudes have a lifestyle that renders them more susceptible to a toxin(s) which may be of importance in developing ALS. The issue of geographic variation in ALS incidence is worthy of further investigation. If such a relationship can be firmly established, it would support an environmental role in ALS, or a role of different geographic racial groups, some with a greater abundance of susceptibility genes for ALS.

Disease duration, prognosis and life expectancy

A question that is frequently asked by newly diagnosed ALS patients and their families concerns the length of their expected survival. Because ALS has such a variable progression, this question is difficult to answer for any given individual when initially seen. Disability scores, which include manual muscle testing as well as computerized measures of isometric muscle strength (Tufts Quantitative Neuromuscular Exam, TQNE), can be used to assess the rate of disease progression. These assessments indicate that over much of its course the clinical decline of ALS is linear and it is possible to predict an individual's rate of progression by

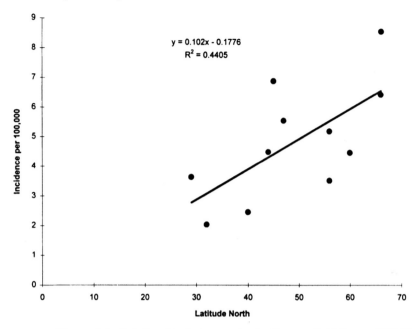

Figure 1.6. Relationship between the incidence of ALS per 100 000 population and the latitude in degrees north. The data are derived from epidemiological studies in the literature that were considered to have near-complete ascertainment. The incidence of ALS is significantly higher in northern climes. The relationship is given by:

$$\text{incidence} = \text{latitude} \times 0.102 - 0.1776 \ (r^2 = 0.4404, \ p < 0.001).$$

calculation of the regression slope obtained from data points using TQNE and other scales. However, to construct and calculate the slope of the regression line which is used to determine the length of survival of an individual, two or more data points must be acquired over several months. This does not allow one to comment on an individual's anticipated survival at the first visit. Appel and colleagues (1987) developed a quantitative measure of clinical function, the Appel Rating Scale. This is based upon the patient's swallowing ability, speech, respiratory function and muscle strength and function. For a given patient, this score has been shown to increase linearly with time, but the rate of progression varies twenty-fold between different patients. However, a change in the score of the Appel Rating Scale of greater than 22 points over 6 months is predictive of death within a year. Jablecki, Berry and Leach (1989) have devised a simple composite predictive score based upon the patient's age at the time of clinical examination, the duration of muscle weakness, and an estimate of the clinical disability. Several electrophysiological measures also correlate to some degree with prognosis and survival of ALS patients. The best and easiest to measure is the amplitude of the compound muscle action potential (CMAP). The presence of low-amplitude CMAPs is associated with a poor prognosis, especially when they are recorded from several different muscles that are segmentally distinct and in a multi-myotomal pattern (Daube, 1985).

There are other factors that might determine the rate of progression of ALS and the length of survival. These include the site of initial clinical involvement, referral patterns and the patient's age at the time of disease onset. A bulbar onset is often considered to be associated with a shorter survival (Salemi *et al.*, 1989; Tysnes, Vollset and Aarli, 1991). However, patients having a bulbar onset are usually older than those with a spinal onset, and when age of onset is factored into the equation bulbar onset is not a significant prognostic index (Eisen *et al.*, 1993c). Referral selection may also predict survival in ALS. Lee *et al.* (1995) followed two cohorts of ALS patients. The first cohort consisted of non-referred ALS cases from Harris County, Texas, diagnosed between 1985 and 1988. The second comprised patients from a tertiary care centre in Houston, Texas, diagnosed between 1977 and 1989. Three-year survival was similar in the two groups (29 per cent and 32 per cent respectively). However, five-year survival was only 4 per cent in the incident cohort compared to 21 per cent in the referral cohort. The difference could not be explained by the distributions of prognostic factors in the two cohorts and was considered to be due to stronger, unfavourable effects of prognostic factors (older age at diagnosis, bulbar onset, positive family history of ALS) in the incident cohort.

The age at which clinical deficit becomes noticeable is probably one of the best predictors of survival. Younger patients live longer (Christensen *et al.*, 1990; Strong *et al.*, 1991; Eisen *et al.*, 1993c; Lee, Annegers and Appel, 1995). This is also true for hereditary ALS (Strong *et al.*, 1991). The mean disease duration determined from our cohort of patients is 3.6 ± 3.1 years. It is slightly, but not significantly, longer for men compared to women (4.0 ± 3.8 years and 3.2 ± 2.5 years respectively). Figure 1.7 shows the second-order exponential relationship, for men and women, which best fitted the data relating onset age and disease duration. It also shows the 75th and 95th upper prediction bounds on disease duration at each age, and the corresponding life expectancy for the population of British Columbia for the years 1993–1995.

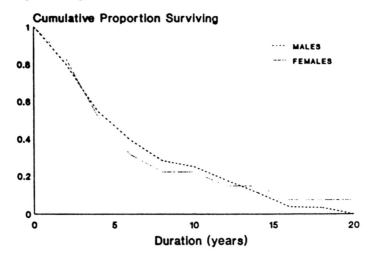

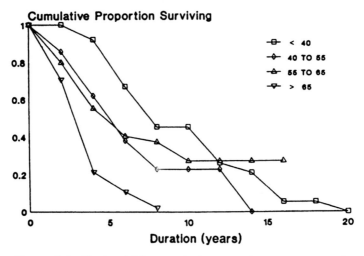

Figure 1.7. Kaplan–Meier survival curves by sex (top) and age (bottom). The survival curves are not significantly different for men and women. Age has a significant effect on survival of ALS, with patients who have a young onset living longer. Survival for the group aged 40 years or less is significantly longer than for those aged 40–55 years and 55–65 years (p = 0.02). The three survival curves for ages ⩽40 years, 40–55 years and 55–65 years are significantly better than for patients who are older than 65 years (p < 0.0001). (From Eisen *et al.* (1993b). *Muscle & Nerve*, **16**; 27–32. Reproduced with permission.)

Table 1.2. *Predicted survival (years) in ALS*

	Onset age (years)	Expected survival (years)	Percentile 75th	Percentile 95th	Life expectancy (years)
Women	30	11.5	27.4	48.7	51.5
	40	6.5	13.4	23.4	41.9
	50	4.1	7.8	13.5	32.5
	60	2.9	5.5	9.5	23.7
	70	2.0	4.6	8.0	15.8
	80	2.0	4.7	8.2	9.1
Men	20	14.1	37.4	74.2	55.4
	30	8.4	19.8	38.9	46.2
	40	5.4	11.9	23.2	36.9
	50	3.8	8.1	15.8	27.8
	60	2.9	6.3	12.2	19.6
	70	2.3	5.5	10.7	12.6
	80	2.1	5.4	10.7	7.4

After Eisen *et al.* (1993c).

This relationship is given by (Eisen *et al.*, 1993c):

$$\text{Disease duration} = \exp (3.93 - 0.07 \times \text{onset age} + 0.0004 \times \text{onset age}^2) \text{ (for men, p = 0.06)}$$

$$\text{Disease duration} = \exp (4.86 - 0.098 \times \text{onset age} + 0.0006 \times \text{onset age}^2) \text{ (for women, p = 0.12)}$$

For men who were 40 years of age or younger at onset, disease duration is significantly longer compared to all other age groups ($p < 0.001$) (Table 1.2). Even though disease duration in young women also appears longer than in other age groups, the numbers were too few for the difference to reach statistical significance. Table 1.2 shows that the differences in survival are significantly affected by age but not by sex. For patients who were 40 years or younger at onset, survival was significantly longer than for ages 41–55 and 56–65 ($p = 0.02$). All three of these age groups had a significantly longer survival compared to patients older than 65 years ($p = 0.0001$). Taken together, men and women below the age of 50 years have a disease duration significantly longer than those aged 61 years or older ($p < 0.001$). Survival analysis by Cox's proportional hazards model jointly by age and sex confirmed that age was a significant factor ($p \leqslant 0.0001$, coefficient 0.035 ± 0.008).

Risk factors for developing ALS

Age and gender are the only indisputable risk factors for sporadic ALS (Nelson, 1996). With the growth of an ageing population, it can be predicted that the incidence of ALS and other neurodegenerative diseases will significantly increase. If the incidence of ALS increases with age, the implication is that there must be a decrease in competing mortalities, but it is unclear how their decline impacts on age and a group of ageing individuals who are susceptible to developing ALS. Gender is a less certain risk factor. Our own data indicate that men have approximately a 30 per cent greater risk of developing ALS than do women. Some studies report data that indicate men have double the risk of developing ALS compared to women. However, as discussed above, the gender difference in the risk of developing ALS lessens with increasing age and by about 65 years of age both sexes are equally at risk (see Fig. 1.2).

In the 'old old', defined as patients over 85 years of age, it is likely that women will have a greater risk of developing ALS by virtue of their greater longevity. There is not a good explanation for the greater number of younger men developing ALS. However, the motoneuron is an androgen target tissue and the density of androgen receptors may be greater on those neurons that are preferentially affected in ALS. The possible role of DHEA in the development of ALS in younger men has already been discussed above. Women developing ALS often have a later menarche and an earlier menopause than usual, making a shorter reproductive period, which could suggest that oestrogens may be relatively protective.

There have been numerous epidemiological studies designed to identify specific risk factors for developing ALS (Brooks, 1996). Approaches that can be used are:

1. Cross-sectional prevalence studies, in which a sample of the general population is identified as to whether or not they have ALS and the risk factor of interest. This type of study provides relatively weak evidence with respect to causality and is not practical in ALS because of its low prevalence rate.
2. Cohort studies, which may be prospective or retrospective. In prospective studies a cohort would be defined having been exposed to a risk factor for a given period and followed for a fixed period to see if they develop ALS. In a cohort retrospective study, a group of ALS patients who have been exposed to a

potential risk factor are compared to a second ALS group of patients who have not been exposed to the factor. Each member of the two samples is then classified as to whether or not ALS developed during the period during which the sampled individuals were observed. This approach is also not practical because of the low incidence of ALS.

3. Case control studies. In a rare disorder such as ALS, these are ideally suited to determining the significance of a particular risk. A group of patients with and another group without ALS are identified and each of the members of the two groups is classified with respect to exposure of the possible risk factors(s). This is usually on the basis of an interview, or information from medical records. The size of the groups does not have to be large, and testing for multiple risk factors can be performed simultaneously. Problems can arise in case control studies because of bias in the selection of cases and controls. Furthermore, these studies depend on the recall of information of previous toxic exposures, which may be different in controls and patients with ALS. In a rare disease, such as ALS, case control studies are the best approach available when multiple exposure factors need to be considered.

The measure of disease risk is expressed as the 'odds ratio', which is the odds of exposure in the diseased cases, divided by the odds of exposure in control cases:

$$(a/c)/(b/d) = (a \times d)/(c \times b)$$

where a = has the disease and is exposed, b = does not have the disease but is exposed, c = has the disease but is not exposed, d = does not have the disease and is not exposed.

In ALS, which is a rare disease, the odds ratio is a reasonable estimate of the relative risk. This is expressed as a ratio of the incidence of ALS in the exposed group divided by the incidence in the unexposed group. A relative risk of 1 indicates that the particular exposure does not increase the risk of developing the disease. A relative risk of 2 indicates that the particular exposure is twice as likely to cause the disease. The precision of the relative risk can be defined in terms of confidence intervals. To date, age and gender are the only risk factors for ALS having significant effects (Norris *et al.*, 1992; Eisen *et al.*, 1993c). However, Table 1.3 lists some

Table 1.3. *Statistically significant industrial, occupational and other risk factors for ALS*

Factor	Number of ALS patients	Number of controls	Relative risk (odds ratio)
Trauma	841	791	5.9
Electrical injury	611	890	5.25
Welding, soldering	118	420	4.4
Heavy labour	175	319	2.3
Active sports	25	25	2.3
Solvents	46	92	2.2
Farming	2033	2416	1.8

Based on worldwide studies after Brooks (1996).

other risk factors, in order of their relative risk, that may be of relevance in the aetiopathogenesis of ALS.

In a recent pilot case control study, Strickland and colleagues (1996) estimated the odds ratios of several occupational and industrial exposures in 25 patients with ALS. Two control groups were used. They included 25 subjects from the community and 25 patients with other neuromuscular diseases, mainly myopathies, from the same centre as the ALS patients. The strongest association with ALS was exposure to welding or soldering materials (odds ratio 5.0). Other industrial exposures that showed large, non-significant differences included paint or pigment manufacturing, the petroleum industry, the printing industry and shipbuilding. An unproven, but potential, common candidate toxin for some of these could be lead or mercury.

Heavy metals

The possibility that heavy metal intoxication may be a risk factor for ALS has been raised for over half a century. Many elements have, at one time or another, been considered as aetiopathogenic candidates for ALS (Mitchell, 1997). Those that have raised the greatest interest include: lead, mercury, copper, iron, aluminium, calcium, magnesium, manganese and selenium. Removal of lead and other putative toxic substances by the use of chelation therapy has not been beneficial in ALS. However, if metal intoxication plays a role in ALS, the damage it induces is likely to be irreversible by the time symptoms have developed. Measurements of serum, cerebrospinal fluid, muscle and brain concentrations of most metals have not been different in ALS patients compared to normal controls. In a recent prospective study, Vinceti and colleagues (1996) analysed a cohort of 5182 residents from Reggio Emilia, Italy, who had been accidentally exposed to drinking water with a high selenium content. Over a nine-year period, four cases of ALS were diagnosed, giving a standardized incidence ratio of 4.22 (95 per cent confidence interval = 1.15–10.8). The standardized ratio was even higher when the analysis was limited to a subcohort with the longest exposure period. However, there are other studies which have shown that ALS patients were exposed to a low selenium content (Hockberg *et al.*, 1997).

Despite the fact that the association between metal toxicity and ALS is tenuous, there remains an attraction to a cause–effect relationship. A recent population-based case control study of the association of PD with exposure to iron, copper, manganese, mercury, zinc or lead reported a significant association with PD and occupational exposure to manganese and copper and a marginally significant association with lead. Exposure to all three of these metals was for more than 20 years (Gorell *et al.*, 1997). Occupational exposure for more than 20 years to two metals was also analysed. The associations were greatly increased, with the odds ratios for developing PD adjusted for age, gender, race and smoking history exceeding that for any exposure to one metal alone. Thus the odds ratio for lead with copper was 5.25 (p < 0.006), and for iron with copper was 3.69 (p < 0.008). It may be that these metals, especially in combination, promote oxidative stress by means of free radical generation (Olanow and Arendash, 1994). This study is the first to document PD and the association of metal exposure after 20 years. It is also the first to consider exposures to combinations of metals. Similar findings could be applicable to ALS, and epidemiological studies directed to long-term exposure are certainly warranted.

The latency period of exposure that is required to induce ALS might explain why animals which have been exposed to metals often do not develop the disease. Animal models using metal intoxication have not been very helpful in replicating neurodegenerative disease typical of humans. It is very difficult to maintain a long-term exposure of metal toxicity in animals that could begin to approach the 20 years or more of exposure that may be needed in humans. Sometimes the results are at odds with findings in humans dying of ALS. For example, chronic low-dose intracisternal administration of aluminium in rabbits produces upper and lower motoneuron deficits and pathological changes in anterior horn cells similar to those seen in human ALS (Wakayama *et al.*, 1996). These include perikaryal inclusions similar to hyaline inclusions and axonal spheroids. However, concentrations of aluminium in the spinal cords of patients dying of ALS are not increased compared to normal (Deibel *et al.*, 1997). Using instrumental neutron activation analysis of trace elements in the spinal cord, Markesbury and colleagues (1995) found significant elevations of iron, selenium and zinc compared to controls. There was no correlation between disease duration, clinical severity or lumbar neuronal counts and the elemental concentrations. This suggests that accumulation of the different elements occurs early and late in the disease and is not simply a result of end-stage pathology.

Clustering of ALS

A cluster of ALS has not been clearly defined but is generally considered to comprise a number of persons developing ALS who shared a restricted geographic territory, such as an apartment building, street or block. A cluster may also include individuals who have worked, for example, in the same factory, ship or football team. Such clustering of ALS has rarely been reported. A cluster of affected individuals would provide evidence for a causative environmental factor(s), but none of the cited studies has shown convincing statistical relationships. Clusters that have been reported include cases living in the same street or block, three members of the same American football team, cases of spousal ALS and a possibly greater incidence of ALS amongst Canadian naval personnel serving during the Second World War. In a retrospective study, Gunnarsson and colleagues (1996) identified 168 cases of ALS (107 men) in the county of Skaraborg, Sweden. Ascertainment was between 1961–1990 and during the five-year period 1981–1985, 70 men with ALS were identified, giving an average annual incidence of 4 per 10 000 person-years, statistically much higher than in the other five-year periods and higher in comparison with a neighbouring county, even when adjusted for multiple comparisons. Agricultural work was significantly more common amongst the cases compared to the rest of the population.

Trauma

Physical injury is so common as to make it an almost invariable antecedent to disease, and its significance is difficult to interpret. Nevertheless, antecedent trauma has been implicated in many neurological diseases (Riggs, 1993). Occasionally, there is a clear relationship between trauma and disease. Pugilistic encephalopathy, subsequent to a career of boxing, is a good example. However, most of the time it is difficult to implicate trauma as a specific risk factor. Given that ALS develops most frequently after 50 years of age, it is almost invariable that some form of antecedent physical injury will have been sustained, often several times. The relationship between trauma and ALS remains statistically controversial. There is no satisfactory analysis of severity, affected areas or type of trauma. For example, there have been several reports of ALS occurring following an electrical injury. The timing between the injury and developing ALS has been very variable and can only be related to the onset of symptoms. This takes no account of a likely 'incubation' period. There have been several positive, but poorly structured, retrospective case control studies showing that prior trauma appears to be a risk factor for ALS (Riggs, 1996). There have also been negative prospective cohort studies. These studies have been small and difficult to interpret. As age is an established risk factor for ALS, the relative significance of other risk factors (including trauma), when combined with age, may diminish with increasing age. Gompertzian risk analysis suggests that only in a young susceptible individual could the age-dependent risk be low enough to relate the development of ALS to preceding trauma. Riggs (1993, 1995) described three young men who developed ALS within two years of trauma, and, more recently, a further six young men were reported who developed ALS after trauma that was sufficient to induce focal axonal injury. Axonal injury induces cell death in selectively vulnerable neurons of immature animals and this provides some support for the idea that antecedent trauma in susceptible individuals may result in ALS. However, the relationship between ALS and trauma remains debatable.

Poliomyelitis and ALS

Hokkaido, which is the northern-most island of Japan, had a very high incidence of poliomyelitis during the 1940–1950 epidemic. Over 2000 cases were seen between 1949 and 1958, and ALS was confirmed in 389 patients over the same period (Moriwaka *et al.*, 1993). There was no correlation between ALS and poliomyelitis in terms of geographic distribution. Mortality rates from ALS have increased, not declined, in populations that have been vaccinated against poliomyelitis (Swingler, Fraser and Warlow, 1992).

Guamanian ALS–PD

Three population groups in the western Pacific had previously epidemic levels of ALS–PD complex. They are the Chamorros of Guam and Rota in the Mariana Islands, peoples of the Kii peninsula of Honshu Island in Japan, and the Auyu and Jaqai speaking people of western New Guinea. The reason why these regions had a previous incidence of ALS that was many times greater than that of the rest of the world remains intriguing but awaits a satisfactory explanation. It is likely that the disorder in these endemic areas is unique and distinctly different from sporadic ALS in ways that are not yet understood. Nevertheless, understanding why the western Pacific incidence was so high and what has caused its decline may have great relevance to western ALS. The Chamorros on Guam refer to the disease as 'lytico-bodig'. The incidence of lytico (ALS) for males peaked in about 1960 when it was 179 per 100 000. For women the incidence was about 60 per 100 000 (male:female ratio = 2.98:1). These values compare to an average incidence of about 1.5 per 100 000 for ALS in the Western world. Since 1960, there has been a steady decline of new cases of lytico-bodig, and by 1985 the incidence for both men and women had dropped dramatically and now is only slightly greater than the highest reported incidence levels of ALS in other parts of the world (see Fig. 1.8, taken from Zhang *et al.*, 1996).

One of the authors (AE) visited Guam in 1989 and performed physiological studies in patients with ALS. All of the cases seen had long-standing disease (average 12.6 years, n = 15), which is much longer than the mean survival of patients developing ALS in British Columbia, Canada (4.0 ± 3.8 years for men and 3.2 ± 1.4 years for women) (Eisen *et al.*, 1993c). This does not necessarily indicate that ALS on Guam has a longer duration; it is more likely that the surviving patients are those who had a more slowly progressive disease. Also, as pointed out above, the disease in the western Pacific is probably fundamentally different from sporadic ALS. New cases on the island seem to occur with equal frequency in all of the ethnic populations of Guam, suggesting that ALS developing at this time is more like sporadic ALS. This possibility awaits pathological confirmation. Guamanian ALS differs pathologically from sporadic ALS by the presence of widespread Alzheimer neurofibrillary tangles, which are prominent in the hippocampus, substantia nigra, locus ceruleus and spinal cord, where they are seen in about 20 per cent of anterior horn cells (Rodgers-Johnson *et al.*, 1986).

Over 35 years ago, Marjorie Whiting, a nutritionist, suggested that

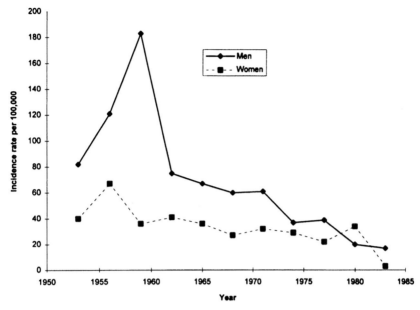

Figure 1.8. Declining incidence of ALS–PD on the island of Guam. The average age-adjusted annual incidence rate for men reached a maximum between the years 1959 and 1961 at 179 per 100 000. The peak incidence for women was 61 per 100 000 and occurred between 1956 and 1958. Since then, there has been a steady decline in the incidence for both men and women. The present incidence is similar to that of the rest of the world. (From Zhang *et al.* (1996). *Acta Neurologica Scandinavica*, **94**; 1–9. Reproduced with permission.)

ALS–PD of Guam was the result of toxic ingestion of the cycad plant (*Cycas circinalis*, false sago plant) (O'Gara, Brown and Whiting, 1964). Before westernization, and with it the construction of large military bases after the Second World War and urbanization of the local island communities, 'fadan' was a staple in the Chamorro diet. This flat bread, not unlike Mexican tortilla, was prepared from the cycad nut by grinding it to a fine pulp. Those indigenous to the island had appreciated that the food was potentially lethal in the 1800s. During the preparation of fadan, the nut was washed in water for several days, after which time its safety was checked by feeding the absorbent water to chickens. The role of cycad as a causative, toxic ingestant in Guamanian ALS was discarded on several counts.

1. The apparently high familial incidence of lytico-bodig seemed to point to a hereditary disorder. However, epidemiology of the

disease is inconsistent with Mendelian inheritance (Kurland and Molgaard, 1982). Even so, a susceptibility gene could be present among the Chamorros. Mutations of the copper/zinc–superoxide dismutase (Cu/Zn–SOD) gene have not been described in Guamanian ALS (Chen, 1995).

2. Feeding some of the several active ingredients of the cycad plant such as β-N-methylamino-L-alanine (BMAA) or cycasin (methylazoxymethanol b-D-glucoside) to animals has not induced motoneuron disease. However, recent studies indicate there is a highly significant correlation between the average annual age-adjusted incidence rates of Guamanian ALS and the flour content of cycasin (Kisby *et al.*, 1992). Also, chronic BMAA intoxication in monkeys induces a motor system disorder akin to ALS.

3. Exposure to cycad in other regions of the western Pacific where ALS was endemic did not appear to be relevant. Spencer and colleagues (1991, 1993), who have devoted considerable effort to understanding the toxic nature of the cycad nut and its chemical composition, have argued powerfully that exposure to cycad and western Pacific ALS are causally related. However, there are many other locally grown vegetables, starchy roots and reef fish which were and are staple to the island diet. How they may interact with cycad is not known.

An alternative hypothesis for ALS–PD in the western Pacific, originally proposed by Garruto (1987), revolved around the geochemical environment. The endemic areas of western Pacific ALS–PD (Kii peninsula of Japan, Marianas and west New Guinea) share a geochemical environment in which the soil and drinking water are poor in calcium, magnesium and zinc but have high concentrations of aluminium, manganese, selenium and iron (Chen, 1995). It is speculated that chronic, lifelong deficiency of calcium, magnesium and zinc promoted excessive absorption of divalent cations, which in turn might accelerate oxidative neuronal stress. The geochemical constellation might also explain the unique pathology of Guamanian ALS in which neurofibrillary tangle-containing neurons accumulate calcium, aluminium and silicon (Perl *et al.*, 1982). However, in recent studies Zhang *et al.* (1996) could not confirm that there was a relationship between soil concentrations of calcium, magnesium and aluminium and the incidence of ALS on Guam. The incidence of ALS did correlate significantly with the iron concentrations in water samples, which is more likely to generate free radicals, oxidative stress and neurodegeneration (Olanow and Arendash, 1994; Beal, 1995). The iron-binding protein lactotransferrin, which also transports aluminium (and other heavy metals), has been shown to be present in the pathological lesions of various neurodegenerative disorders. Lactotransferrin is strongly immunoreactive with Betz cells (and other pyramidal cells in normal primary motor cortex). The same lactotransferrin-immunoreactive cells are severely affected in ALS. It has been hypothesized that these cells take up or synthesize lactotransferrin at an elevated rate, resulting in the excessive accumulation of iron and aluminum (Leveugle *et al.*, 1994). These findings suggest that increased deposition of iron could be pathogenic in ALS. Since the Second World War, there has been considerable change to the environment on Guam as a result of vast construction, urbanization of the villages, deep well water supplies, electrification and construction of sewage systems. This has altered the geochemical environment and the soil and drinking water sufficiently to account for the dramatic change in the incidence of ALS–PD on Guam in the last two to three decades.

Both the cycad toxicity theory and the role of the geochemical environment are attractive. They are not necessarily mutually exclusive, but it is difficult to conceptualize a role that is common to both. It has been speculated that the pathogenesis of Guamanian and possibly other western Pacific ALS is dependent on the interaction of one or several susceptibility genes predisposing to environmental neuronal toxicity from cycads and a deleterious geochemical environment (Roman, 1996).

The epidemiology of the Cu/Zn–SOD gene mutations

About 5–10 per cent of ALS is hereditary (FALS). The clinical picture in these cases is largely similar to that of sporadic ALS, although phenotypes with some specific characteristics are being gradually identified. The onset of symptoms, on average, commences about a decade earlier than for the sporadic form, but there is considerable heterogeneity amongst different families. Most cases of FALS have a limb onset, with less than 20 per cent having a bulbar onset. Many FALS patients have an onset at less than 50 years of age. Although younger onset ALS is usually associated with a longer survival, the mean survival of FALS is shorter than that of sporadic ALS (Strong *et al.*, 1991; Eisen *et al.*, 1993c). This contradiction may relate to a paucity of numbers of patients with FALS who have been well studied, with a skew due to phenotypes with larger numbers that have a genetically determined short disease duration (Fig. 1.9). Unlike sporadic

Mean Survival of 3 SOD1 Mutations

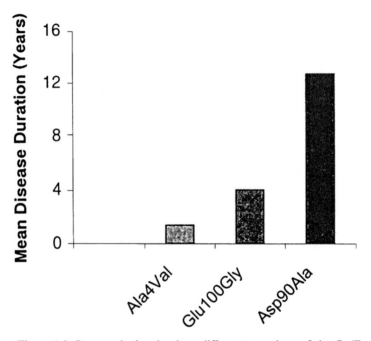

Figure 1.9. Bar graph showing how different mutations of the Cu/Zn–SOD1 gene influence the duration of ALS. More than 50 mutations have been discovered, but the three shown are the most common. The information about these mutations (Ala4Val, Glu100Gly and Asp90Ala) is sufficient for comparisons to be made. The Asp90Ala mutation has a slow progression. It is inherited as an autosomal recessive trait.

ALS, FALS is more evenly distributed amongst men and women and in some families with Cu/Zn–SOD mutations women are affected more often than men. This may reflect the bias of small numbers of patients. In 1993, Rosen *et al.* reported linkage between a subgroup of FALS and 11 different missense mutations in the gene encoding the Cu/Zn–SOD enzyme in 13 North American families. Since then, some 47 different missense and some deletional mutations in the Cu/Zn–SOD gene, which is linked to the long arm of chromosome 21q21, have been described in over 120 families world wide (Radunovic and Leigh, 1996; Siddique, Nijhawan and Hentati, 1996). The majority have come from North America and Europe, but this is probably because genetic analyses are more readily available in these areas. The mean onset of FALS associated with all Cu/Zn–SOD mutations is 45.5 $\pm$ 8.9 years and the mean disease duration is 3.4 $\pm$ 4.5 years (Juneja *et al.*, 1997). However, most of the mutations of the Cu/Zn–SOD gene have been identified in asymptomatic family members and the majority of patients with FALS (>85 per cent) do not appear to have either deletion or mutation of the Cu/Zn–SOD gene. In some families which carry a given mutation, the majority of members are asymptomatic, indicating a low penetrance of the mutant gene. The clinical details of the few that are affected are often still sparse, which makes numerical data difficult to interpret. Mutations have not been found in normal people but have been reported in a few cases of sporadic ALS.

Some of these cases may eventually turn out be similar to the Asp90Ala mutation described in families from Finland and northern Sweden (Andersen, 1997). This particular mutation is the only homozygous mutation associated with familial ALS and has a recessive inheritance. Several of the affected members have been believed to be cases of sporadic ALS (Andersen *et al.*, 1996). Cu/Zn–SOD mutations have not been found in the ALS–Parkinson–dementia complex of Guam, or familial or sporadic PD.

The Ala4Val mutation has been the most commonly reported but it is restricted to North America. It is largely associated with rapidly progressive disease, having a mean duration of 1.0 $\pm$ 0.4 years (see Fig. 1.6) with a mean onset of 47.0 $\pm$ 13.7 years (Siddique *et al.*, 1996; Juneja *et al.*, 1997). The Glu100Gly mutation has a mean onset of 48.6 $\pm$ 12.7 years and a mean duration of 5.1 $\pm$ 3.3 years, much more like sporadic ALS. The Glu100Gly and the Ile113Thr mutations have been found widely (in the UK, North America, Australia and New Zealand). Maybe they have a common ancestory, possibly originating in the UK. The Ile113Thr mutation has been reported in four cases of sporadic ALS but, as mentioned earlier, some may really be familial. The His46Arg mutation has a very slow disease progression with a mean of 17.4 $\pm$ 6.4 years (Aoki *et al.*, 1993; Juneja *et al.*, 1997), but there are too few cases to be statistically meaningful. The most recently identified Cu/Zn–SOD mutation, Asp90Ala, is also slowly progressive with a mean disease duration of 12.7 $\pm$ 6.3 years and mean age of onset of 43.5 $\pm$ 13.8 years. Most of the cases of 'sporadic' ALS in which Cu/Zn–SOD mutations have been described are of the Asp90Ala type. Its recessive inheritance is more likely to have cases mistakenly designated as being sporadic. The majority of FALS associated with Cu/Zn–SOD mutations are of limb onset, and the Asp90Ala mutation starts with dominant upper motoneuron signs, starting with leg paresis, progressing to the arms and finally involving bulbar muscles. Difficulty in micturition is also a common feature of this rather distinct phenotype (Andersen *et al.*, 1996). Also, a number of patients had preparetic symptoms, sometimes lasting several years, consisting of an insidious sense of stiffness, leg cramping, unsteadiness and fatigue. Some patients had burning and aching in the low back and buttocks, often unresponsive to simple analgesics. Electrophysiolgy in a few that were tested in this stage of the disease was normal. One of the cases reported by Andersen *et al.* (1996), patient 4 in family T, was originally seen in our clinic and thought to have sporadic ALS.

Case report 1.1

The patient was initially seen in 1989 when she was 45 years old. She was born in Finland and moved to Canada in 1963. Slowly progressive, generalized, but asymmetrical, muscle weakness began when she was about 43 years old. Muscle cramping and fasciculation were major complaints. However, for several years before that she had been aware of 'some difficulties with her legs'. There were no complaints referable to bulbar dysfunction. Examination showed there was modest muscle weakness in the arms and legs ranging between Medical Research Council (MRC) 3.5 and 4.5. Deep tendon reflexes were diffusely brisk and there were bilateral extensor plantar responses. Sensory examination was normal. Needle electromyography (EMG) studies already showed changes indicating a diffuse, chronic, neurogenic process. Transcranial magnetic stimulation (TMS) elicited a small-amplitude, very dispersed, motor-evoked potential (MEP) from the thenar complex. Its latency and central conduction times were normal. By 1991, her voice had become dysphonic and she complained of frequency of micturition. Her jaw jerk and facial reflexes had become brisk and limb muscle wasting was very apparent. Bulbar symptoms progressed and she finally died of ALS in 1996, aged 53 years. Her disease had lasted approximately 10 years. After her death it was discovered that she had a brother living in Finland who had developed ALS. Both she and her brother were homozygous and two other normal siblings were heterozygous for the Asp90Ala Cu/Zn–SOD mutation described above.

This case, considered throughout the course of the patient's disease to be sporadic ALS, is very interesting from two aspects. It underscores that there are a number of different clinical phenotypes of ALS. It also stresses that what appears to be a sporadic disease may not be so, this particular one being characterized by long duration, starting in the legs and having a disturbance of micturition. There are other rare recessively inherited 'motoneuron diseases' occurring mainly in Tunisia (Ben Hamida chronic juvenile amyotrophic lateral sclerosis) (Ben Hamida *et al.*, 1990). They are not linked to chromosome 21 and they are not associated with mutations of the Cu/Zn–SOD gene. It is also likely that there is a genetic component to sporadic ALS, and that one or several susceptibility genes are needed before the disease will manifest.

When was ALS first recognized?

Dating the earliest descriptions of a disorder may have implications in its aetiopathogenesis. For example, the AIDS epidemic is new, having been first recognized in the 1970s. A new disease of this sort with a rapidly rising incidence invariably spells the introduction of a toxin or transmittable agent into the environment, or survival of a population which might have succumbed to another disorder. It seems that the earliest descriptions of ALS are relatively recent, having been first reported about 150 years ago. This implies that either the disease had not previously occurred, or if so, very rarely. It is possible that it may not have been recognized by the neurologists of the mid-1880s but, given the considerable observational skills of the physicians of the early and middle nineteenth century, this seems unlikely. ALS is so devastating a disease it is difficult to imagine it was overlooked, even if it was not recognized as ALS. Although Charcot has been credited with having first described ALS, there were prior, albeit less definitive, reports of the disease (Bell, 1830; Aran, 1850; Duchenne, 1853). Nevertheless, Charcot was the first to define clearly the clinical and pathological characteristics of ALS (Charcot, 1874).

There are at least two possible explanations for the apparent rarity, or absence, of ALS prior to about 1850. The first relates to longevity. The incidence of ALS peaks at about 55–60 years of age. This has not substantially changed since the earliest descriptions of the disorder, although there has been a rising incidence of the disease and maybe more younger people with it are being recognized (see below). However, over the one and a half centuries since ALS was first recognized and described, longevity has steadily risen from a mean survival of about 45 years in 1850 to a mean approaching 80 years in 1996. Epidemiological studies in the early 1950s indicated that more than 75 per cent of deaths from ALS were in patients who were older than 54 years of age (Kurland, Choi and Sayre, 1969). Case reports from Charcot's time also indicate that ALS generally occurred in patients over 50 years of age. We suspect that because of the shorter mean lifespan, few individuals survived to an age which would have put them at risk for developing ALS. The lifespan of most mammals is much shorter than that of humans, and survival beyond 50–60 years of age seems to be a prerequisite for the development of ALS and other neurodegenerative disorders. This is probably one reason why there are no naturally occurring animal models which completely mimic ALS. Those mammals that do live a long time do not have a well-developed cortico-motoneuronal system, which is the prime target of ALS. The great apes (chimpanzees, gorillas and orangutans) do have a fairly well-advanced corticomotoneuronal system, but they have a relatively short lifespan. None of the common neurodegenerative diseases (ALS, PD and AD) has been described in them whilst living in their natural habitat. There is an isolated description of PD developing in a female gorilla who was kept in captivity all of her life.

It is well established that the incidence of AD rises sharply with age. This is also true of PD. Crude incidence rates of ALS decrease after the age of 70 years, but age-adjusted mortality rates continue to rise significantly with age (see Fig 1.1). The role of ageing in neurodegeneration is unclear. There is a decline in the number of anterior horn cells and corticomotoneurons with age (McComas, 1994; W. F. Brown, 1994; Eisen, Entezai-Taher and Stewart, 1996). Presumably this cell loss places additional demands on the surviving neurons, which then renders them more susceptible to external and internal environmental stresses. In this way a positive feedback cycle could be set up, resulting in an ever-greater loss of neurons. There is also growing evidence that metals and free radicals accumulate in brain regions which are affected in neurodegenerative disease, including ALS. Metal-induced oxidant stress can damage critical biological systems, initiating a cascade of events that includes mitochondrial dysfunction, excitotoxicity and excess cytosolic free calcium over many years, which in turn result in receptor degradation and dysfunction (Olanow and Arendash, 1994). These issues are discussed in greater detail in Chapter 4. Ageing alone cannot be the only predisposing factor for ALS. There are some data indicating that younger people develop the disease more frequently than formerly.

A change in the environment is one explanation for the emergence of a new disease. This might include the appearance of a new transmittable agent, or toxins which were previously non-existent or at low levels. Some of these issues are reviewed in this chapter, but it is intriguing that the first recognition of ALS seems to have coincided with the rise of the Industrial

Revolution. Undoubtedly, since that time there have been large amounts of toxic materials added to our environment.

Summary

It is possible that ALS did not predate the mid-nineteenth century. This is most easily explained by the dramatic change (doubling) in lifespan between 1850 and 1990 as ALS is unlikely to develop in individuals with a short lifespan. Age is the most established risk factor for ALS, and a continued increase in longevity dictates that there will be an increasing incidence in ALS in the twenty-first century. Proportionally, the prevalence of ALS may increase even more as drugs are used that can 'slow down' the disease but do not cure it. It is also possible that toxicity from a number of environmental agents has become sufficiently chronic as to now be of importance, when they previously may not have had time or potency to cause sufficient neuronal damage.

Young-onset disease is the most important predictor of longer survival once ALS has developed. Sex is a relative risk factor, with men being at significantly greater risk for ALS up to about age 55 years. After age 65–70 years, the male:female ratio approaches one. There are many other possible risk factors for ALS, including trauma and chronic elemental toxicity, especially with lead, iron, copper, manganese and mercury. Trauma and selected occupations in which the common denominator may be chronic elemental toxicity are also risk factors. However, statistically, most studies have been negative or marginal. A firm relationship between ALS and the risk factors cited, which presumably are only effective in a genetically disposed population, remains unproven. It is likely that the disorders that were endemic in Guam and other regions of the western Pacific are different from sporadic ALS. It is very probable that Guamanian ALS (lytico) and Parkinson–dementia (bodig) only rarely affect the same person and for the most part occur independently of each other. The dramatic fall in the incidence of these disorders strongly favours a changed environment. Whether this represents a changed geochemical composition of the drinking water and the soil, especially as it relates to the concentrations of calcium, aluminium and magnesium, and/or the decline in use of 'fadan' prepared from the cycad nut is not clear.

The epidemiology of mutations involving the Cu/Zn–SOD gene now number more than 50. These mutations have been described in over 120 families throughout the world, and are beginning to reveal clinical phenotypes. These phenotypes are characterized by their different disease durations but also by some clinical characteristics. At least one mutation the (Asp90Ala) has a recessive inheritance, so that members of a family with this mutation may initially masquerade as sporadic ALS.

2

The clinical spectrum of ALS

Diagnostic criteria

There is presently no diagnostic marker for ALS, and therefore the diagnosis of this disease depends upon the recognition of a characteristic clinical constellation of symptoms and signs with supportive electro-physiological findings. An additional requirement for the diagnosis of ALS is the exclusion of other disorders which may have similar clinical features. The constellation of weakness and muscle wasting which crosses both a peripheral nerve and myotomal distribution, and is associated with fasciculations and hyper-reflexia, is nearly always due to ALS. From the point of view of therapy, it would be ideal to be able to identify cases of ALS in a pre-symptomatic phase before neural death has occurred. It is probable that by the time clinical deficits appear and the diagnosis is more evident, the possibility of reversing the progression of the disease is less feasible. Diagnosis of ALS during the pre-symptomatic period must await the identification of a biochemical or other biological marker for ALS with proven specificity and sensitivity that has been assessed in prospective studies.

Once the disease has been present for a few months, the diagnosis of ALS can usually be made with a reasonable degree of confidence and is normally straightforward. The combination of painless, progressive but asymmetrical muscle weakness with wasting, fasciculation (and cramps), associated with upper motoneuron signs, a normal sensory examination, and normal sphincter and ocular function in a middle-aged patient is almost always due to ALS. As an additional support for the diagnosis, it is necessary to exclude other causes for the symptoms, especially those producing a cervical cord syndrome. These include syringomyelia, arterio-venous malformations, spinal cord tumour and cervical spondylotic myelopathy. The last diagnosis is by far the most common. It can cause

Table 2.1. *Presentations of ALS*

Multi-limb upper motoneuron
Multi-limb lower motoneuron
Hand dysfunction
Fasciculation
Shoulder dysfunction
Weak foot
Spastic gait
Respiratory insufficiency
Cognitive impairment

Multi-limb may include bulbar dysfunction.

particular difficulty because some degree of degenerative disc disease is almost invariable at an age when ALS has its greatest frequency. In this chapter the differential diagnosis of ALS is discussed, viewed from the perspective of the variety of ways that the disorder may present (Table 2.1).

At its onset, classical ALS is quite heterogeneous in presentation. The current dogma is that in spite of differences in age, sex, rate of progression and pattern of onset (whether bulbar or limb) in ALS patients, the underlying disorder has the same mechanisms. Time may prove this view to be incorrect, in that we may be erroneously 'lumping' a variety of disorders that closely mimic each other. However, their differences may reflect heterogeneity of defective gene products, some or several of which may turn out to be associated with a particular clinical phenotype. The spectrum of Charcot–Marie–Tooth neuropathies is a good example of several distinct disorders that are largely indistinguishable on clinical grounds but are associated with different genetic abnormalities. When patients with ALS are first seen, there is a need to establish certainty about the diagnosis because once patients are informed of this possibility they envisage a short survival. If there is any doubt about the diagnosis, it is better to review the situation in a timely fashion rather than jump to the wrong conclusion. Diagnostic uncertainty became the impetus for a classification system to estimate the probability of having ALS. These diagnostic criteria also became important for use in clinical drug trials, in which patient homogeneity should be a prerequisite. Table 2.2 classifies the certainty of diagnosing ALS according to the El Escorial criteria. This classification was developed by the World Federation of Neurology Subcommittee on Motor Neuron Diseases (Brooks, 1994). The clinical criteria have recently been validated in a clinicopathological study in

Table 2.2. *El Escorial diagnostic criteria for ALS*

Definite
UMN and LMN signs in bulbar and two spinal regions
or
UMN and LMN signs in three spinal regions
Probable
UMN and LMN signs in two regions (spinal or bulbar) and UMN signs in a region
  that is rostral to LMN signs
Possible
UMN and LMN signs in one region (spinal or bulbar)
or
UMN signs in two or three regions (spinal or bulbar)
Suspected
LMN signs in two or three regions (spinal or bulbar)

UMN, upper motoneuron; LMN, lower motoneuron.

which the likelihood of the patient having ALS by the diagnostic criteria
was correlated with the frequency of ubiquitin-immunoreactive intraneuronal inclusion bodies. The presence of these inclusions, although not
entirely specific for ALS, is a very frequently observed pathological
characteristic of the disease (Chaudhuri *et al.*, 1995).

In addition to these criteria, which are needed to make a firm diagnosis
of ALS, there are several other clinical features that the committee
considered as being inconsistent with the diagnosis of ALS. These are
sensory dysfunction, sphincter impairment, autonomic dysfunction,
abnormalities of eye movements, movement disorders and cognitive
dysfunction. These exclusion criteria hold true for the majority of patients
with ALS, throughout much of the course of their disease, but there
are well-reported exceptions to all of them that have been verified by
both electrophysiological and pathological examination. The exclusion
criteria should be relative not absolute. For example, pathological studies
reveal that Onuf's nucleus, which innervates the urethral and external
anal sphincters, is frequently involved in ALS (Bergmann, Volpel and
Kuchelmeister, 1995). Cytoskeletal abnormalities, including axonal
spheroids, Bunina bodies and ubiquitin-immunoreactive material, typical
of those seen in the spinal alpha-motoneurons in ALS, are also frequent in
the neurons of Onuf's nucleus; however, neuronal loss does not occur
(Bergmann *et al.*, 1995; Pullen, 1996). The findings suggest that sparing of
Onuf's nucleus reflects a relative, and not absolute, protection of its
neurons from the disease process. Needle EMG has demonstrated that
there is an increased fibre density in the external anal sphincter muscle in

Table 2.3. *Clinical clues raising concern about the diagnosis of ALS*

Clinical clue	Alternative diagnosis
Symmetrical deficit	Progressive muscular atrophy or inclusion body myositis
Absence of clinical or electrophysiological fasciculation	
Weakness without muscle wasting	Multifocal motor neuropathy with conduction block
Depression or loss of reflexes in weak myotomes	Chronic idiopathic demyelinating polyneuropathy

patients with ALS in the absence of bowel dysfunction, indicating that this muscle also is not spared by disease, despite the absence of clinical symptoms (Carvalho, Schwartz and Swash, 1995).

Eye movement abnormalities are also rare in ALS. However, they are being reported more frequently in patients who have had the disease a long time and in particular after prolonged respiratory support. Hayashi, Kato and Kawada (1991) studied 30 ALS patients, all of whom were at least five years from the date of onset of the ALS. These patients were remarkable for ophthalmoplegia, reductions in the number of neurons in the substantia nigra, and widespread tract degeneration at autopsy. Ophthalmoplegia in these patients was initially believed to be supra-nuclear, based on the presence of intact oculocephalic reflexes. The gaze abnormalities are initially relatively restricted to up and down gaze. With time, nuclear and segmental disorders of gaze occur, with attenuated vestibulo-ocular reflexes and other changes. These observations are of interest in view of the usual lack of involvement of the oculomotor system in ALS. Potentially, these oculomotor abnormalities could be related to ventilator use, but this appears unlikely. These data also complement other literature suggesting that abnormalities in oculomotor function can occur in ALS patients who are not on a respirator.

As listed in Table 2.3, there are other clinical clues that should raise concern that the diagnosis is *not* ALS.

Clinical presentation of ALS

Upper and lower motoneuron signs

The combination of upper and lower motoneuron signs is essential for the diagnosis of ALS and most patients have readily discernible upper and lower motoneuron features at the time of presentation. However, either the upper or the lower motoneuron component is frequently more dominant than the other. Upper motoneuron abnormalities may be subtle and difficult to recognize or interpret. This prompted Rowland and colleagues (Younger *et al.*, 1990, 1991) to introduce the concept of possible upper motoneuron signs (PUMNS). The concept is useful and refers to patients who do not have overt or obvious upper motoneuron signs such as a Babinski sign or clonus, but who do have the combination of incongruously active tendon jerks in weak, wasted, fasciculating limbs. Questionable lower motoneuron impairment can usually be confirmed by EMG since abnormalities of needle EMG are frequent in clinically strong muscles and frequently predate obvious muscle wasting. Providing re-innervation keeps pace with denervation, a large number of motor units (up to 80 per cent) can be lost before muscle weakness and wasting become evident. Some patients will have upper or lower motoneuron signs in isolation for several months, but persisting, isolated upper without lower motoneuron signs (primary lateral sclerosis, PLS) (Pringle *et al.*, 1992) or lower motoneuron signs without upper motoneuron signs (progressive muscular atrophy, PMA) are worrisome and a diagnosis other than ALS needs to be considered. The syndromes of PLS and PMA may represent diseases distinct from classical ALS (Eisen, Kim and Pant, 1992). Nevertheless, a recent report describes three men with PLS who developed typical ALS after intervals of 8, 9 and 27 years (Bruyn *et al.*, 1995). If PLS does progress to ALS, one can predict a median survival that is four to five times longer than for ALS commencing with both upper and lower motoneuron signs.

Case report 2.1: primary lateral sclerosis

A 45-year-old man had developed insidious, progressive weakness of the right leg, with dragging of the right foot, when aged about 38 years. A year before our initial examination, when he was aged 44, he began to notice difficulty using his right arm. There was loss of dexterity of the right hand and difficulty raising the arm above the shoulder. He considered that the function of the left arm and leg were normal and there were no bulbar symptoms. He had not noticed cramps or fasciculation. Examination showed marked hyper-reflexia in the right arm and leg, with an extensor plantar and Hoffman's response. There was no evidence of lower motoneuron disease on needle EMG, nor of motor conduction block on electrophysiological testing. Magnetic resonance imaging (MRI) of both the cerebral cortex and cervical spinal cord was normal. Haematology, blood chemistry, immunology and thyroid function were also normal.

This case is an example of PLS progressing over at least seven, but probably more, years. It remains to be seen if he develops lower motoneuron signs at some future time.

The other main diagnostic considerations in patients presenting with purely upper motoneuron symptoms and signs are listed in Table 2.4. Sometimes, MRI may be helpful in patients with mainly upper motoneuron features. In approximately 40 per cent of cases there are bilateral, well-defined, round, symmetrical, T2 increased signal intensities seen along the corticospinal pathways and most readily visualized at the level of the middle or lower internal capsule (Cheung *et al.*, 1995). In some patients there may also be low signal intensities within the motor cortex. These abnormalities are not specific and if symmetric can also be seen in some normal subjects.

Cervical spondylotic myelopathy is common in the same age range in which ALS occurs. Usually it is not symptomatic, but may be responsible for brisk reflexes, especially in the legs. When this scenario is combined with modest 'neurogenic' EMG abnormalities in leg muscles, it can cause concern about early ALS. Furthermore, high level (C3, C4) spondylosis sometimes results in, or even presents with, hand wasting in the absence of sensory abnormalities or pain and it can closely mimic ALS (Goodridge *et al.*, 1987). The problem one faces is to decide how relevant abnormalities seen in the computed tomography (CT) scan or MRI of the cervical region are for the clinical features. Over 50 years of age, abnormalities seen with these imaging techniques are very common. If there are clinical or electrophysiological indications of lower motoneuron disease involving myotomes that are several, or better still, many segments, caudal to the cervical spine (i.e. legs or chest wall), then ALS is more likely to be responsible for the overall disorder. On the other hand, if there is obvious cord compression, especially associated with myelomalacia of the cord on MRI, and unclear evidence of lower motor involvement caudal to the cervical cord, it is likely that the neurological deficit can be ascribed to the structural deformity. If there is doubt about the diagnosis of ALS, it is worth considering surgery even if the lesion does not explain the whole clinical picture.

Brain tumours, other cerebral mass lesions and multiple sclerosis (MS) occurring in the elderly are readily confirmed by MRI, and unless the patient has definite ALS as defined by the El Escorial criteria, we suggest that patients suspected of having ALS have a CT scan or MRI of the head and cervical spinal cord to rule out a structural lesion. Multiple cerebral infarcts (multi-infarct state), which can closely mimic PLS, are also readily

Table 2.4. *Diagnostic considerations in ALS presenting with upper motoneuron deficits*

Cervical spondylotic myelopathy
Multi-infarct state
Brain tumours
Other system degenerations:
progressive supranuclear palsy
Shy–Drager syndrome
olivopontocerebellar atrophy
multiple system atrophy
diffuse Lewy body disease
Gerstmann–Straussler–Scheinker syndrome
cortical basal ganglionic degeneration
Creutzfeld–Jakob disease
Multiple sclerosis
Lathyrism
Konzo

confirmed by CT scan or MRI. On the other hand, single, silent infarcts are quite commonly visualized radiologically in patients with ALS. Their site, size and an estimate of their age are important determinants of whether or not they have any role in the presenting clinical picture. There are other system degenerations listed in Table 2.4 which may be confused with bulbar onset ALS (Mathias and Williams, 1994; Cardoso and Jankovic, 1994; P. Brown, 1994). They all result in variable bulbar dysfunction, predominantly dysarthria and an associated brisk jaw jerk. In the disorders listed, the dysarthria may be pyramidal, extrapyramidal or cerebellar in origin, or any combination of these. Pseudobulbar affect with emotional incontinence occurs in some of the conditions listed, but usually does so late in these disorders, as do long-tract signs. Many of these degenerations have predominant abnormalities of eye movement, Parkinsonian features, cerebellar dysfunction, dementia and disturbances of autonomic function. These are all rare events in typical ALS.

Lathyrism

Lathyrism is due to toxicity from the consumption of *Lathyrus sativus* (the chickling pea). The responsible ingredient, β-N-oxalylamino-L-alanine (BOAA), is an excitotoxic amino acid. Lathyrism is endemic in geographic areas subject to famine and drought such as Bangladesh, China, Ethiopia and India. The chickling pea is a drought-resistant crop, and at times of famine it may become the only source of nutrition. For unknown reasons, the disease affects men more frequently than women and characteristically induces leg weakness in a pyramidal distribution. The arms are typically much less involved (Spencer *et al.*, 1991). Use of transcranial magnetic stimulation in lathyrism has demonstrated prolonged central conduction from the cerebral cortex to the lumbar spine in patients in whom a leg MEP could be recorded. In many patients this is not possible. MEPs recorded from hand muscles are usually normal (Hugon *et al.*, 1989).

Konzo

Konzo has many similarities to lathyrism. It too causes an acute onset of spastic paraparesis, particularly in young, malnourished males during dry seasons in Tanzania, Zaire and other parts of East Africa (Howlett *et al.*, 1990; Tylleskar *et al.*, 1992). The disease spectrum varies from lower extremity hyper-reflexia to severe spastic paraparesis with weakness in the arms. There is good evidence that konzo results from the ingestion of insufficiently processed cassava roots used to make flour. Short-soaking of the cassava root leads to residual cyanohydrins in the flour and it is likely that these are responsible for the neurological deficit (Tylleskar *et al.*, 1992). Long-standing high cyanide levels result in reactions between cyanide and cysteine residues in albumin yielding aminothiazolidine carboxylic acid, which has structural similarities to BOAA (Rosling, 1986). A recent study from Uppsala (Tylleskar *et al.*, 1992) involved extensive electrophysiological testing in two patients with konzo disease who were previously seen in Tanzania (Howlett *et al.*, 1990). In both patients, motor and sensory nerve conductions, EMG, including single fibre EMG (SFEMG), autonomic testing, somatosensory, visual and auditory brainstem evoked potentials and electroencephalography (EEG) were all normal. However, repeated efforts to stimulate the motor cortex with the magnetic coil at 100 per cent output, with and without facilitation, failed to elicit any MEPs from either hand or leg muscles. Stimulation of the cervical roots with the coil elicited normal responses.

Based upon the clinical findings and the results of MEP studies, lathyrism and konzo appear primarily to involve the motor cortex, and they might be better referred to as toxic disorders of the motor pathways since it seems that it is the corticomotoneuron that is primarily involved. The exact site of the lesion could be further elucidated by comparing the ability to evoke responses by electrical versus magnetic stimulation. If the lesion is truly one of the corticomotoneuron, then it should be possible to

Table 2.5. *Diagnostic considerations in ALS presenting with lower motoneuron deficits*

Adult-onset spinal muscular atrophies
Monomelic amyotrophies
Motor neuronopathy with conduction block
Kennedy's syndrome (bulbospinal neuronopathy)
Inclusion body myositis

elicit a response by electrical (i.e. distal to the cell body) but not magnetic stimulation. On the other hand, if the lesion is one of the motor tracts, then both magnetic and electrical stimulation of the cortex will fail to elicit a response.

ALS commencing as a lower motoneuron syndrome

ALS commencing as a purely lower motoneuron syndrome is more frequent in young-onset disease, especially amongst young men. However, this may simply reflect the fact that, overall, young-onset ALS is much more common in men than women (see Chapter 1). In these cases there may be an interval of several years before obvious upper motoneuron signs become readily appreciated and it is easy to conclude erroneously that the patient has one of the PMAs. There are several other conditions in which lower motoneuron features occur in isolation and which can mimic ALS (Table 2.5).

Adult-onset spinal muscular atrophies

The adult-onset spinal muscular atrophies (SMAs) comprise the largest group of conditions that may be confused with ALS when it presents with purely lower motoneuron deficit. The clinical spectrum of these conditions is large and they have been previously classified according to their mode of inheritance, age of onset and rapidity and severity of progression. They are genetically heterogeneous, including autosomal dominant, recessive and sex-linked modes of inheritance. In the majority of cases the pattern of inheritance is autosomal recessive (Hausmanowa-Petrusewicz, 1991); this is also true for adult-onset cases, in which < 30 per cent are autosomal dominant. In adult-onset cases, the disease may begin between the fourth and the sixth decade and progress rapidly, with death from respiratory failure within two years in the absence of corticospinal tract dysfunction

Table 2.6. *Gene linkage of some hereditary neurogenic diseases that might be confused with ALS*

Disease	Mode of inheritance	Gene linkage	Gene product or protein receptor
FALS	AD	21q22	CuZn–SOD1
Kugelberg–Welander	AR	5q11-q13	SMN, NAIP
SMA, scapuloperoneal	AD	7p	SMN, NAIP
SMA, adult onset (proximal)	AD/AR	5q11-13	SMN, NAIP
SMA, adult onset (distal)	AD/AR	5q11-13	SMN, NAIP
Kennedy's disease	XR	Xq21-22	Androgen
Charcot–Marie Tooth			
Type 1a	AD	17p11.2	PMP22
Type 1b	AD	1q21-23	PMP0
Type 2	AD	1p35-36	?
X-linked	XR	Xq13	Connexin
Spastic paraplegia	XR	Xq21-22	Proteolipid protein

After Kaplan, J-C. and Fontaine, B. (1996). Neuromuscular disorders: gene location. *Neuromuscular Disorders*, 6:1–1X.
AD: autosomal dominant; AR: autosomal recessive; XR: sex-linked recessive; SOD1: superoxide dismutase; SMN: survival motoneuron protein; NAIP: neuronal apoptosis inhibitory protein; PMP: peripheral myelin protein.

(Jansen *et al.*, 1986). This picture is then very similar to, and can be readily confused with, ALS. Features that differentiate the SMAs from ALS include (1) the pattern of inheritance, (2) the generally younger age of onset, (3) the symmetrical distribution of motor deficits, and (4) the absence of fasciculations and upper motoneuron abnormalities.

In 1990, linkage was established for SMA types 1, 2 and 3 to markers on chromosome 5q12-q13 (Melki *et al.*, 1990; Brzustowicz *et al.*, 1990). The responsible gene, the survival motoneuron gene (SMN), was recently discovered and found to be absent or truncated in >98 per cent of both childhood and adult cases of SMA (Table 2.6). Deletions in another gene, the neuronal apoptosis inhibitory protein (NAIP) gene, have also been identified in significant numbers of patients (Morrison, 1996). Programmed death of motoneurons is a normal phenomenon during embryogenesis and one model of SMA invokes an inappropriate persistence of motoneuron apoptosis. The NAIP gene is responsible for the timely cessation of apoptosis (Roy *et al.*, 1995). It is unclear whether deletions of both the SMA and NAIP (or other unidentified) genes are needed for developing SMA. The function of the protein product(s) of the

SMA gene and how it alters the biology of the anterior horn cell in the spinal muscular atrophies remain to be determined. This will eventually result in a logical classification scheme and, it is to be hoped, useful therapeutic advances in the SMAs.

X-linked recessive bulbospinal neuronopathy (Kennedy's syndrome)

This is the first example of a motor system degeneration to which a specific gene mutation of the androgen receptor was linked (Kennedy, Alter and Sung, 1968; Harding *et al.*, 1982). Gene linkage is to Xq21-22 (see Table 2.6). The disease has clinical characteristics making it clearly distinguishable from other SMAs. They include X-linked inheritance, so that only males are affected, generally older age of symptom onset (usually older than age 30–40 years), diffuse, often marked fasciculations, and involvement of bulbar as well as spinal musculature. The bulbar deficits are lower motoneuron in type. Early 'puckering of the chin' is common. Gynaecomastia and testicular atrophy are present in many patients. We have performed magnetic stimulation studies in five cases from three different families, recording from a variety of muscles that are innervated through motor cranial nerves (facial, masseter, tongue and sternomastoid). In all cases the only abnormality was a reduced or small amplitude MEP. The findings suggest that the central motor pathways in this disease are intact. If this is correct, it is of interest because it is the only example of a SMA in which fasciculations are usually very widespread. Even though sensory complaints are unusual and clinical sensory examination is largely normal, sensory nerve action potentials (SNAPs) are small or absent (Trojaborg *et al.*, 1995; Li *et al.*, 1995). Deep tendon reflexes are usually depressed or absent; this is considered to be the result of dorsal root ganglion involvement. There are endocrine abnormalities which include testicular atrophy and gynaecomastia, oligospermia or azoospermia, slightly elevated serum gonadotrophin levels, glucose intolerance, and feminization of the skin. Kennedy's syndrome can be diagnosed by DNA analysis of blood or muscle. There is an increased number of repeated trinucleotide sequences (CAGs) within the exon 1 coding regions of the androgen receptor gene which correlate with the severity of the phenotype. In recent years, several quite different diseases have been identified that are characterized by an increase in DNA triplicate repeats. The number of repeats is often proportional to the severity of the disease. Kennedy's syndrome is usually slowly progressive and compatible with normal longevity. Post-mortem material is lacking. Cases have been described with a very similar clinical picture but without the DNA abnormalities. On the basis of the available evidence, this disease is probably a combined motor neuronopathy and sensory ganglionopathy.

Case report 2.2: Kennedy's syndrome

A 64-year-old man presented with walking difficulty, a nasal voice and occasional choking on dry foods. These symptoms had been present over at least three to four years. He had been previously well and there was no family history of a neuromuscular disorder. Examination showed moderate gynaecomastia and testicular atrophy. There was modest, diffuse and relatively symmetrical muscle weakness and wasting. Fasciculation was seen in proximal muscles and over the chest wall. He also had a mild facial diplegia and obvious fasciculations in the tongue and chin. His gait was quite ataxic – more than one would have expected for the degree of weakness – but proprioceptive sensory loss was modest. There was also modest weakness of the shoulder girdle muscles. Deep tendon reflexes were uniformly absent.

Median, ulnar and peroneal motor conduction velocities were normal and F-waves were not prolonged. Sensory nerve conduction velocities in the same nerves were normal but SNAPs were much reduced in amplitude. Needle EMG showed fasciculation potentials and reduced recruitment of motor unit potentials (MUPs). The motor units were large, of increased duration, increased fibre density and often unstable. These changes are in keeping with an active proximal neurogenic process. DNA testing for triplet repeat expansion of the androgen receptor gene was positive. It is likely that the gait ataxia was due to the sensory ganglionopathy.

Particular patterns of clinical onset and their diagnosis

The previous sections consider diagnostic concerns in ALS as they relate to relatively global upper or lower motoneuron disease. However, it is common for weakness or painless wasting in ALS to commence in any muscle group or combination of groups. Muscles are not usually affected in isolation, or in a peripheral nerve distribution, but rather, the wasting or weakness has both an upper and lower motoneuron component, and tends to follow a 'functional pattern', meaning it affects muscles responsible for specific activities such as thumb opposition or flexion. This suggests, if not a cortical origin for the disease, then at least a close relationship between the involvement of upper and lower motoneurons. This issue is discussed in further detail in Chapter 5. Some particular

Table 2.7. *Initial clinical presentation of ALS*

	Percentage of total presentations
Dysarthria	32.8
Painless hand dysfunction	19.7
Weak/wasted shoulder	13.6
Foot drop	12.5
Fasciculations – cramps	11.4
Spastic gait	4
Respiratory failure	4
Cognitive impairment	2

Frequency is based on 664 patients seen at the Vancouver ALS Clinic between 1980 and 1996.

presentations are more frequent than others and serve as a means for distinguishing ALS from other diseases (Table 2.7).

Dysarthria and bulbar onset

Approximately one in four patients with ALS has a bulbar onset. This type of onset is more common in women than in men. In our clinic the female:male ratio of patients with a bulbar onset is 2:1. Bulbar onset is rare under age 50 years and the mean age of patients with a bulbar onset is older than those with a spinal onset (63.8 + 8.7 years compared to 55.6 + 14.8 years). The difference probably reflects the larger number of young men with ALS whose disease most frequently starts with limb onset. Up to age 75 years, there is a linear, or possibly an exponential, increase in the frequency of bulbar onset cases with age. In contrast, the age of patients with spinal onset ALS is much more evenly distributed. The most frequent bulbar symptom is dysarthria. Usually the upper motor component is much more marked than is the lower motoneuron component, so that when the speech deficit becomes obvious it is spastic more than dysphonic. In the context of ALS, spastic dysarthria is frequently associated with pathological, or inappropriate, laughing and crying and a brisk jaw jerk. It is very rare for patients with ALS to have other bulbar-related symptoms (choking, excess salivation) in the absence of dysarthria.

For weeks or months the dysarthria may be mild and is frequently intermittent, only becoming obvious toward the day's end when patients

Table 2.8. *Differential diagnosis of ALS presenting with hand wasting or weakness*

Intramedullary spinal cord lesions
Cervical spondylotic radiculopathy
High level cervical stenosis (C3–C4)
Non-traumatic lower trunk brachial plexopathies
Monomelic amyotrophies (Hirayama disease)
Multifocal motor neuropathy with conduction block
Carpal tunnel syndrome

---

are tired. It is often interpreted by the patient as a hoarseness of the voice, sometimes related to a recent respiratory infection. Mild dysarthria may not be appreciated outside the immediate family and it is common for patients presenting with dysarthria to be initially investigated for a vocal cord problem through an ENT facility. There are not many diagnostic considerations in the differential diagnosis of slowly progressive dysarthria outside ALS. Other system degenerations, including PD, may present with impaired vocalization. A previously silent cerebral infarct followed by another one involving the contralateral hemisphere, or subcortical structures, will result in dysarthria. The onset is usually sudden, severity is maximum at onset and does not vary or progress with time. Kennedy's syndrome and myasthenia gravis may result in a nasal voice from lower motoneuron impairment. In myasthenia gravis the speech impediment is dysphonic rather than dysarthric and rarely if ever occurs without accompanying oculomotor impairment, such as ptosis or double vision.

Hand weakness and wasting

In about 20 per cent of patients with classical ALS, unilateral and, less frequently, bilateral hand dysfunction is the presenting complaint. Some diagnostic considerations for this symptom other than ALS are listed in Table 2.8. Intrinsic (intramedullary) spinal cord disorders affecting the lower cervical segments (C8, T1), such as syringomyelia and ependymoma result in loss of anterior horn cells and wasting of the small muscles of the hand. This is usually associated with sensory deficit, pain and reflex loss in the involved spinal segments, and increased reflexes in segments caudal to the lesion.

Intramedullary lesions are readily identified on MRI. The issue of high level cervical spondylotic stenosis and how it can produce hand wasting have already been discussed. The mechanism involved is uncertain. One possible explanation involves venous stasis and secondary anterior horn cell loss (Goodridge *et al.*, 1987).

Non-traumatic brachial plexopathies are usually painful and associated with sensory symptoms and a sensory deficit. Lower trunk plexopathy due to a cervical rib or fibrous band is an exception and typically presents as painless thenar wasting (Gilliat *et al.*, 1978). This condition almost invariably affects young women, whereas ALS occurring in young adults has a predilection for men. Painless thenar wasting is also a feature of carpal tunnel syndrome affecting elderly people; they seldom have sensory complaints, even though there usually is an objective deficit to sensory testing. Conduction studies confirm that the wasting is due to a mononeuropathy affecting the median nerve at the wrist.

The monomelic amyotrophies

Monomelic amyotrophies comprise a heterogeneous group of disorders characterized by clinical deficit restricted to one limb, most frequently the upper, with prominent hand wasting. The best-defined type of this group of disorders is Hirayama's disease (Hirayama, 1991). Like the other types of monomelic amyotrophy, it is insidious in its onset and predominantly affects young men aged 15 to 25 years. Progression is very slow and frequently the disorder is self-limiting. Almost all cases are sporadic and the largest series have come from Japan and India, but Hirayama's disease has been recognized in many countries. There is weakness of the fingers with painless wasting of hand and forearm muscles affecting the C7 through T1 myotomes. More rostral spinal segments (C5/C6) are usually spared. The initial symptoms are characteristically temperature dependent and patients often first become aware of their hand weakness in winter. One arm is very predominantly affected, while there is variable, usually minimal, involvement of the contralateral limb. Unlike with ALS, fasciculations are absent and stretch reflexes are not increased. Very rarely, a disease indistinguishable from that seen in the upper limb affects a lower limb (DiMuzio *et al.*, 1994). Electromyography shows chronic neurogenic changes in affected muscles, without evidence of active denervation (fibrillation and positive sharp waves). In most patients, homologous muscles in the non-affected limb show similar abnormalities. Imaging, including MRI, is normal. However, with neck flexion the MRI shows marked anterior–posterior distortion of the lower cervical spine (Toma and Shiozawa, 1995). These radiological abnormalities led Hirayama to coin the term 'amyotrophic cervical myelopathy in adolescence' for the disease he first described in 1959 (Hirayama, Toyokura and Tsubaki, 1959).

Case report 2.3: monomelic amyotrophy of the upper limb

An 18-year-old Japanese man developed weakness and wasting of his left upper limb over a period of three years. He had not noticed any recent progression. The small hand muscles, with relative thenar sparing, were primarily involved. The right hand was mildly involved in a similar distribution. There were no sensory complaints and sensory examination was normal. The hand weakness was aggravated in cold weather. Tendon reflexes were very depressed in both arms but they were normal in the legs. Conduction studies were normal; there was no conduction block. Needle EMG showed bilateral neurogenic changes, more apparent on the left. The abnormalities were restricted to myotomal segments C7, C8 and T1. There was evidence of acute denervation in paraspinal muscles of the same myotomes. Transcranial magnetic stimulation studies were also normal. MRI of the cervical spinal cord was normal.

This case is typical of those described by Hirayama (1991). At recent follow up the young man's clinical state was unchanged.

Case report 2.4: monomelic amyotrophy of the lower limb

A 28-year-old Asian man presented with a slowly progressive wasting of the right lower leg which had developed over several years and was brought to his attention by a friend. He did not think there had been any progression of the problem and had maintained his work in construction without difficulty. The major wasting involved the gastrocnemius; the tibialis anterior was much less involved. There was good muscle bulk of S1-innervated muscles in the foot. All reflexes were easily obtained except the right ankle jerk, which was absent. Despite the marked gastrocnemius wasting, plantar flexion was strong. Conduction studies were normal and there was no evidence of conduction block, even after root stimulation with a monopolar needle. The amplitude of the CMAP of the abductor digiti minimi muscle in the foot was normal. Needle EMG of the leg muscles showed surprisingly little abnormality given the extent of wasting. The abnormalities seen were clearly neurogenic. MRI of the spinal cord was normal.

We have seen two other almost identical cases, also in young men. One has been followed for 12 years without substantial disease progression. These cases are examples of monomelic amyotrophy affecting the leg, in particular the gastrocnemius muscle. The focal nature of the amyotrophy, which spares some muscles sharing the same peripheral and myotomal

Table 2.9. *Characteristics of 11 patients with multifocal motor neuropathy*

Sex M/F	10/1
Mean age of onset (years)	44.1 ± 8.1
Disease duration (years)	9.45 ± 7.3
Progressive course	7/11
Static course	4/11
Fasciculation*	10/11
Cramps*	7/11
Hyporeflexia or arreflexia*	9/11
Upper limb onset	9/11
Lower limb onset	2/11

* In distribution of affected nerve(s) – see Table 5.2.
With grateful appreciation to our colleague Dr Gillian Gibson.

innervation, makes it difficult to localize the lesion anywhere but within the spinal anterior horn. It is possible that this disorder is the equivalent of Hirayama's disease but affects the lower extremity. However, the very focal nature of the amyotrophy could reflect excessive motoneuron loss due to prolonged programmed neuronal death. The disorder is considered to be benign and hence the importance of its recognition.

Multifocal motor neuropathy with persistent conduction block

Multifocal motor neuropathy with persistent conduction block (MMN) is an interesting and unusual condition. This syndrome was only recognized about a decade ago, but undoubtedly existed prior to the first descriptions (Kornberg and Pestronk, 1995; Parry, 1996). MMN is easily mistaken for ALS; it is important to distinguish between the two because MMN has a much better prognosis and is compatible with normal longevity. About half of the patients respond quite dramatically to intravenous immuno-globulin (IVIg) therapy (Bouche *et al.*, 1995; Azulay *et al.*, 1997). However, most busy neuromuscular centres see fewer than two to three cases a year so that cumulative experience, especially in terms of long-term response to therapy, is limited. We have seen 11 cases over the last seven years (Table 2.9).

The diagnosis of MMN requires electrophysiological confirmation of conduction block in one or more nerves. In some cases there is a focal increase in signal intensity which can be seen on T_2-weighted MRI imaging. This is most frequent in the brachial plexus, either in the neck or the axilla (Van Es *et al.*, 1997). However, MRI abnormalities which are indistinguishable from those seen in MMN may also be visualized in chronic inflammatory demyelinating polyneuropathy (CIDP) (Kuwabara *et al.*, 1997).

Once appreciated, the clinical picture of MMN is very stereotyped. Initially there is focal weakness, which can usually be traced to an individual peripheral nerve. A proximal distribution with involvement of the brachial plexus or musculocutaneous nerve is common. Sites that are typically involved in entrapment neuropathies are rarely affected, and lower limb nerves are much less frequently involved than upper limb nerves. Fasciculations and cramps are frequently associated with the clinical deficit, which usually remains restricted in its anatomical distribution for many years. Symptoms begin and progress indolently over years or decades and durations of over 20 years are well documented. A major clinical clue is the presence of normal muscle bulk together with paresis or paralyis which is the result of conduction block in the motor nerve innervating the muscle. The pathological substrate for this is demyelination. Conduction block is confirmed by the ability to evoke a CMAP below the site of the block whereas above the block the response is usually < 10 per cent of the amplitude evoked by distal stimulation (Fig. 2.1). Motor nerves are affected much more than are sensory nerves, and objective sensory deficit is rare. There is no good explanation for the motor nerve predilection.

The disease appears to be immune mediated and about 20–30 per cent of patients have high (> 1:6000) titres of serum autoantibodies directed against GM1 ganglioside. A further 40–50 per cent have titres between 1:4000 and 1:400. However, these levels also occur in a number of other polyneuropathies, classical ALS and even normal subjects. Negative titres do not rule out the diagnosis of MMN. Pestronk *et al.* (1997) have recently identified patients with MMN whose serum has selective IgM binding for the GM1 ganglioside-containing lipid mixture of galactocerebroside and cholesterol but not for GM1 alone. Debate continues as to whether or not MMN is a specific entity or merely one end of a spectrum of conditions usually labelled as CIDP. Pathological material is sparse and suggests that at least there is considerable overlap between MMN and CIDP. It is likely that some cases of monomelic amyotrophy, indistinguishable from those described by Hiryama, may have been due to focal demyelination in the brachial plexus or, rarely, the lumbosacral plexus with weakness of the lower limb.

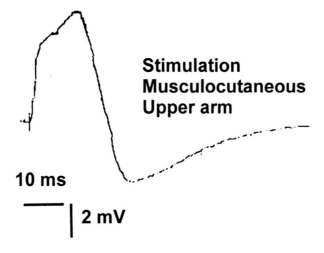

**Stimulation
Musculocutaneous
Upper arm**

10 ms

2 mV

**Stimulation
Erb's point**

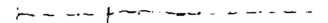

Figure 2.1. Multifocal motor neuropathy with persistent conduction block (see Case report 2.5). The patient had a weak, fasciculating right biceps of near-normal bulk even after four years of deficit. The biceps jerk was absent and there were no sensory abnormalities. A normal CMAP was recorded from the weak biceps brachii after stimulation of the musculocutaneous nerve in the axilla (top). Stimulation of the upper trunk of the brachial plexus at Erb's point failed to evoke any recognizable response (lower). This represents a conduction block approaching 100 per cent.

Azulay *et al.* (1997), have analysed the long-term outcome of treating MMN with IVIg. The mean follow-up period was 25.3 months and the median time between onset of the disease and treatment was 5.8 years. About 70 per cent of patients improved. There was no good correlation between improvement and length of disease or extent of neurological deficit. Most patients required maintenance therapy at regular intervals. The effects of IVIg are transient and the treatment is expensive. A few patients who do not respond to IVIg do show improvement with cyclophosphamide.

Case report 2.5: motor neuropathy with persistent conduction block

A 50-year-old man first noticed muscle twitching in the right arm, particularly affecting the biceps muscle, when aged 45 years. There was insidious development of weakness of flexion at the elbow, despite which he maintained a relatively normal lifestyle. There were no other complaints. On examination, there were fasciculations seen in the right arm, particularly the biceps muscle. This muscle was only slightly wasted and there was a disproportionate loss of strength. Otherwise motor power was normal in the right arm, left arm and both legs. Deep tendon reflexes were depressed in both upper limbs and difficult to obtain in the legs. The plantar responses were downgoing and the remainder of the examination was normal.

Electrophysiology showed > 90 per cent conduction block in the right musculocutaneous nerve (see Fig. 2.1). Other motor and sensory conduction studies were normal. Needle EMG confirmed the presence of complex fasciculations in the biceps. Motor unit recruitment was greatly reduced in this muscle and the motor units were of large amplitude and complex, with increased fibre density and unstable. These are features of a chronic neurogenic process. Muscles other than the biceps muscle were normal. MRI of the right brachial plexus showed a hyperdense focal lesion, several centimetres in length, predominantly affecting the upper trunk. After three courses of intravenous hyperimmune globulin, there was considerable improvement in the clinical deficit and he remains well, but still has neurological deficit.

Morphological information from nerve biopsy is sparse and has come mainly from the brachial plexus, usually inadvertently. The biopsies have shown there is a mild loss of myelinated nerve fibres and the formation of rudimentary onion bulbs. There is endoneurial oedema that accounts for the nerve enlargement and increased signal sometimes seen on MRI. Occasionally, there is sparse lymphocytic infiltration around epineurial blood vessels (Parry and Sumner, 1992; Parry, 1996). These pathological changes are identical to those that characterize CIDP and support the notion that MMN results from immune-mediated demyelination. However, they do not explain the strange predilection for involvement of motor axons. Two recent reports (Veugelers *et al.*, 1996; Kinoshita, Kaji and Akiguchi, 1997) raise concern that MMN may not always be benign. A patient with classical sporadic ALS was found at autopsy to have characteristic pathological features of proximal nerve demyelination. The other patient, a 53-year-old man, had progressive weakness of the left arm spreading to other limbs. There was diffuse muscle wasting and fasciculations. Electrophysiologically there was multiple conduction blocks and anti-GM1 antibodies were elevated. He was given cyclophosphamide but died of respiratory failure. Autopsy showed a combination of patchy demyelination but also changes characteristic of ALS (Veugelers *et al.*, 1996).

Foot drop and impaired gait

There are several ways in which difficulty in walking presents in ALS before muscle weakness or wasting is overt. They include exercise intolerance and fatigue, rubbery or heavy leg(s), and loss of leg control. These symptoms are usually due to upper motoneuron dysfunction even though evidence of this, such as increased tone, hyper-reflexia and a positive Babinski sign, is frequently lacking. As discussed above, cervical spondylotic myelopathy is the most frequent alternative diagnosis and the presence of multisegmental degenerative disc disease often confounds the early diagnosis of ALS.

A partial foot drop is usually due to lower motoneuron disease. Lumbar (L5) radiculopathy, peroneal palsy and progressive lumbar plexopathy all need to be considered in the diagnosis. Lumbar radiculopathy is not always painful or the pain may be modest and considered simply as a nuisance. Similarly, subjective or objective dermatomal sensory deficits may be mild or non-existent. Peroneal palsies are usually acute in onset and the motor deficit is more complete than usually occurs with a radiculopathy or anterior horn cell disease. Progressive lumbosacral plexopathies are most frequently due to diabetes, vasculitis or secondary carcinomatous infiltration. They are typically painful and associated with a sensory deficit. Monomelic amyotrophy rarely affects the leg, compared to the arm (see Case report 2.4 above); when it does do so, the disease course and characteristics are identical to those of the commoner upper limb monomelic amyotrophy. Multifocal motor neuropathy with conduction block rarely starts in the leg (Nobile-Orazio, 1996); when this happens, the predominant weakness is proximal.

Painless, weak, wasted shoulder

Shoulder muscle wasting or weakness is a common early feature of ALS, often first becoming noticeable when the patient is shaving, combing the hair or brushing the teeth. Some of the myotomes involved are also those commonly affected by degenerative disc disease, particularly the C5/C6 myotomes. Abnormalities of routine radiographs and CT scans are almost invariable in the age group having the peak incidence of ALS. Sometimes, disc degeneration is painless, even when causing considerable muscle wasting; this adds to difficulty in diagnosis. Clues pointing to ALS as being the cause of impaired shoulder function include fasciculation involving the pectoralis muscle with preservation of tendon reflexes in weak myotomes, such as an easily elicited pectoralis tendon reflex. Weakness and atrophy of the pectoralis muscle are an ominous clinical feature because the innervation of this muscle is shared with that of the diaphragm. Needle EMG of the diaphragm, in the face of pectoralis muscle weakness, is often abnormal, even in the absence of respiratory distress. Motor neuropathy with conduction block is another diagnostic consideration in the context of painless shoulder weakness. As previously discussed, weakness without wasting and loss of reflexes in the affected myotome are important clues pointing to MMN, which is readily confirmed by demonstrating proximal conduction block (see Case report 2.3).

Three particular nerve palsies, of the accessory nerve, serratus anterior and suprascapular nerve, can occur as isolated palsies. They all cause motor deficits around the shoulder joint, often without pain. As a result they may not be noticed by the patient at onset, but are often first detected by relatives or during a routine physical examination. Furthermore, idiopathic brachial neuritis (neuralgic amyotrophy) may be painless and restricted in distribution. The three palsies are then misinterpreted as being progressive in nature.

Spontaneous accessory nerve palsy

This syndrome is akin to neuralgic amyotrophy and results from a lesion at an accessory nerve branching point, usually as it exits from the posterior margin of the sternomastoid (Eisen and Bertrand, 1972). The site of the lesion is probably distal to the motor branch of the sterno-cleidomastoid, since this muscle is spared. Unlike typical neuralgic amyotrophy, the onset may not be painful and others rather than the patient may first notice the motor deficit. The weakness in the wasted shoulder might be assumed by the patient or physcian to be progressive in nature. Weakness of the upper portion of the trapezius muscle predomi-nates and weakness of shoulder elevation is the main functional deficit. Initially, pain in the shoulder may be severe, but sensory deficits are never encountered. In most cases the upper trapezius muscle fibres atrophy so that the scapula becomes unstable. This produces a 'droopy shoulder' which leads to variable, chronic, low-grade discomfort, probably related to traction on the brachial plexus and changes in the glenohumeral joint. The upper trapezius fibres insert into the lateral end of the clavicle, the acromion and the spine of the scapula. Unlike scapula winging due to serratus anterior nerve palsy, the winging of accessory nerve is brought out by lateral movement of the arm. The angle of the scapula is shifted laterally and downwards, whilst in a serratus anterior palsy the angle of the scapula moves medially and upwards. Conduction time through the accessory nerve can be measured by stimulating the nerve as it exits from behind the sternomastoid and recording over the upper trapezius. Conduction is invariably normal, but the upper trapezius CMAP amplitude is often very reduced, indicating an axonal mononeuropathy. Needle EMG of the upper trapezius fibres shows variable amounts of fibrillation and positive sharp waves. Recovery is the rule but may take many months.

Serratus anterior nerve palsy

When occurring spontaneously, the disorder also forms part of the spectrum of neuralgic amyotrophy. The nerve to serratus anterior may be involved in isolation or with other nerves, which arise from the brachial plexus. Scapula winging is the only clinical deficit, accentuated by forward extension of the arms. The angle of the scapula moves upward and medially towards the midline. The lesion is best confirmed by demonstrating abnormalities on needle EMG. Needle examination of the serratus anterior is a little tricky. The easiest approach is with the patient lying prone with the arm dangling over the bed. The needle is inserted under the scapula just below and lateral to its inferior angle.

Suprascapular nerve palsy

The suprascapular nerve (C4–C6) innervates the supraspinatus and infraspinatus, which are external rotators of the shoulder. The supraspinatus is also a shoulder abductor, in particular for the first 30° of lateral elevation of the arm. Abduction from 15° to 70° is maintained by the deltoid, but abduction between 70° and 120° is also often markedly impaired because the short leverage imparted by the deltoid is not sufficient to elevate the extended arm. Weakness of the supraspinatus and infraspinatus never completely abolishes external rotation because the posterior deltoid and teres minor have the same function.

The suprascapular nerve is frequently involved in neuralgic amyotrophy. Chronic compression of the nerve is rare but occurs with repetitive

Table 2.10. *Causes of fasciculation raising the possibility of ALS*

Cause	Comment
Benign fasciculation	Intermittent, long periods of time without fasciculations
Kennedy's disease	Sex-linked, lower motoneuron signs only, DTRs absent
Motor neuropathy with conduction block	Limited to muscles innervated by involved nerve(s), good bulk in weak, areflexic muscles
Radiculopathy	Limited to one, rarely two, myotomes
Cramp–fasciculation syndrome	Usually legs only, cramping more prominent
Phosphate and parathyroid disorders	Settle down with treatment of underlying disease

forward traction of the shoulder. Occasionally, this seems to happen spontaneously (Berry *et al.*, 1995). In chronic compression of the supra-scapular nerve, pain is deep-seated and throbbing, located along the superior border of the scapula and extending towards the shoulder. Wasting of the infraspinatus is more easily detected because, unlike the supraspinatus, it is not covered by the trapezius muscle. It may be possible to document conduction slowing through the suprascapular nerve stimu-lating the brachial plexus at Erb's point and recording from either the supraspinatus or infraspinatus. Using a monopolar needle as a recording electrode is advantageous because it reduces the confounding effects of volume conduction from other shoulder girdle muscles.

Fasciculations and cramps

Fasciculations are seen in many normal subjects and a variety of neuromuscular disorders (Table 2.10). However, in ALS they are particu-larly striking and so often diffuse. They are frequently prominent in clinically strong muscles. Kennedy's disease may be the only other condition in which fasciculations are so pronounced. Fasciculations in ALS are frequently accompanied by muscle cramps, but the two do not necessarily occur in the same muscle. The origin of both fasciculation and cramps must be an aetiopathogenic clue to the disorder; this issue is reviewed later. However, it is likely that they are a common expression of several quite different mechanisms.

When fasciculations are associated with multimyotomal muscle weakness and upper motoneuron signs, the diagnosis is virtually always ALS. We suggest that fasciculation is such an essential component of ALS that its absence on clinical or EMG examination makes the diagnosis suspect. Fasciculation may be moderately or sometimes dramatically reduced in patients taking riluzole (Rilutek) and other glutamate antagonists such as lamotrigine or neurontin. Before concluding that fasciculation is truly absent, one needs to inquire about treatment with any of these recently introduced medications. Fasciculation of the tongue is the most sensitive clinical indicator of ALS that is presently available. Unfortunately, fasciculations are not readily recognized in the tongue unless it is maintained very still. Tongue fibrillation, often confused with fasciculation, is easier to identify. The confusion probably developed in the late 1930s, when the terms fibrillation and fasciculation were used interchangeably. However, fasciculation reflects the spontaneous, intermittent activation of some or all of the muscle fibres innervated through one or possibly more motor units (Howard and Murray, 1992; Kaji, 1997), and fibrillation is the spontaneous activity of a single muscle fibre which cannot be seen clinically in muscle covered by skin. The tongue is the only 'skinned' muscle and fibrillation may be seen in it as a fine, continuous shimmering.

Fasciculations occurring in the absence of other symptoms, for example muscle weakness or wasting, are usually regarded as being of little consequence (Reed and Kurland, 1963; Blexrud *et al.*, 1993). The results of a mail survey of 121, mostly young, adults who were initially seen because of fasciculations but with a normal neurological examination revealed that after a mean follow-up period of about seven years, none had developed a serious neurological disease, in particular ALS. However, the same conclusion should not be made for patients aged 45 years or older who develop fasciculations for the first time. In our experience, and that of others (Cambier and Serratrice, 1995; Swash, 1995), fasciculations may predate other clinical abnormalities of ALS by many months. Out of a total of 258 patients with ALS examined by one of the authors (AE) over a five-year period between 1987 and 1992, 36 (14 per cent) had fasciculation, usually associated with muscle cramping, as the initial manifestation of their disease. The mean time interval between developing fasciculation and other clinical manifestations of ALS was 7.6 ± 3.4 months (3 to 11 months) (Eisen *et al.*, 1992). In two patients, fasciculation was initially noted in the abdominal musculature and the diaphragm. Both patients were women who later developed marked bulbar dysfunction. In three patients we were able to perform serial EMG studies over several months which showed an absence of motor unit abnormalities at the time that the fasciculations first started. Chapter 5 describes how, on electrophysiological grounds, fasciculations can usually be recognized as not 'benign' when they occur in non-wasted, strong muscles. However, there are no definite clinical clues to indicate that the fasciculation is benign or otherwise. Fasciculation occurring in small hand or foot muscles often causes movement of the digit, but this too can happen in benign fasciculation. One possible clue, observed about 30 years ago by Norris, is the synchronous occurrence of fasciculations in antagonists and homologous muscles innervated through several adjoining spinal segments. If this observation is correct, and it can really only be proved by sophisticated physiological studies, it would be clear evidence that in ALS fasciculations must arise at least as proximal as the anterior horn cells and can involve more than one motor unit (Norris, 1965).

Benign fasciculation occurring in normal subjects, although extremely common, is largely of no concern to those who experience it (Reed and Kurland, 1963). Onset is usually before age 30 years and the fasciculations continue for months or years, but do so intermittently. There may be long periods lasting many months when the fasciculations, which are mainly felt at night, become quiescent. Their frequency is increased by exercise, fatigue, over-indulgence in alcohol, caffeine ingestion, stress and, as personally experienced, long air flights. These factors have little effect on the fasciculations of ALS. Cramps are commonly associated with fasciculation in ALS but are rare in benign fasciculation. Fasciculation in Kennedy's disease may be very prominent. However, the sex-linked inheritance, lack of upper motoneuron signs, depressed or absent deep tendon reflexes and small or absent SNAPs easily distinguish it from ALS. Fasciculation occurring in association with a radiculopathy is limited to one or two myotomes with depressed or absent reflexes in the same distribution. Even if pain or subjective sensory complaints are absent, some objective sensory deficit is nearly always detectable in radiculopathies. When fasciculation is prominent in MMN with conduction block it is restricted to muscles innervated by a single or several nerves. The weak muscles have normal bulk for many years, which serves as a clinical clue to the presence of conduction block. Cramp–fasciculation syndrome, although usually sporadic, may be recessively inherited. The fasciculations are most prominent in the legs, particularly the gastrocnemius muscle. Neurological examination is otherwise normal. There may be a mild elevation in serum creatine kinase, and muscle biopsies may show mild abnormalities or neurogenic atrophy. Repetitive nerve stimulation at rates of 0.5 to 5 per second evoke showers of electrical activity that follow the compound muscle action potential. Fasciculations and the evoked electrical discharges are abolished by regional curare, but not by nerve block. This strongly suggests that the origin of the activity is at the postjunctional level and is distal to the nerve terminal. Most patients will respond to therapy with carbamazepine (Tahmoush *et al.*, 1991).

Onset with respiratory failure

Respiratory insufficiency, leading to exercise intolerance and shortness of breath, occurs commonly as ALS progresses, and respiratory difficulties are frequently the cause of death. However, severe respiratory failure needing ventilation is sometimes the presenting feature of ALS (Hill, Martin and Hakim, 1983; Chen *et al.*, 1996). The correct diagnosis is not usually appreciated until after the patient is unable to be weaned off the respirator and becomes dependent upon home ventilation, either using BIPAP or a mechanical ventilator. The usual course of events is for the patient to be admitted to the intensive care unit (ICU) and for respiratory investigation to fail to find a satisfactory explanation for hypercapnic respiratory failure, which is usually attributed to pneumonia, chronic obstructive pulmonary disease (COPD) or sleep apnoea. Thirteen (2.1 per cent) of our 624 patients presented with respiratory difficulties. Clinical examination in all of them showed poor chest expansion and paradoxical indrawing of the abdomen during inspiration indicative of bilateral diaphragmatic weakness. Electrophysiological examination in these patients is important because it shows disproportionate involvement of the diaphragm, and to a lesser extent the intercostal muscles, compared to the limb musculature. Active denervation with profuse fibrillation or positive sharp waves is seen in the diaphragm or intercostal muscles.

An important new source of information about ALS and its interrelation with other diseases has come from analysis of the clinical and pathological features of ALS patients who have been maintained for long periods on respiratory support. These patients provide a view of what signs would become manifest if patients did not succumb to respiratory insufficiency. This has given rise to the designation 'total manifestations of ALS'. An important limitation of these studies is the possibility that some signs could be a complication of respiratory support, such as episodes of hypoxia or ischaemia.

ALS presenting with respiratory failure raises particularly challenging ethical issues given that the disease is previously undiagnosed and yet the patients are precipitated into lifetime dependency on respiratory support. The nature of the disease should be carefully explained and the option of home ventilation should be introduced impartially and without bias. The patient should be given ample time to arrive at a decision for long-term ventilation.

Cognitive impairment in ALS

The issue of cognitive impairment in ALS is interesting and is discussed further in Chapter 8. Overt dementia is rare in ALS and in our experience less than 5 per cent of patients demonstrate progressive cognitive decline in association with their disease. When it occurs, cognitive impairment may be the presenting feature. The nature of the cognitive impairment, especially how it may differ from that seen in AD, was formerly uncertain and confused (Hudson, 1981). However, recent studies have shown that it tends to have the characteristics of a frontal lobe dementia, consisting of impaired shifting from one line of thinking to another, perseveration, emotional disinhibition and impaired judgement. In addition there are parietal deficits of design, verbal fluency, visual attention and performance on the Wisconsin Card Sorting Test. In the presence of significant bulbar involvement and spasticity, some of the cognitive deficits may be difficult to appreciate and interpret.

Cognitive dysfunction has been demonstrated in non-demented ALS patients using a variety of tasks. It is most easily revealed using verbal fluency or word generation paradigms, which place demands on executive functions. Abnormalities are also detected using other psychometric measures. Positron emission tomography (PET; Gallassi et al., 1989; Ludolph et al., 1992; Kew et al., 1993; Abrahams et al., 1996) and, more recently, functional MRI have also demonstrated abnormalities of the frontal and prefrontal cortex in ALS patients who are not clinically demented. It remains to be seen if ALS patients with cognitive impairment, which is especially linked to pseudobulbar palsy, represent a distinct phenotype of the disease or simply reflect a part of the clinical spectrum that has not previously been fully appreciated. In any event, these abnormalities which result from lesions that are outside the primary motor cortex suggest that the 'selective vulnerability' of the motor pathways in ALS is relative and not absolute.

Of our total patient database (664 patients) 16 (2.4 per cent) had significant cognitive decline occurring simultaneously with the characteristic motor deficits of ALS or preceding them by several months and occasionally a year or two. At autopsy, in addition to the typical lesions of ALS, there are widespread pathological changes involving much of the neocortex, limbic cortex and hippocampus (Kato *et al.*, 1994). Neuronal loss, gliosis and sponginess are present in the involved areas. This particular combination suggests an overlap between ALS and AD. The issue of overlapping of the neurodegenerative disorders is revisited in Chapter 8.

Case report 2.6: ALS with frontal lobe dementia

A 69-year-old retired radiologist, who had been previously well and physically very active, noticed diffuse fasciculation involving the arms, legs, chest wall and back for about 12 months. Over the same period he had developed difficulty articulating. He had no limb weakness at the time of initial examination, but was short of breath when lying down. There was paucity of tongue movement, associated dysarthria and fasciculation in the tongue. Reflexes were moderately brisk, but there were no overt upper motoneuron abnormalities. His attitude to his complaints was somewhat facile, despite his advanced medical knowledge. He insisted that his symptoms were due to multilevel spondylosis. Over the next 18 months his bulbar symptoms progressed and he eventually needed a percutaneous endoscopically placed gastrostomy (PEG) and use of intermittent and then continuous BIPAP. Diffuse muscle weakness and wasting also developed. He became increasingly demented. His behaviour was frequently inappropriate, irrational and combative and he continued to deny the existence of serious disease until shortly before his death. The personality changes and features of cognitive decline were subsequently recognized by a number of different physicians with whom he had previously worked.

Case report 2.7: ALS with frontal lobe dementia

A 29-year-old woman died of a progressive neurodegenerative disorder which had lasted four to five years. Her initial symptom was difficulty in speaking: 'I can think of the words but can't speak them'. Her slurred speech eventually required her to leave her job as a legal secretary. There was a general decline in her function and eventually she could no longer take care of her children or the household. The family noted loss of inhibition with inappropriate behaviour. Her speech became restricted to single words. When examined about 15 months before her death, she was alert with impaired grooming. The combination of dementia and severe dysarthria precluded assessment of mental content. Her affect was flattened and pseudobulbar with inappropriate laughter and crying. She could only follow one-step commands. She was moderately bradyphrenic and bradykinetic. There was no voluntary conjugate eye movements. When asked to look up or down, right or left, she had to turn her head. Brainstem reflexes were intact. She was spastic and hyper-reflexic in her extremities and had bilateral up-going toes. She had a snout and sucking reflex and bilateral palmomental and grasp reflexes and a very brisk jaw jerk. Cerebellar testing was normal and there were no sensory abnormalities. Extensive laboratory investigations, to rule out vasculitis, Wilson's disease, liver disease, mitochondrial disorders, heavy metal intoxication, chronic infection and MS were unhelpful. A bone marrow aspiration was normal. Two MRIs were normal. The EEG showed diffuse slowing and low-voltage activity maximum in the frontal and central regions. There were no periodic discharges.

Pathology On gross inspection of the brain, there was marked gyral atrophy confined to the frontal convexities (Fig. 2.2A). On serial coronal sectioning, there was enlargement of the lateral ventricles and marked atrophy of the caudate nucleus. The cortical grey ribbon of the frontal lobe was thinned and showed spongiosis and gliosis of the neuropil. There was considerable neuronal dropout. Remaining neurons frequently contained pale eosinophilic cytoplasmic inclusions that were eccentric to the nucleus and were strongly ubiquitin immunoreactive. Staining for senile plaques, neurofibrillary tangles and Pick bodies was

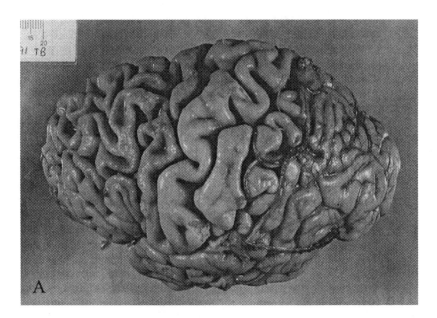

Figure 2.2. Pathological findings from Case report 2.7. (A) There is marked gyral atrophy of the motor, prefrontal and orbitofrontal cortices. There was no significant loss of neurons in the spinal cord, but degeneration of the lateral corticospinal tracts was very marked (B). (C) Ubiquitin-reactive inclusions are shown in the anterior horn cells within the spinal cord. (Scale in centimetres.)

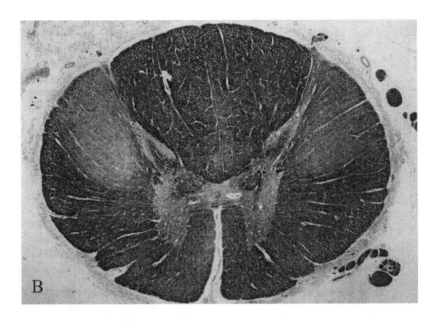

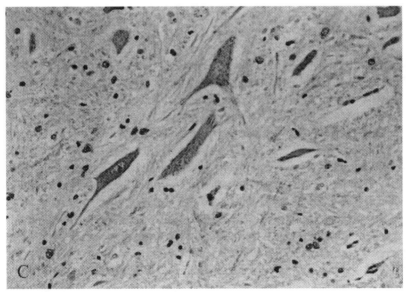

Figure 2.2. *Continued.*

negative. The cytoplasmic inclusions stained negatively for antibodies to neurofilament protein. Similar, less severe, changes were present in the precentral and postcentral gyri, inferior and middle temporal gyri and angular gyrus. The occipital lobe was normal. There were decreased numbers of Betz cells in the primary motor cortex. There was not significant loss of neurons in the spinal cord, but degeneration of the lateral corticospinal tracts was marked (Fig. 2.2B). Ubiquitin-reactive inclusions were also present in the amygdala, hippocampus, thalamus, caudate nucleus and medial part of the putamen. These structures showed severe neuron loss and gliosis. Ubiquitin-reactive inclusions were also present in the trochlear and hypoglossal nuclei and anterior horn cells within the spinal cord (Fig. 2.2C).

Comment The clinical features, pattern of neuronal degeneration and character of the cytoplasmic inclusions are typical of ALS with dementia of the frontal lobe type. This case is unusual because of the young age of the patient. This, the severe dementia, ophthalmoplegia, lack of apparent muscle wasting and absence of clinical fasciculations probably accounted for the failure to think of ALS–dementia. As a result, an EMG was never done.

(This patient was seen at the University of British Columbia, Department of Psychiatry. We are indebted to Drs T. A. Hurwitz and T. G. Beach (neuropathology) for allowing us to publish the details.)

ALS and neoplasm

The first case of cancer occurring with ALS was described in 1961 (O'Doherty, 1961). The patient had lung cancer and a rapid neurological decline, due to motoneuron disease, with death within four months. Autopsy showed pathological changes typical of ALS with no nervous system metastases. Subsequently, Brain, Croft and Wilkinson (1965) and Norris and Engle (1965) described a further 24 patients between them with cancer and ALS. Not all of the cases had typical pathological changes of ALS and in many there were no upper motoneuron signs. Since then there have been several reports, both positive and negative in terms of a significant relationship between cancer and ALS. The incidence of a positive relationship has ranged from 0 per cent to 10 per cent of ALS patients (Rosenfeld and Posner, 1991). As both the incidences of ALS and of cancer peak in the same age groups, they are likely to occur together in some patients by coincidence. In one study the frequency of malignancy amongst nearly 4000 patients with ALS was 2.0 per cent, which is not statistically different from the population at large. At present there is no proven significant increase in the incidence of either ALS in patients with cancer or cancer in patients with ALS. However, as pointed out by Rowland (1995), in Israel, where it is possible to collect data on all cases of ALS, thus removing ascertainment bias, the frequency of malignancy amongst patients with ALS is 4.5 per cent, which is more than double that of controls (Gubbay *et al.*, 1985). In our own ALS population we have had 2 (0.3 per cent) patients with otherwise typical ALS who had associated cancers, one with pancreatic cancer and the other with non-Hodgkin's lymphoma. Treatment of the cancers did not change the course of their ALS. Alteration of the natural history of ALS by treating a concomitant malignancy would be an important indication that there is a meaningful linkage, presumably autoimmune, between the cancer and ALS. There are published reports of eight patients whose ALS was improved or 'cured' after effective treatment of the tumour (Rosenfeld and Posner, 1991; Rowland *et al.*, 1994). The issue, then, of solid organ cancer and ALS is not entirely settled, but if there is a true, non-coincidental relationship, it must be extremely rare (Forsyth *et al.*, 1997).

The association of ALS with lymphoproliferative disease appears to be more definite than that with solid organ malignancies (Rowland, 1997). There have been descriptions of this association in 56 patients (most frequently Hodgkin's disease) (Rowland, 1995). However, most cases have had lower motoneuron signs only and thus were not typical of classical ALS. Others had both definite upper and lower motoneuron abnormalities and some had PUMNS. Half of the patients who have had autopsies had abnormalities of the corticospinal tracts and all but one of the indexed patients have died of their neurological disorder. There is a spontaneously occurring mouse disorder, due to a retrovirus, in which lymphoma is associated with progressive muscular atrophy. It is possible that the murine virus causes lymphoma followed by antibody production that attacks the anterior horn cell. How this might relate to the human disease is uncertain.

Monoclonal paraproteinaemia and motoneuron diseases

There has been interest in monoclonal proteins and how they relate to motoneuron diseases for about 15 years. The described relationships to ALS are confusing, but can, as suggested by Rowland (1995), be considered under four categories of motoneuronal immunopathy: antibodies to GM1, MMN with persisting conduction block, lymphoproliferative disease, and paraneoplastic motoneuron disease with other tumours. The monoclonal protein is most often of the IgM class, and

Table 2.11. *Incorrect diagnoses of ALS amongst 664 patients seen at the University of British Columbia ALS Clinic*

Diagnosis	Number (%) of patients
Cervical spondylotic myeloradiculopathy	14 (2.1)
Painless radiculopathy	4 (0.6)
Progressive spinal multiple sclerosis	4 (0.6)
Monomelic amyotrophy	7 (1.1)
Motor neuropathy with conduction block	12 (1.8)
Chronic inflammatory demyelinating polyneuropathy	3 (0.5)
Progressive bulbospinal neuronopathy (Kennedy's syndrome)	2 (0.3)
Inclusion body myositis	1 (0.2)
Total	47 (7.1)

reacts with glycolipids or other neuronal antigens. The frequency of observations of such monoclonal peaks is about 10 per cent in ALS, 30 per cent in patients with multifocal conduction block, 40 per cent in patients with lymphoproliferative disease, and 80 per cent in patients that have a cerebrospinal fluid protein content of > 75 mg/dl.

Accuracy of diagnosis of ALS

A false-positive diagnosis of ALS by neurologists is uncommon. If patients with ALS and without dementia or Parkinsonian features are excluded, diagnostic accuracy is greater than 90 per cent (Davenport *et al.*, 1996). Diagnostic accuracy is greater when patients attend large ALS clinics where the neurologists are more familiar with the nuances of the disease. Accurate and early diagnosis is essential to allay anxiety in the setting of a universally fatal disease, often of short duration. Public awareness of ALS has escalated considerably and many patients suspect they have the disease prior to being diagnosed with ALS. Accurate diagnosis is essential to rule out other illnesses that have a better prognosis than ALS, and which may respond to therapy. Therapeutic efforts in ALS are now more encouraging than ever, and if advantage is to be taken of these advances, the diagnosis must be made as early as possible. On the other hand, patients should not be informed that they have ALS until the diagnosis is considered secure. If after complete investigation (including imaging if indicated and electrophysiology) the diagnosis is still in doubt, it is better to follow the patient's clinical course for a few months, after which the picture usually becomes clearer. The most common errors in diagnosis are listed in Table 2.11.

Summary

The constellation of weakness and muscle wasting in a pattern of functional movement rather than a peripheral nerve or a myotomal distribution associated with fasciculation and hyper-reflexia is nearly always due to ALS. The El Escorial diagnostic criteria are now reasonably well established and, even though they may be modified over time, they should be used to classify ALS into definite, probable, possible and suspected categories. ALS starting with limb or bulbar onset, affecting the young or old or having rapid versus slow progression should not be assumed to represent a single disease. ALS in the young is more common in men and usually has a limb onset. Fasciculation is an integral part of ALS; when clinically or electrophysiologically absent, the diagnosis becomes doubtful. Fasciculation occurring for the first time in patients aged over 45 years must be considered seriously; this may be the presenting feature of ALS. Degenerative disease of the cervical spine is a very frequently associated with ALS. Determining how much neurological deficit should be attributed to cervical myelopathy or ALS may be challenging. Important differential diagnostic considerations for ALS include:

1. High cervical cord compression which causes hand wasting.
2. Hirayama's monomelic amyotrophy: this usually affects young men, one arm and is self-limiting.
3. Multifocal motor neuropathy with persisting conduction block: the weakness is in the distribution of a peripheral nerve, and muscle bulk is maintained in the face of marked weakness.
4. Kennedy's syndrome (X-linked bulbosinal neuronopathy) which does not have an upper motoneuron component and is associated with a variable sensory ataxia and absent reflexes.

Whereas ALS usually presents with limb or bulbar dysfunction, it may rarely present with respiratory failure. In this setting patients are admitted to hospital or the intensive care unit for investigation of a primary lung disease. In about 5 per cent of patients with ALS there is an overt dementia; frontal lobe dementia may be a presenting feature.

3

The pathology of ALS

Introduction

This chapter examines some neuropathological features of ALS.
Formerly, neuropathological studies of this disease described the pattern
of neuron loss. However, more recent studies have revealed that ALS
tissue possesses a wide array of cytoplasmic abnormalities. These
abnormalities have become much better understood with immunohistochemical and electron microscopic analysis. For instance, the observation
that neurofilaments accumulate within motoneurons and other cells has
raised the possibility that this neurofilamentous change could be a cause
or consequence of impaired axonal transport. The observation of
ubiquitin immunoreactivity has also generated considerable excitement
as it is possible that the inclusions may represent a protein that is
involved in the pathogenesis of ALS, or a marker of a distinct patho-
physiologic process ultimately resulting in the specific pattern of involvement seen in the disease. The role of neuropathological studies in ALS is
undergoing a transformation. These studies are no longer purely descrip-
tive but have become a means of validating the importance of various
animal models of ALS. This is particularly the case for transgenic mice,
in which manipulation of the genome of the animal results in a different
phenotype. To evaluate how closely a transgenic mouse model
approaches human ALS requires a thorough neuropathological evaluation to describe the distribution and type of cell loss. Conversely,
neuropathological studies of mutant animals have provided insights into
possible neuropathological features of human ALS which were formerly
unrecognized. It is for this reason that descriptions of pathological
features of a number of mutant and transgenic animals are included in
this chapter. These animal models can be used to determine the conditions under which intracellular inclusions can be seen, or when

motoneuron death will occur. As is discussed in Chapter 7, pathological studies using animal models can also be used to evaluate therapeutic strategies to prevent motoneuron loss.

In this chapter, the term ALS is used as a general definition to describe a disorder characterized by progressive involvement of motoneurons as well as descending motor tracts. Traditionally, ALS has been subdivided into relatively distinct clinicopathological syndromes (see Chapter 2). The term ALS itself has also been used to identify the syndrome associated with loss of both bulbar and spinal motoneurons in addition to motor pathways within the central nervous system. PMA comprises cranial and spinal motoneuron involvement exclusively, without evidence of degeneration of 'upper motoneurons'. Progressive bulbar palsy identifies a syndrome with bulbar and pseudobulbar features, but without more extensive upper or lower motoneuron dysfunction. The generally accepted view is that ALS, PMA and progressive bulbar palsy are different manifestations of the same disease process.

Neuropathologically, the diagnosis of ALS is based upon the demonstration of spinal and bulbar motoneuron loss as well as variable reductions in the numbers of descending corticospinal projections. These general changes result in well-defined gross and microscopic features which include atrophy of brain, spinal cord, peripheral nerve and muscle. This is also accompanied by microscopic evidence of neuron loss, cellular changes and other effects.

In general, macroscopically evident changes in ALS are usually limited to atrophy of motor nerves, ventral roots and skeletal muscle. Cerebral atrophy is unusual, although occasional patients may have atrophy of the precentral gyri. These macroscopic observations have been supported by recent imaging studies which have found normal volumes of cortical and subcortical tissue in ALS patients compared to controls (Kiernan and Hudson, 1994; see also Chapter 6). Examination of the spinal cord reveals shrunken ventral roots, which contrast with normal-appearing dorsal roots. The spinal cord itself usually appears normal on external examination; however, transverse sections demonstrate shrinkage and whitish discoloration in the lateral aspect of the lateral funiculi, in regions which correspond to the corticospinal tracts (Brownell, Oppenheimer and Hughes, 1970; Rossi, 1994). Atrophy of the hypoglossal nerves can be seen with brainstem involvement and may also be observed in patients with more generalized disease. Skeletal muscle is atrophied, pale and fibrotic.

Table 3.1. *Microscopic findings in ALS*

(A) Neuronal changes that are invariably present
   (i)   Neuronal loss
   (ii) Simple atrophy
   (iii) 'Senescent' changes
(B) Neuronal changes that are frequently seen but are absent in some cases
   Cellular inclusions
   (i)   Neurofilament accumulation
       spheroids
       phosphorylated neurofilaments
       nitration of neurofilaments
   (ii) Ubiquinated inclusions
   (iii) Bunina bodies
   (iv) Basophilic inclusions
   (v) Hyaline inclusions
   Pattern of involvement
   (vi) Involvement of interneurons
   (vii) Tract degeneration
(C) Uncommonly observed features
   (i)   Lewy bodies
   (ii) Heterotopic neurons
   (iii) Astrocytosis
   (iv) Microglial activation
(D) Neuronal changes in related conditions
   (i)   ALS with dementia
   (ii) ALS with Parkinsonism–dementia
   (iii) Guamanian ALS
   (iv) Familial ALS
   (v) ALS with prolonged survival

Microscopic findings in ALS

Microscopic examination of the nervous system reveals a wide range of cellular changes in ALS. The distribution of neuron involvement is relevant in terms not only of which cell groups are affected, but of which are spared. For instance, although motoneuron loss can be prominent in bulbar and spinal motoneuron pools, the nuclei of the extraocular muscles and the sacral sphincteric motoneurons (nucleus of Onufrowicz) are conspicuously spared (Pullen, 1996). Involvement of these motoneuron pools can occur, but it is often late in the course of the disease (Swash and Schwartz, 1992).

Microscopic neuronal changes in ALS may be classified into four categories (Table 3.1): (A) neuronal changes which are invariably present, (B) neuronal changes that are frequently seen but absent in some cases, (C) uncommon neuronal changes, and (D) neuronal changes reported largely in special groups of ALS cases (Hirano and Iwata, 1979).

Neuronal changes invariably present in ALS

Neuronal loss

Neuronal loss, especially in the ventral horns and precentral cortex, is a defining feature of ALS. However, the reduction in the number of neurons is difficult to quantify and is seldom uniform and symmetric (Brownell *et al.*, 1970; Tsukagoshi *et al.*, 1979; Chou, 1994). Loss of the large pyramidal neurons (Betz cells) is seen; however, the axons of these cells constitute only a small fraction of the pyramidal tract and neuron losses are not restricted to this cell type. In the spinal cord, the neuron loss may be more prominent in cervical regions than in other areas. Many of the remaining ventral horn cells exhibit different stages of atrophy, including a reduction in cell volume, increased pigmentation and nuclear displacement. Certain motoneuron nuclei are more often involved than others. In the brainstem, the nuclei of XII and the motor nuclei of V and VII are more often involved than the other bulbar motoneurons. In the spinal cord, the dorsolateral motoneuron pool is often more affected than the ventromedial pool (Chou, 1994).

Quantitation of neuron loss in ALS has been performed by several groups. Tsukagoshi and colleagues (1979) found that large motoneurons were lost more commonly than smaller motoneurons, and this loss was diffuse rather than focal in the C6 cervical segment. The number of surviving motoneurons correlated with the number of normal-sized muscle fibres in the corresponding biceps muscle (Tsukagoshi *et al.*, 1979). The 'diffuse' nature of the motoneuron loss found in this autopsy study contrasts with clinical reports suggesting that involvement of the contralateral lower limb after unilateral leg involvement may occur more frequently than upper limb involvement. This suggests that the motoneuron loss is not diffuse and random within motoneuron pools (Brooks *et al.*, 1994). There is also abundant clinical experience indicating that ALS tends to affect motoneurons innervating distal extremity muscles, rather than proximal muscles. This selectivity might arise as the motoneurons of distal muscles have a more extensive innervation by corticospinal tract axons than motoneurons innervating proximal muscles. How corticospinal tract loss might translate into motoneuron death is unknown, but it could involve aberrant exchange of trophic substances between these neuron pools. Both α and γ motoneurons disappear in ALS (Tsukagoshi *et al.*, 1979). Neuron loss in spinal cord is not restricted to motoneurons and also includes interneurons (Swash *et al.*, 1986), neurons of Clarke's column (Averback and Crocker, 1982) and sensory neurons (Kawamura *et al.*, 1981). However, the loss of sensory neurons and interneurons in the spinal cord is modest when compared to the extensive loss of motoneurons.

Simple atrophy

Simple atrophy (neuronal atrophy) is the most common cellular change seen in ALS. The atrophic cells appear shrunken and dark, with nuclear pyknosis and corkscrew deformities of the dendrites. The distribution of atrophic neurons includes the large motoneurons of the brainstem and spinal cord as well as cortical neurons (Chou, 1994). Studies of the

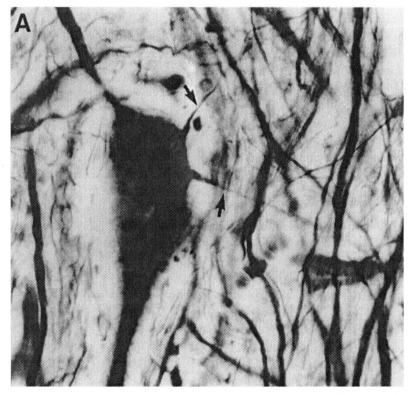

Figure 3.1. (A) and (B) Dendritic atrophy (arrows). Holmes stain. (Courtesy of Dr S. Carpenter.)

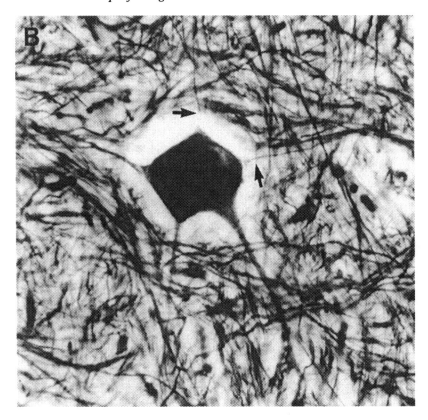

Figure 3.1. *Continued.*

pyramidal tract neurons in ALS have revealed that the somata of Betz cells are swollen, with a reduction in the size and complexity of the dendritic arbour (Hammer, Tomiyasu and Scheibel, 1979). Dendrites are fragmented and irregular, with a reduction in calibre (Fig. 3.1).

'Senescent' changes

Various cellular changes are almost invariably present in ALS which overlap with morphological alterations seen in tissue from normal, aged individuals. These cellular changes include the possible accumulation of lipofuscin, as well as dendritic fragmentation and loss. An unresolved issue is whether the observation of these 'senescent' changes merely reflects the age of the patients examined at autopsy, rather than any other feature of the disease. Lipofuscin accumulation involves the intra-cellular deposition of yellow or orange, acid-fast granules, which are often

Table 3.2. *Cellular inclusions in ALS*

Inclusion	Site	LM appearance	Component proteins
1. Spheroids	Axons and MNs	Rounded hyaline swellings 10–100 μm (diameter) eosinophilic, argyrophilic	NFs, (P+, P−) ubiquitin
2. Hyaline bodies	MNs	Homogeneous, eosinophilic, argyrophilic conglomerates	NFs, (P+, P−)
3. Bunina bodies	MNs	Eosinophilic, rounded or elongated, single or multiple masses (1–10 μm diameter)	Ubiquitin + and −
4. Basophilic bodies	MNs	Basophilic, 'globoid' or 'asteroid' shapes (3–4 μm diameter)	Not known
5. Lewy body-like inclusions	MNs; occasionally extracellular in spinal grey matter	Eosinophilic concentric bodies with dense core and lightly staining halo (7–20 μm diameter)	NFs, (P+, P−) ubiquitin
6. Tubular particles	Axons and MNs in spinal grey matter	Not detected	Not known
7. Pericapillary bodies	Capillary wall in spinal cord	Eosinophilic, single or multiple (0.5–8 μm diameter) ovoid bodies	GFAP+
8. Hirano bodies	Perikarya and dendrites of MNs, axons in spinal grey matter	Eosinophilic, rod-shaped bodies (4–6 μm diameter)	Actin, α-actinin, tau, tropomyosin; vinculin
9. Granulovacuolar degeneration (Guam ALS)	MNs	Clear vacuoles (3 μm diameter), containing 1 μm granules	NFs, (P+) tubulin

Table modified and reproduced from Leigh and Swash (1991) with permission.
MNs, cranial and spinal motoneurons; NFs, neurofilaments; P+, phosphorylated; P−, non-phosphorylated epitopes; GFAP, glial fibrillary acidic protein.

seen in large neurons. On electron microscopy, these granules are lobulated and membrane bound. As the accumulation of lipofuscin is believed usually to be an age-related phenomenon, it is difficult to determine whether the prominence of these granules is due to greater accumulation of this product, or to a decrease in the volume of neurons. The reduction in cellular components may make the lipofuscin more conspicuous. Microdensitometric analysis of lipofuscin granules in spinal motoneurons from ALS tissue has been reported to be unchanged compared to control tissue (McHolm, Aguilar and Norris, 1984). Lipofuscin-bearing cells have also been reported to be strongly immuno-reactive for the oncoprotein bcl-2 in ALS tissue (Migheli *et al.*, 1994). This oncoprotein is believed to be protective and its presence may lead to improved survival of lipofuscin-bearing neurons. Dendritic fragmentation of Betz cells has been reported in ALS but, like lipofuscin accumulation, this finding is often seen in normal ageing (Hammer *et al.*, 1979).

Neuronal changes frequently seen in ALS

A number of neuronal inclusions are seen in ALS. These are summarized in Table 3.2. The frequency with which these inclusions are seen is open to debate, with some authors claiming the almost universal finding of ubiquinated inclusions in ALS (Leigh, 1994).

Neurofilament accumulation

A conspicuous neuropathological feature in some patients with ALS is the accumulation of neurofilaments (NFs) in the cell bodies and proximal axons of motoneurons and other cell types (Carpenter, 1968; Delisle and Carpenter, 1984). The neurofilamentous accumulation in ALS is distinct from other neurodegenerative disorders in that the abnormal filaments are only found intracellularly. Although the accumulations of NFs are not cytoplasmic inclusions in a strict sense, they are associated with the abnormal deposition of axoplasmic components in two general patterns of involvement. The most striking is a focal deposition of NFs giving rise to cell body or proximal axonal enlargement. Alternatively, diffuse accumulation of NFs can be seen in cell bodies, axons and dendrites. Morphologically, the focal accumulations constitute swollen segments of axons with diameters of greater than $20 \, \mu m$, which contain normal-appearing NFs, so-called spheroids (Carpenter, 1968; Fig. 3.2A). Focal perikaryal lesions are variable and may be a component of hyaline inclusions (Chou, 1994).

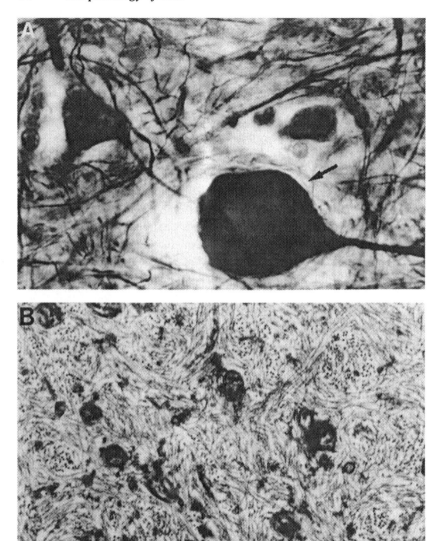

Figure 3.2. (A) Axonal swelling (arrow). Bodian stain. (Courtesy of Dr S. Carpenter.) (B) Portion of a spheroid showing accumulation of randomly arranged neurofilaments. × 26 600. (Courtesy of Dr S. Sasaki.) (C) Neuritic swelling in cultured motoneurons following activation of PKC (arrow). Dissociated cultures of murine spinal cord were exposed to 10 μm of the synthetic diacylglycerol, diC8, for 10 minutes. After 24 hours, the culture was fixed and immunolabelled with mouse anti-NF-H (phosphorylation independent) antibody. Scale bar 20 μm. (Courtesy of Dr H. Durham.)

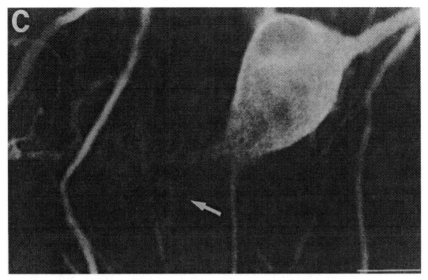

Figure 3.2. *Continued.*

Motoneurons, like other neurons, contain large numbers of NFs, which are the most abundant structural proteins present. These NFs are composed of three polypeptide subunits of low (60–70 kDa, NF-L), medium (95 kDa, NF-M) and high (115 kDa, NF-H) molecular weight (Bruijn and Cleveland, 1996; Julien, 1997). The subunits are encoded by different genes but contain a conserved central domain of about 300 amino acids which is involved in α-helical rod assembly. Neurofilaments in vivo are believed to consist of a core of low molecular weight NF (NF-L) subunits with medium molecular weight NF (NF-M) and heavy molecular weight NF (NF-H) incorporated onto the NF-L backbone, exposing the long carboxy-terminal tail region of these heavier subunits (Hirokawa, 1991; Bruijn and Cleveland, 1996). The side-arm projections of NFs appear to cross-link NFs to each other and to other structures such as intracellular organelles. Both NF-M and NF-H contain charged amino acids which probably regulate NF spacing depending on the phosphorylation state of the carboxy domain. This phosphorylation is thought to modify the spacing between NFs and the strength of the NF cross-linkages (Julien, 1997).

Spheroids Axonal spheroids, initially reported to be present only rarely in ALS (Carpenter, 1968), may be seen in over half of ALS cases

(Delisle and Carpenter, 1984). They are more common in patients with ALS than in normal individuals and are located particularly in the ventral horns of spinal cord. The absence of spheroids in ALS cases has been associated with more severe neuronal loss in spinal cord (Delisle and Carpenter, 1984). Immunochemical studies have indicated that spheroids contain proteins which can be labelled with antibodies against phosphorylated NFs (Munoz et al., 1988). Antibodies to the intermediate filament protein, peripherin, also label spheroids in a manner similar to the distribution of immunostaining against NF protein. A few spheroids demonstrate immunoreactivity to α-internexin, another intermediate filament protein. All NF subtypes appear to be represented in the spheroid. Electron microscopically, spheroids contain interwoven bundles of 10–15 nm NFs oriented in different directions (Fig. 3.2B). They also have characteristic small side arms which can be found in normal axons. Organelles such as mitochondria, vesicles and fragments of smooth endoplasmic reticulum are found among the bundles of NFs. The neurofilamentous accumulation is not entirely specific for ALS in that a similar pattern of involvement has occasionally been seen in autopsies from patients without ALS (Hirano, 1996).

The mechanism behind the disrupted NF organization and accumulation of spheroids in ALS is unclear. Simplistically, the accumulation of NFs could be due to increased synthesis of NFs, an impaired transport of these proteins, or reduced degradation of NF subunits (Xu et al., 1993). Neurofilamentous accumulation within proximal axons may lead to more substantial neuronal injury than a comparable accumulation of NFs within the cell body (Eyer and Peterson, 1994). Whether this is due to a greater impairment of axon transport by a damming effect of NFs is unclear (Julien, 1995).

The effects of overexpressing NF protein in transgenic mice have been investigated by several groups. Fourfold overexpression of NF-L results in substantial accumulations of NFs, swollen neuronal perikarya and displaced, eccentric nuclei, with proximal axonal swelling, axonal degeneration and atrophy of skeletal muscle (Xu et al., 1993). Neuropathological examination of transgenic animals showing twofold overexpression NF-H demonstrates eccentrically placed nuclei with perikaryal and proximal axonal swellings (Côté, Collard and Julien, 1993). These swellings consist of densely packed NFs which displace mitochondria, vesicles and other structures. Axonal atrophy is present as well as atrophy of skeletal muscle (Côté et al., 1993). Thus, the neurofilamentous changes seen in these transgenic mice have similarities to those in

ALS patients. Also of relevance to the possible involvement of NFs in ALS are observations of codon deletions in the carboxy-terminal tail region of the NF-H gene. This tail region has multiple repeats of lys-ser-pro (KSP) that serve as phosphorylation sites and are probably involved in cross-bridge formation. There is evidence that changes in the phosphorylation of these residues could regulate neurofilament spacing and axonal calibre (Julien, 1997). Two deletion mutations in the gene encoding for the KSP region of NF-H have been reported in five of 356 patients with sporadic ALS (Figlewicz *et al.*, 1994). More recent studies have shown two other deletion mutations in the same NF-H tail region in two of 196 sporadic ALS patients (Julien, 1997). No mutations of the NF-H gene have been reported in more than 100 cases of familial ALS or 300 control subjects.

The mechanism by which the KSP deletion mutations produce disease is unknown. However, several of these mutant NF-H proteins will convert the phosphorylation sequence from one which is activated by the cdk5 kinase, to a sequence activated by a stress-activated protein kinase (Julien, 1997). Furthermore, activation of some isoforms of the stress-activated kinase can cause abnormal phosphorylation of NF-H in cultured neurons (Julien, 1997).

It has been hypothesized that the accumulation of NFs could impair the intracellular transport of NFs and other proteins by additional subunit cross-linkages or by impeding a slow transport (Côté *et al.*, 1993). Evidence for impaired axonal transport has been demonstrated in transgenic mice overexpressing NF-H (Collard, Côté and Julien, 1995). In motor axons of NF-H-overexpressing animals there is a substantial reduction in the transport rates for all NF subunits, as well as for tubulin, actin and mitochondria. Although NF transport is impaired in both ventral and dorsal horn neurons, the large amounts of NFs in motoneurons may make them more vulnerable than other neurons. Unfortunately, it is not known whether aggregation of NFs is a critical event in motoneuron death or a non-specific response to neuronal damage.

An association between mutations in the SOD1 gene and neurofilamentous pathology has been examined in one case report (Rouleau *et al.*, 1996). A patient with a substitution mutation of SOD at Ile 113 had proximal axonal swelling and disordered arrays of NFs, especially in motoneurons. Some transgenic mice with mutations in the Cu/Zn–SOD1 gene also exhibit neurofilamentous changes similar to those in ALS patients (Tu *et al.*, 1996).

Phosphorylation of NFs ALS is characterized not only by an accumulation of NFs in motoneurons and other cells, these focal collections of NFs are often abnormally phosphorylated. This has been established by immunocytochemical analysis using antibodies to phosphorylated NF epitopes (Munoz *et al.*, 1988). In contrast, tissue from control subjects usually does not demonstrate such immunoreactivity. Neurofilament proteins are phosphorylated by a wide range of protein kinases in vitro including protein kinase A (PKA), protein kinase C (PKC), cdc2 or cdc2-like kinases, calcium/calmodulin-dependent protein kinases and tau protein kinases, among others (Nixon and Sihag, 1991). It also appears likely that the kinases responsible for protein phosphorylation at the amino-terminal head domains of NFs are different from those at the carboxy-terminal tails (Nixon and Sihag, 1991). Potentially, the reversibility of phosphorylation reactions may permit the rearrangement of the cytoskeleton, especially in dividing cells. Observations on cultured spinal cord neurons have demonstrated that activation of PKC in these cells results in the fragmentation of NFs. Neurons have massive swelling of their proximal extensions and a progressive increase in their immunoreactivity for antibodies directed to hyperphosphorylated NFs (Fig. 3.2C) (Doroudchi and Durham, 1996). This raises the possibility that PKC could be the protein kinase primarily responsible for abnormal NF phosphorylation in ALS. Furthermore, when transfected neuronal cells having abnormally phosphorylated NFs are exposed to a PKC inhibitor, a re-establishment of the normal filamentous network occurs (Carter *et al.*, 1996).

Some of the neurofibrillary changes in ALS resemble those seen following chronic intrathecal administration of aluminium into rabbits (Strong, 1994). In these animals, aluminium intoxication leads to the cellular aggregation of NFs, which have been shown to be phosphorylated within the carboxy-terminal domain of NF-H and NF-M, leading to dephosphorylation resistance, suggesting an impairment of protein phosphatase activity. Although aluminium is not the cause of ALS, this model may be of value in the further evaluation of NF phosphorylation in neurofilamentous pathology.

The aluminium intoxication model raises the issue as to whether protein phosphatase activity is normal in ALS. Protein phosphorylation is controlled by two major reciprocal enzyme systems involving the addition or removal of phosphate groups from amino acids. Protein kinases are responsible for the addition of phosphate groups to protein, whereas the protein phosphatases act to dephosphorylate proteins. Evidence that ALS

Table 3.3. *Factors potentially leading to neurofilament accumulation*

Factor	Evidence and references
Impaired regulation of neurofilaments	Transgenic mice overexpressing NF-L, NF-M, NF-H (Côté *et al.*, 1993; Xu *et al.*, 1993)
Neurofilament gene mutations	Codon deletions in the gene for NF-H of ALS patients (Figlewicz *et al.*, 1994)
	Severe motorneuron disease in transgenic mice expressing a NF-L assembly-disrupting mutant (Lee *et al.*, 1994)
SOD1 mutations	Neurofilamentous inclusions in FALS patients and in transgenic mice expressing SOD1 mutants (Rouleau *et al.*, 1996; Tu *et al.*, 1996)
Altered neurofilament phosphorylation	Aggregation of neurofilaments modulated by PKC inhibitor (Carter *et al.*, 1996)
	Neurofilamentous accumulation with PKC stimulation (Doroudchi and Durham, 1996)
Aluminium intoxication	Neurofibrillary pathology in rabbits (Strong, 1994)

ALS, amyotrophic lateral sclerosis; NF, neurofilament; PKC, protein kinase C; SOD, superoxide dismutase.

could be associated with an impairment of protein phosphatase activity is derived from a single report which claimed that there are differences between the binding of an N-methyl-D-aspartate (NMDA) receptor ion channel ligand in tissue from ALS patients and controls. Several characteristics of the binding could be modified differently in ALS and control patients, with protein phosphatase inhibitors suggesting that differences in the activities of protein phosphatases occurred in ALS (Wagey, Krieger and Shaw, 1997). This evidence is very indirect and requires further substantiation using direct measurement of protein phosphatase activity in ALS and control tissue.

As described in Chapter 4, there is evidence that the activity of PKC is increased in spinal cord tissue of ALS patients compared to controls. It is possible that the elevations of PKC activity are related to the impaired NF accumulation and abnormal phosphorylation found in autopsy studies. A list of factors that could lead to neurofilamentous accumulation is given in Table 3.3 (Julien, 1997).

Nitration of NFs Although the abnormal phosphorylation of NFs could be important for NF accumulation in ALS, it need not be the only explanation for the post-translational modifications of NFs.

Beckman and his colleagues (1993) have suggested that nitration of tyrosine residues in NF-L could interfere with NF assembly through either phosphorylation or another means. Support for this hypothesis derives from a recent histochemical analysis showing that immunoreactivity for nitric oxide synthase (NOS) and Cu/Zn–SOD1 co-localizes to motoneurons, where they can be found in neurofilamentous accumulations (Chou, Wang and Komai, 1996). Nitric oxide synthase is an important enzyme responsible for the generation of nitric oxide (NO) from arginine. Nitirc oxide, in turn, can generate peroxynitrite. Nitration of NF-L can disrupt the assembly of normal NFs (Beckman *et al.*, 1993).

Ubiquitinated inclusions

A number of distinct intraneuronal deposits, variously described as 'skein-like', 'globose', 'small rounded bodies', or having other appearances, have been observed in nervous system tissue in ALS (Leigh and Swash, 1991; Lowe, 1994). Some of these deposits demonstrate immunoreactivity to ubiquitin, a highly conserved, low molecular weight (8.5 kDa) heat shock protein implicated in the non-lysosomal degradation of protein. The presence of ubiquitin-immunoreactive structures suggests that proteins of these inclusions are resistant to proteolysis through the ubiquitin pathway. Ubiquitin immunoreactivity is seen in a number of different types of inclusion, some containing intermediate filaments including Lewy bodies and neurofibrillary tangles (see Table 3.2). The presence of ubiquitin immunoreactivity in these inclusions is not specific for ALS because ubiquitin is detected in a wide range of neurodegenerative disorders. However, ubiquitin-immunoreactive structures are only rarely observed in control material (Leigh and Swash, 1991).

Detailed morphological studies have demonstrated that ubiquitin-immunoreactive neurons are seen especially in spinal and cranial motoneurons, but are not seen in neurons of Clarke's column, the intermediolateral cell column, or Onuf's nucleus, nuclei which are rarely involved in ALS (Leigh and Swash, 1991). Inclusions have sometimes been detected in oculomotor neurons and large pyramidal neurons, as well as in the inferior olivary nucleus. The most common ubiquinated inclusion is an aggregate of thread-like structures which probably corresponds to an area of rarefaction in the neuronal cytoplasm. Thread-like inclusions can be fine or thick (coarse skein), where the extent of filamentous aggregation may represent a progressive process within motoneurons. The density and proportion of filaments within the inclusion may account for the variation in the light microscopic appearance of inclusions, which can vary from rounded bodies (with a few, thick filaments) to hyaline inclusions (with many, thick filaments) (Lowe, 1994). Although skein-like inclusions are often seen in ALS, these are not specific and have been reported in atypical Parkinsonism and other circumstances (Hirano, 1996). Less commonly observed ubiquinated inclusions are solid or dense bodies, which may correspond to hyalin or Lewy-like inclusions (Lowe, 1994). Bunina bodies do not generally demonstrate ubiquitin immunoreactivity, but immunoreactivity is commonly seen in axonal spheroids. Quantitative evaluation has suggested that ubiquitin-immunoreactive inclusions are often seen in ALS cases of short duration and are thus probably generated early in the disease.

Ubiquitin conjugation is frequently associated with neurofilamentous inclusions and it has been claimed that the substrate for ubiquitin immunoreactivity is a degradation product of NF. The specific protein involved has not been identified.

Bunina bodies

Among the most frequently observed and specific inclusion in ALS is the Bunina body (see Table 3.2). These inclusions are small (1–10 μm), granular, cytoplasmic bodies which are eosinophilic when stained with haematoxylin and eosin and are sometimes surrounded by a halo (Fig. 3.3). They are usually found in the cytoplasm of large motoneurons where they may be seen in the vicinity of proximal axonal spheroids near the cell surface. They occasionally can also be observed in the cytoplasm of large cortical neurons. However, they are never seen extracellularly, within the neuropil. Bunina bodies are typically seen in 50–75 per cent of sporadic ALS cases (Chou, 1994), as well as in the familial and Guamanian forms of the disease. Multiple Bunina bodies can fuse into beaded chains up to 20 μm in length. Bunina bodies are best detected in thin sections from well-fixed spinal cord and are never seen in pyknotic neurons. Failure to see these inclusions may be a consequence of poor fixation.

Ultrastructurally, Bunina bodies are composed of amorphous granular material surrounded by filaments, vesicles, fragments of endoplasmic reticulum, dense bodies, mitochondria and lipofuscin (Fig 3.3B) (Hirano, 1996). The nature of these inclusions is unknown. They are seldom labelled by antibodies to ubiquitin or neurofilaments, although they may be associated with ubiquitin-immunoreactive material (Leigh and Swash, 1991). To date, eosinophilic inclusions with ultrastructural features consistent with Bunina bodies have been reported only in ALS (Hirano, 1996). Thus, this inclusion is possibly a specific cytopathological marker

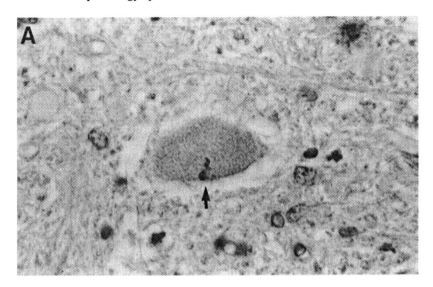

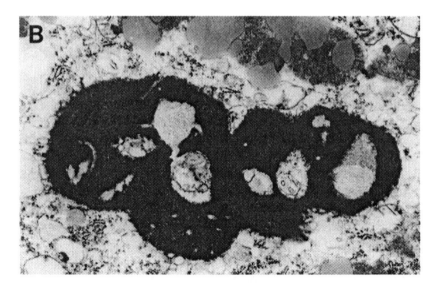

Figure 3.3. (A) Bunina body. Haematoxylin and eosin stain. (Courtesy of Dr S. Carpenter.) (B) Bunina body consisting of electron-dense material with vesicles and tubular structures containing neurofilaments. × 12 730. (Courtesy of Dr S. Sasaki.)

of ALS. Bunina bodies are seen only in neurons which are mildly affected, suggesting that they represent an initial response of the motoneuron to an insult.

Basophilic inclusions

Although infrequently observed in ALS, ventral horn neurons will some-times have mildly basophilic globoid inclusions in their cytoplasm (Chou, 1994). The inclusions are homogeneous but may vary in shape and size (4–16 μm) (Chou, 1994). Like Bunina bodies, they are best observed in well-preserved motoneurons and are seen in sporadic and familial ALS. Occasionally, Bunina bodies and basophilic inclusions are seen in the same neuron. Electron microscopic examination of these inclusions demonstrates aggregated microtubules associated with endoplasmic reticulum and ribosomes (Chou, 1994).

Hyaline inclusions

This intracytoplasmic inclusion is usually 4–6 μm in size, poorly staining and hyaline-like in appearance. Occasionally, the inclusions possess a central core which is round or oval, and may be surrounded by a halo. Chou (1994) maintains that there is little histochemical difference between these inclusions and Bunina bodies or basophilic inclusions and that homogeneous, hyaline-like inclusions might be considered a variant or an advanced stage of basophilic inclusion. It may be that some of these inclusions form a continuum of features occurring as a consequence of an impairment of axonal transport, as is shown in Fig. 3.4.

Involvement of interneurons

As indicated above, spinal neuron involvement in ALS is not limited to motoneurons. Neurons of Clarke's nucleus are occasionally reduced in number (Averback and Crocker, 1982; Swash *et al.*, 1986) and may contain Bunina inclusions, axonal spheroids or other cytological changes. Large sensory neurons in the dorsal spinal ganglia are often reduced in ALS (Kawamura *et al.*, 1981). Detailed neuron counting in ALS and control subjects has demonstrated reductions in interneuron numbers. However, the delineation of these changes has proved to be difficult. Neuron losses in cell groups having longer axons, such as dorsal root ganglion neurons and spinocerebellar neurons, have been suggested as being due to an impairment of axonal transport in these neurons (Chou, 1994).

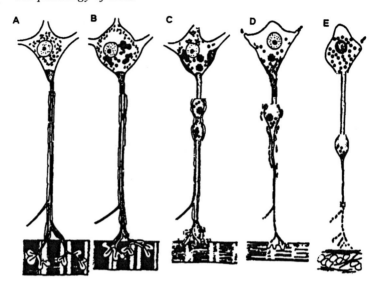

Figure 3.4. A hypothetical scheme of the interrelations between different intracellular inclusions in ALS as a consequence of impaired axonal transport. In panel A, a normal motorneuron is shown schematically. The earliest change in ALS shown in B may involve shrinking of the nerve terminal with development of basophilic inclusions. In C, hyaline and conglomerate inclusions become manifest, with nerve terminal retraction and distal axonal atrophy. In D, Bunina bodies and axonal swellings become evident, with further nerve terminal retraction. Further axonal atrophy is evident in E, with loss of dendrites, pigmentary atrophy and distal axonal swellings. (Adapted from Chou, 1994.)

Tract degeneration

Changes in the white matter are commonly seen in ALS but are variable in distribution. In the series of Brownell and colleagues (1970), no degeneration was seen in the white matter in approximately 25 per cent of sporadic cases. In another 25 per cent, degeneration was confined to regions which were thought to constitute the pyramidal tract, and this involvement could be asymmetric. Myelin and axonal degeneration can be traced to the midbrain or cerebral hemispheres where loss of fibres can be detected in the posterior limb of the internal capsule, corpus callosum and other regions (Brownell *et al.*, 1970). In approximately 50 per cent of ALS patients, white matter involvement included both lateral and anterior white columns. This pattern of white matter involvement is distinct from cases attributed to a selective loss of corticospinal tracts secondary to cerebral infarction or hemispherectomy and follows the distribution of degeneration seen with pontine gliomas or transverse myelopathy. These results suggest that loss of fibres from the lower brainstem frequently occurs in ALS and not just selective pyramidal tract loss. Demyelination is usually most apparent in the cervical spinal cord and, to a lesser degree, the medulla. The degeneration of pyramidal and other descending tracts is more marked at lower rather than at higher spinal levels. The demyelination is thought to be secondary to axonal loss; however, this is difficult to establish. In possibly 10 per cent of cases some degeneration is seen in the posterior columns (Brownell *et al.*, 1970). Generally, loss of descending tracts does not result in 'secondary' degeneration of anterior horn cells, although this has been seen in some cases. Recent studies using MRI have supported and extended these pathological findings by demonstrating signal changes consistent with demyelination in descending tracts within living patients (see Chapter 6).

Uncommonly observed pathological features of ALS

Lewy bodies

Lewy bodies are rarely seen in sporadic ALS patients, even those with Parkinsonism and dementia. Typically, they are not seen in Guamanian ALS patients. Lewy-like inclusions consist of an eosinophilic core and a distinct halo (Fig. 3.5A). Ultrastructurally, they consist of focal accumulations of randomly oriented 10-μm NFs intermingled with ill-defined fibrillar or neurofilamentous material (Fig. 3.5B) (Hirano, 1996). Lewy-like inclusions can be seen in motoneurons from FALS and sporadic ALS patients and a recent report claims that these inclusions are seen in approximately 50 per cent of ALS patients, especially within spinal motoneurons (Shibata *et al.*, 1993). Some of these inclusions demonstrate immunoreactivity to Cu/Zn–SOD and Mn–SOD (Shibata *et al.*, 1993).

Heterotopic neurons

The presence of neurons within the white matter of the brain and spinal cord has been interpreted as evidence for disordered neuronal migration during embryogenesis. Kozlowski and colleagues (1989) examined the presence of neurons within the white matter of the spinal cord using immunocytochemical markers and claimed that neurons were heterotopically located in ALS. A more recent report by Martin *et al.* (1993b) has refuted these claims. This group examined the frequency of heterotopic neurons in ALS compared to controls and patients with poliomyelitis or

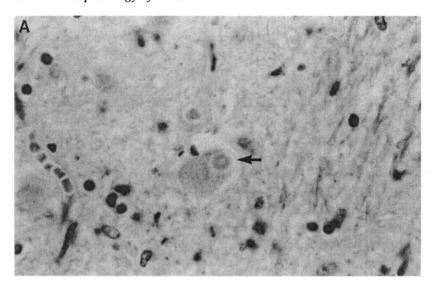

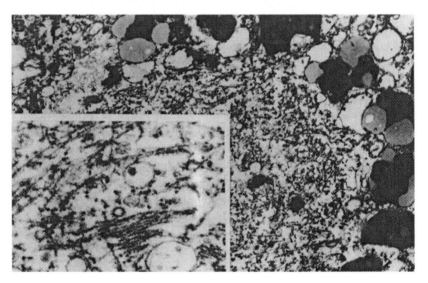

Figure 3.5. (A) Lewy-like body (arrow) within neuron. Haematoxylin and eosin. (Courtesy of Dr S. Carpenter.) (B) Lewy body-like hyaline inclusion consisting of a network of linear structures associated with ribosome-like granules having electron-dense material. × 15 200. (Inset) Higher magnification of Fig. 3.5b. Each filament has a diameter of approximately 20 nm. × 51 300. (Courtesy of Dr S. Sasaki.)

spinal muscular atrophy and no significant differences in the numbers of heterotopic neurons were found.

Two other unusual pathological features of ALS include chromatolysis and vacuolation. Neuronal chromatolysis is not regarded as a usual feature of ALS, except in cases which run a rapid course. Vacuolation is only very rarely observed in humans, whereas this finding is not infrequent in a number of animal models of motoneuron disease (see Table 3.4).

Astrocytosis

Although ALS is characterized by neuronal death, glial proliferation in spinal cord and brain occurs frequently, but is variable in extent. Foci of astrocytosis have been observed in motor, premotor and sensory cortices (Hammer *et al.*, 1979; Rossi, 1994), as well as in other cortical regions (Kushner, Stephenson and Wright, 1991). Marked astrocytosis has also been noted in subcortical regions, especially in the superficial white mater, in a widespread distribution (Kushner *et al.*, 1991). Reactive, hypertrophic astrocytes can be identified along the border between grey and white matter, although such changes are also seen in aged controls (Chou, 1994). Some of these astrocytes express histocompatibility glycoprotein human leucocyte antigen-DR (HLA-DR), and these cells have been identified using double immunostaining against glial fibrillary acidic protein (GFAP) and HLA-DR (McGeer and McGeer, 1994). Unfortunately, only a limited number of studies have examined the properties of astrocytes in ALS. Kushner and her colleagues have reported a decrease in SOD1 immunoreactivity in spinal cord astrocytes in ALS tissue compared to controls (O'Reilly *et al.*, 1995). It is also possible that the close association between astrocyte processes and the motoneuron soma may be altered in ALS. Astrocytes are known to be responsible for buffering glutamate and are involved in the regulation of glutamate-induced cytotoxicity. Thus, glial involvement may be of particular relevance in view of observations demonstrating an impairment of the high-affinity glial transporter in ALS (Rothstein, 1996a).

Microglial activation

In addition to astrocytosis, reports have indicated that activated microglia are present in the precentral gyrus, spinal cord and pyramidal tracts in ALS tissue (McGeer and McGeer, 1994). These activated microglia are believed to be derived from circulating monocytes. In response to the presence of foreign proteins, monocytes and microglia digest the protein and present these antigens to T cells with major histocompatibility complex (MHC) markers. The expression of HLA-DR has been used as a marker of reactive microglia and astrocytes. The significance of increased numbers of reactive microglia is unclear because the appearance of these activated cells is noted in a large number of conditions which are not neccesarily linked by a common pathophysiological mechanism. McGeer and McGeer (1994) have claimed that the observation of reactive microglia suggests that these cells may contribute to an active, cell-mediated immune response, although the reasons for the initiation of this process are unclear. Potentially, free radical generation by reactive microglia could lead to oxidative stress.

Microglia have been demonstrated to participate in the response to motoneuron degeneration produced by toxins, axotomy and other agents. In animal experiments, the number of activated microglia peaks within the first month following the insult and then returns towards normal levels. The current literature on this subject appears too limited to draw firm conclusions about the role of microglia in sporadic ALS.

Neuronal changes in specific related conditions

ALS with dementia

Some patients with ALS will also exhibit dementia, which has been reported to occur in up to 5 per cent of patients (Hudson, 1981). Clinically, this is manifest as the appearance of typical ALS but with a superimposed dementia (see Chapters 2 and 7). Neuropathologically, the changes found in typical ALS are seen. The posterior columns of spinal cord and Clarke's column are usually, but not always, spared (Hudson, 1991b). In the cerebral hemispheres, degenerative changes are more marked in demented patients. Loss of neurons and gliosis is seen in the frontotemporal cortex, especially in more superficial layers. Occasionally, a spongiform appearance of the cortex is noted (Rossi, 1994). Subcortical structures including the caudate, putamen, globus pallidus, thalamus, substantia nigra, red nucleus, inferior olive and dentate nuclei of cerebellum may also demonstrate degenerative changes. Neuritic plaques, neurofibrillary tangles, granulovacuolar degeneration and Pick bodies are usually absent (Hudson, 1991b). This topic is discussed in greater detail in Chapter 7.

Parkinsonism–dementia in sporadic ALS

ALS is rarely associated with Parkinsonism, this association appearing far less often than that between ALS and dementia (Hudson, 1991b). There are probably too few autopsy reports of this association to make general statements about the neuropathology of this condition. More common are patients having Parkinsonism, dementia and ALS, where ALS, the Parkinsonian features and dementia usually occur within several years of one another. The neuropatholological features of this overlap syndrome are similar to those of ALS–dementia, and subcortical involvement is prominent, especially degeneration of the substantia nigra. As in the ALS cases associated with dementia, neurofibrillary tangles and granulovacuolar degeneration are not seen. Lewy bodies are sparse, or absent.

Guamanian ALS

The high prevalence of ALS on the islands of Guam and Rota in the Marianas chain in the western Pacific has led to continued surveillance of the affected population. Clinical, epidemiological and neuropathological studies have indicated that Parkinsonism and dementia could occur with a high incidence in families of individuals affected with amyotrophy (Rodgers-Johnson *et al.*, 1986). Neuropathologically, Guamanian ALS patients exhibit Alzheimer neurofibrillary tangles in both the brain and spinal cord (Hirano *et al.*, 1966). Neurofibrillary tangles are found in the cerebral cortex, hippocampal gyrus, amygdaloid nucleus, hypothalamus, substantia innominata, substantia nigra, locus ceruleus and other regions. Granulovacuolar changes are also seen in the pyramidal neurons of Ammon's horn. These neuropathological features are similar to those seen in patients from the Kii peninsula of Japan. Neuropathological features of this disorder are discussed more fully in Chapter 7.

Familial ALS

The majority of patients with familial ALS have neuropathological features which are indistinguishable from those of the sporadic disease (Williams, 1991). Although it has often been argued that involvement of posterior columns and spinocerebellar tracts is the major distinguishing feature between sporadic and familial disease, it has become clear that degeneration of these pathways is seen only in a minority of FALS cases (Hirano *et al.*, 1966). Furthermore, the same neuropathological findings may be seen in sporadic ALS. In patients with FALS, variation in posterior column and spinocerebellar tract loss is so great that classification based on these findings has been virtually impossible. Variation in neuropathological involvement has been seen even within the same family (Williams, 1991). Apart from these distinctions, the neuropathological features of FALS demonstrate the same variability as those of sporadic ALS and can comprise cases where pyramidal tract degeneration is prominent or relatively mild (Chou, 1994). It has also been claimed that involvement of cerebral cortex and white matter is more extensive in FALS than in sporadic ALS (Hudson, 1981). It is likely that some of the neuropathological variation may reflect the different phenotypes of Cu/Zn–SOD1 and other mutations. Neuropathologists have recently attempted to correlate genetic findings and neuropathological data in FALS patients. In contrast to studies in transgenic mice, neuropathological studies of patients with mutations in the Cu/Zn–SOD1 gene do not reveal prominent vacuolation or abnormalities in mitochondria (Hirano, 1996).

ALS with prolonged survival

The increased use of ventilators and other means of respiratory support may prolong survival for patients with ALS. Neuropathological studies of patients with severe weakness who have been maintained past the period when they would have succumbed to respiratory failure have demonstrated involvement of posterior columns, spinocerebellar tracts, Clarke's nucleus, substantia nigra and other regions, including the nucleus of Onufrowicz. Nuclei of the extraocular muscles are well maintained but some patients have a supranuclear disorder of extraocular movements. Clinical features seen in these patients with long survival are discussed more fully in Chapter 2. The more widespread pathological changes in these patients suggest that selective vulnerability is only relative.

ALS pathology outside the central nervous system

Spinal nerve roots and peripheral nerves

Among the most common findings in ALS are thinning and discoloration of the ventral nerve roots with preservation of the dorsal roots. Typically, these changes are most apparent at the cervical segments of spinal cord, as well as at the cauda equina. Microscopically, a loss of myelinated axons is evident in the spinal roots, which in some cases may be related to a reduction in the calibre of large myelinated fibres without an actual change in their number (Rossi, 1994). Generally, however, there is a reduction in the number of large axons consequent to the loss of motoneurons in the disorder. A number of studies have indicated a loss of large myelinated fibres in ALS (Bradley *et al.*, 1984). Teased fibre preparations have demonstrated several abnormalities of the peripheral nerve in ALS including axon degeneration, myelin ovoids and other features. Demyelination can occur but is not prominent. A recent report describes a patient who had electrophysiological features of multifocal motor neuropathy with conduction block and pathological evidence of ALS (Kinoshita *et al.*, 1997). Electrodiagnostic findings included moderately delayed terminal motor latencies, absent f-waves and reduced compound muscle action potentials in several nerves. Sensory nerve studies were unremarkable. Neuropathological findings were typical of ALS but included abnormally large myelinated fibres in the ventral roots, often with fusiform swellings. These swellings were composed of abnormal vesicular material including organelles, dense bodies and myelin debris. Notably, myelin sheaths appeared normal and were not thinned. The abnormal debris was believed to derive from the cytoplasm of adnexal Schwann cells. This pattern of involvement is unique in our experience.

Muscle

Muscle atrophy is a well-established observation in ALS, even early in the disease. Muscle biopsy can be useful in the diagnosis, but is not specific and is more helpful to exclude primary muscle disease. Muscle fibres demonstrate features of neurogenic disease such as small, angular fibres or groups of atrophic fibres. There is also evidence of re-innervation with a loss of the usual mosaic pattern of different fibre types and their replacement with large groups of fibres having a homogeneous fibre type (type grouping). Generally, inflammation is uncommon. Studies of motor end-plates in muscle biopsy specimens have shown a higher fraction of small or absent axon terminals than control biopsies. Postsynaptic folds and junctional acetylcholine receptors appear unremarkable (Tsujihata *et al.*, 1984).

Skin

Numerous authors have commented upon the infrequency of bedsores in patients with ALS in spite of the severe degree of atrophy that eventually develops. This effect has been attributed to the preservation of sympathetic vasomotor tone in the skin. Recent studies have indicated that ALS patients differ from controls in having less collagen, as well as increased solubility of collagen in salt solutions. This may be due to a large proportion of immature collagen in ALS, or altered cross-linking of collagen (Ono and Yamauchi, 1992). The skin of ALS patients also exhibits a rapid decline in several components of elastin, as well as in the cross-linking of elastin (Ono and Yamauchi, 1994).

Liver

Several reports have identified swollen hepatic mitochondria with intra-mitochondrial inclusions in ALS patients (Nakano, Hirayama and Terao, 1987). These patients sometimes have impaired liver function tests. Other workers have commented on pancreatic abnormalities in ALS, including impaired glucose tolerance and altered levels of amylase.

Anatomical issues

Trans-synaptic changes in ALS

The presence of motoneuron and corticospinal tract loss in ALS raises the possibility that one of these functionally related systems is affected prior to involvement of the other. The view espoused by Charcot was that the disease initially affected the descending cortical neurons and that loss of motoneurons followed (Charcot, 1865). Also relevant to this view are the observations that several motoneuron populations which are conspicuously spared in ALS (nucleus of Onufrowicz, extraocular motor nuclei) are those without known direct corticomotoneuron connections. This hypothesis has been revisited recently (Eisen *et al.*, 1992, 1995) and has been extensively evaluated using neurophysiological techniques (see Chapter 5). Attempts to examine this hypothesis using neuropathological techniques have employed correlations between numbers of motoneurons and cortical pyramidal cells in ALS. Kiernan and Hudson (1991) have measured motoneuron numbers at the L4 spinal segment and the hypoglossal nucleus, as well as large precentral neurons in the cortical areas thought to innervate these motoneuron pools. There was a clear reduction in the number of motoneurons in the hypoglossal nucleus and lumbar motoneuron pool in ALS. Although reductions in cortical pyramidal areas were also detected in ALS, the extent of these cortical losses were much less than those seen in the brainstem and spinal cord. Furthermore, cases with greater reductions in motoneuron number were not necessarily the same as those with cortical neuron depletion, and losses in these cell populations were not correlated (Kiernan and Hudson, 1991). The authors claim that the absence of correlations between the extent of pathological change in the motor cortex and the spinal cord or brainstem makes it likely that neuronal degeneration occurs independently in 'upper' and 'lower' motoneurons.

Similar findings have been reported by Pamphlett, Kril and Hng (1995). These investigators measured the density of corticomotoneurons in the arm and hand region of motor cortex and compared this to the density of brachial spinal motoneurons in ALS patients and controls. Although reductions were found in the density of corticomotoneurons and spinal motoneurons in patients with ALS, compared to controls, there was a poor correlation between corticomotoneuron and spinal motoneuron densities. This study, like that of Kiernan and Hudson (1991), suggests that the losses of corticomotoneurons and spinal motoneurons proceed at different rates and are independent of each other.

One limitation of these conclusions is that a single descending corticomotoneuron may ramify extensively, making anatomical correlation difficult. Given this limitation, experiments using physiological methods are also critical to assess whether corticomotoneurons are lost prior to motoneurons. This 'corticomotoneuron' hypothesis for the origin of ALS (Eisen *et al.*, 1992, 1995) is discussed further in Chapter 5.

Target dependence of motoneuron ultrastructure

The notion that the ultrastructural inclusions seen in ALS could reflect a loss of muscle-derived trophic factors has some support from experimental models of axotomy. In cat thoracic motoneurons which were axotomized using either nerve crush or nerve transection with proximal ligation, clear differences were apparent in the light and electron microscopic appearance of affected cells (Johnson, 1996). Initially following axotomy, Nissl body ultrastructure is lost, with or without more extensive light microscopic evidence of chromatolysis. Although chromatolysis is rarely seen in ALS, more slowly developing changes in the appearance of the rough endoplasmic reticulum would be difficult to detect. At late stages following nerve crush in cats, re-establishment of normal Nissl body ultrastructure is found, whereas motoneurons subjected to transection and ligation do not regain normal Nissl ultrastructure (Johnson, 1996). Further evidence for persistently impaired ultrastructural changes in motoneurons associated with changes in rough endoplasmic reticulum-derived structures derives from experiments on partial central deafferentation where a persistently elevated frequency of C-type synapses is seen (Pullen, 1996). The C-type synapse has a distinct morphology and is characterized by a 15 nm wide cistern beneath the postsynaptic membrane which extends over the entire length of the presynaptic terminal. The cistern is contiguous with the rough endoplasmic reticulum of an adjacent

Nissl body. The increased frequency and modified ultrastructure of these synapses reflect a proliferation of the postsynaptic lamellae of rough endoplasmic reticulum which may be a compensatory interaction between the interneuron providing the C-type terminal and the postsynaptic motoneuron (Pullen, 1996).

These observations demonstrating changes in the ultrastructure of the Nissl substance of motoneurons following axotomy are relevant for claims that alterations of Nissl substance are an important and specific feature of ALS (Chou, 1994). In the hypothetical schema of Chou (see Fig. 3.4), the earliest pathological feature of ALS may be dissolution and conglomeration of the Nissl substance, potentially reflected at the light microscope level by the presence of basophilic inclusions (Chou, 1994). Basophilic inclusions may be more evident in cases of ALS where survival is shorter and these 'relatively acute' stages of neuronal change may be uncontaminated by further cellular changes at autopsy. The condensed basophilic inclusions may ultimately develop into the deeply staining eosinophilic Bunina body (Chou, 1994; see Fig. 3.4). Evidence for this claim derives from: (i) the morphological resemblance between basophilic inclusions and Bunina bodies, (ii) the presence of inclusions which are intermediate between basophilic inclusions and Bunina bodies, and (iii) similarities in the staining properties of these two types of inclusion. Hyaline inclusions may represent a transitional stage between basophilic and eosinophilic inclusions. The evidence for this is discussed elsewhere (Chou, 1994). Changes in the Nissl substance of motoneurons and the development of inclusions within these cells in ALS could occur as a consequence of an impairment of transport of muscle-derived trophic factors. These trophic substances and their actions upon motoneurons and other cells are described more fully in Chapter 8.

In addition to alterations of Nissl body organization, several studies have suggested that the Golgi apparatus undergoes fragmentation as an early feature in ALS (Hirano, 1996).

Apoptosis in ALS

Recent evidence has indicated that neuron death is associated with either of two general types of morphological change. One type of change, termed necrosis, is characterized by cell swelling leading to the rupture of the plasma membrane with leakage of intracellular contents. A second type of cell death, termed apoptosis, is characterized morphologically by a reduction in cell volume and chromatin condensation, but with the preservation of the plasma membrane. Thus, the loss of membrane integrity is believed to be a late event, and deoxyribonucleic acid (DNA) degradation occurs prior to the development of membrane breakdown. The cleavage of DNA occurs in a relatively stereotyped fashion with the production of oligonucleosomal fragments of approximately 200 base-pairs, which is detected by the appearance of a ladder-like pattern when DNA is isolated from cells and subjected to agarose gel electrophoresis. These distinctive electrophoretic findings are a consequence of enzymatic degradation of the DNA by an endonuclease acting in the internucleosomal linker region. The internucleosomal region may be more available to endonuclease action, as the DNA is weakly associated with histone H1 in this area, permitting better access by the enzyme. This topic has been the subject of numerous reviews (Bredesen, 1995) and it is also likely that the distinctions between necrosis and apoptosis may not be absolute.

The relevance of apoptotic cell death in ALS is unknown. There is evidence that mammalian motoneurons and interneurons undergo programmed cell death during embryogenesis (Oppenheim, 1991) and the early postnatal period (Lawson *et al.*, 1997). Although it is tantalizing to suggest that motoneuron death in ALS represents a 'gene-directed' pattern of cell suicide, very little evidence for this possibility has been presented. Down-regulation of Cu/Zn–SOD1 activity in cultured neurons produces cell death having features of apoptosis (Rothstein *et al.*, 1994). Although the mechanism of cell death associated with FALS cases having mutations in the Cu/Zn–SOD1 gene is unknown, some data support the notion that this effect is produced by programmed cell death because of aberrant Cu/Zn–SOD1 activity or oxidative damage (Bredesen *et al.*, 1996). Bredesen and coworkers have shown that wild-type Cu/Zn–SOD1 exerts an anti-apoptotic effect on immortalized mammalian neural cells. In contrast, FALS-associated Cu/Zn–SOD1 mutants promote, rather than inhibit, apoptosis (Rabizadeh *et al.*, 1995). Morphological evidence for apoptosis has been sought in ALS cases; however, actual support is limited. A brief report claims that in-situ end-labelling of fragmented DNA in several CNS regions revealed labelled cells in ALS tissue, whereas controls did not show as much labelling (Troost *et al.*, 1995). Immuno-cytochemical labelling with bcl-2, an oncoprotein which is believed to be protective, was increased in the postcentral gyrus in ALS tissue compared to control (Troost *et al.*, 1995). Of some relevance may be recent reports that the motoneuron loss in SMA may be due to the loss of function of a mammalian gene related to the baculovirus apoptosis inhibitor, the NAIP gene (Roy *et al.*, 1995).

Table 3.4. *Major genetic and phenotypic features of inherited and sporadic motoneuron disease in mouse, dog and other species*

	Chromosome		Clinical phenotype			
Disease	Gene	Location	Onset	Pattern	Neuropathology
Mouse					
Wobbler	wr	Chr 11	Not known	3–4 w	Lower	Vacuoles, astrogliosis, spermatozoid defect
Muscle deficient	mdf	Chr 19	HSA 11q13	3–8 w	Lower	Vacuoles, astrogliosis, spermatozoid defect
Progressive motor neuronopathy	pmn	Not known	Not known	3 w	Lower	No vacuoles, no astrogliosis, axonopathy, no type grouping in muscles, spermatozoid defect
Motoneuron degeneration 1	mnd1	Chr 8	Not known	5–11 m	Upper, lower	No vacuoles, ubiquitin, ceroid lipofucsinosis accumulation
Motoneuron degeneration 2	mnd 2	Chr 6	HSA 2p13	21–24 d	Lower	No vacuoles, ubiquitin, neurofilament accumulation, no astrogliosis, regression of lymphoid organs
Neuromuscular	nmd	Chr 19	HSA 11q13	2 w	Lower	Fading, no vacuoles, no astrogliosis
Wasted	wst	Chr 2	HSA 20q	14–18 d	Lower	Vacuoles, neurofilament accumulation/immunological disorder

Dog						
Hereditary canine spinal muscular atrophy	HCSMA	Not known	Not known	6–8 w, 6 m–1 y	Lower	Chromatolysis (early form), no vacuoles, no astrogliosis, Brittany spaniel
Hereditary progressive neurogenic muscular atrophy		Not known	Not known	5 m	Lower	Lipid granules accumulation, Pointer dog
Familial spinal muscular atrophy		Not known	Not known	4 w	Lower	Chromatolysis, Rottweiler
Horse						
Equine motoneuron degeneration	EMND	Sporadic		15 m–15 y	Lower	Chromatolysis, inclusions (ubiquitin) neurofilament accumulation, astrogliosis, no type grouping in muscle
Cow						
Bovine spinal muscular atrophy	BSMA	Not known	Not known	3 w	Upper and lower	Vacuoles, neuronophagia, ubiquitin, astrogliosis

Adapted from Blot, Poirier and Dreyfus (1995), with permission of the *Journal of Neurology and Experimental Neuropathology*. Clinical phenotype includes age of onset; involvement of upper and/or lower motoneurons as indicated. d, day; m, month; w, week; y, year.

Animal models of motoneuron degeneration

One approach to the study of motoneuron disease is to identify animal models that reproduce the pathology seen in human ALS. These animal models can be used for investigations to clarify the pathophysiology of the disease. In general, these animal models can be divided into those which are experimentally induced and those which occur on a hereditary basis. Several recent reviews have appeared on this topic (Sillevis Smitt and de Jong, 1989; Mitsumoto and Pioro, 1995). To this list of animal models must be added transgenic mice which are constructed by aggregating embryonic cells from animals with a normal genotype and from animals with a mutant genotype. The logic behind the use of transgenic animals is that genetic diseases generally involve mutations in specific proteins that result from mutations in the gene which encodes for the protein. As the list of candidate genes suspected of being involved in ALS grows, it is possible to construct mutant genes which will then encode for the presumptively abnormal protein responsible for the defect. For instance, transgenic animals have been constructed to investigate the role of genes encoding for subunits of neurofilaments, Cu/Zn–SOD1, as well as other genes (see below).

There have been a number of hereditary animal models of ALS. Because of space considerations, only some murine models of motoneuron disease and SMA will be reviewed. Features of these and other animal models of motoneuron disease are summarized in Table 3.4.

Spontaneously occurring murine models of motoneuron disease

Wobbler mouse The wobbler mouse (wr/wr) is an autosomal recessive mutant in C57BL/Fa mice that develops motoneuron degeneration within the brainstem and spinal cord. This mutant is normal at birth, but by the third to fourth week of life, affected littermates gain weight less rapidly and develop slowly progressive deficits consisting of tremor, forelimb weakness and atrophy as well as extraocular muscle involvement. Disease progression is variable, but by 12–16 weeks of age some affected mice die from the severe muscle weakness. Heterozygous littermates are normal. Neuropathologically, the wobbler mouse is characterized by prominent vacuolation of the motoneurons in brainstem and cervical spinal cord. This vacuolation can be seen prior to clinical evidence of neuronal loss. Electron microscopy demonstrates that vacuoles develop from dilatation of the cisternae of the rough endoplasmic reticulum. Lipofuscin accumulation is also seen. There is no astroglial reaction.

Little is known of the pathophysiology of motoneuron death in wobbler mice. Recent studies have indicated that expression of the human bcl-2 transgene in these mice neither arrests nor delays motoneuron death, even though it protects spinal and bulbar motoneurons from naturally occurring cell death and axotomy-induced motoneuron loss (Coulpier *et al.*, 1996). There is also evidence that lecithinized Cu/Zn–SOD can exert a protective effect on motoneurons in wobbler mice (Ikeda *et al.*, 1995), as can the free radical inhibitor N-acetyl-L-cysteine (Henderson *et al.*, 1996) and various growth factors such as brain-derived neurotrophic factor (BDNF) and ciliary neurotrophic factor (CNTF) (Mitsumoto and Pioro, 1995). Therapeutic studies using these mice are discussed in Chapter 7.

Muscle-deficient mouse In the murine muscle-deficient (mdf) mutation, homozygotes develop a waddling gait with prominent hindlimb weakness beginning at 4–8 weeks of age, with subsequent forelimb weakness (Blot *et al.*, 1995; see Table 3.4). The lifespan of these animals is generally eight months. Pathologically, ventral horn neurons exhibit profound vacuolation with some chromatolysis. Vacuolar changes are seen in dendrites as well as in the neuronal perikaryon. In the brainstem, abnormal motoneurons are evident in the motor nucleus of cranial nerve five, but the nuclei of the seventh and twelfth cranial nerves are spared.

Wasted mouse Homozygotes develop tremor and inco-ordination as well as progressive paralysis. Systemically, the mice have lymphoid hypoplasia with a reduced mass of splenic, thymic and lymph node tissue. Neuropathologically, 'wasted' mice demonstrate degeneration of cerebellar Purkinje cells and demyelination of the cerebellum and spinal cord. These mice have clinical and pathological features that resemble ataxia telangiectasia. However, several researchers have suggested that these animals have some features suggestive of motoneuron disease.

Progressive motor neuronopathy mouse Mice homozygous for the progressive motor neuronopathy (pmn) trait undergo progressive paralysis beginning in the hindlimbs during the third week of life. Forelimb and brainstem involvement follows and death ensues by six to seven weeks. Motoneurons become small and chromatolytic. Axonal degeneration is prominent distally and there is muscle atrophy without re-innervation. This disease most closely resembles a 'dying-back' type of motor neuropathy (Schmalbruch *et al.*, 1991). The lifespan of these mice has been reported to be prolonged by more than 50 per cent by using an adenovirus

Table 3.5. *Animal models of motoneuron disease*

Neurotoxins
Excitatory amino acids
Doxorubicin
Aluminium
Viruses
Polio
Autoimmune
Experimental autoimmune motoneuron disease

delivery system for genes coding for the neurotrophic factors neuro-trophin-3 (NT-3) and CNTF (Haase *et al.*, 1997).

Motoneuron degeneration 1 mouse Motoneuron degeneration 1 (mnd1) mouse is characterized by an accumulation of mitochondrial ATP synthase subunit c. Clinically, these mice develop progressive, severe, spastic weakness without muscle atrophy. Blindness becomes apparent after two months of age. At autopsy, the mice have prominent intraneur-onal inclusions in most regions of the brain and spinal cord. Electron microscopy reveals that these inclusions have laminar profiles reminiscent of ceroid lipofuscinosis. The use of these animals as a model of moto-neuron disease has been questioned as their clinical features and pathol-ogy are so dissimilar from those of human ALS.

Animal models of motoneuron disease (induced)

There is an enormous amount of literature regarding toxin-induced models of ALS in experimental animals, some of which has been reviewed elsewhere (Mitsumoto and Pioro, 1995). In view of the potential role of excitatory amino acid-mediated neurotoxicity, as well as neurotoxicity associated with Cu/Zn–SOD1 mutations, several of these models will be reviewed here, especially with regard to their neuropathological findings. Table 3.5 lists several of these animal models of motoneuron disease. Only the pathology of excitatory amino acid-induced motoneuron disease will be discussed here.

Excitatory amino acids

Following the observations which have suggested involvement of excita-tory amino acids (EAAs) in motoneuron disease (see Chapter 4), numer-ous studies have been undertaken to define the neuropathological consequences of EAA application in the spinal cords of rats (Hugon *et al.*, 1989; Nag and Riopelle, 1990; Ikonomidou *et al.*, 1996), chickens (Stewart *et al.*, 1991), mice (Urca and Urca, 1990) and other animals. It has generally been observed that application of NMDA effects dorsal horn neurons more than ventral horn neurons (Ikonomidou *et al.*, 1996). However, NMDA appears capable of producing morphological changes in the anterior horn of spinal cord (Nag and Riopelle, 1990). The non-NMDA receptor agonists quisqualate and α-amino-3-hydroxy-5-methyl-1,4-isoxazole proprionic acid (AMPA) may produce greater involvement of ventral horn neurons than dorsal horn neurons (Ikonomidou *et al.*, 1996). Cellular changes resulting from EAA exposure include mild astrocytosis and neuronal loss. Surviving motoneurons demonstrate dendritic swelling and cytoplasmic shrinkage, with evidence of cellular necrosis. Motoneuron perikarya are often filled with vacuoles which originate from the rough endoplasmic reticulum and mitochondria. Proximal axonal swelling can occur, with accumulation of vacuoles, organelles and filaments (Ikonomidou *et al.*, 1996). In contrast, presynaptic axon terminals appear to be well preserved. These morphological features are very different from those of ALS and suggest that if EAAs play a role in cell death in ALS, the effects may occur as a result of modestly elevated concentrations of an excitotoxin acting over long time periods.

Transgenic animals

Transgenic animals are constructed by incorporating specific genes of interest (transgenes) and manipulating these genes so that the gene product will be expressed in an animal. This permits the evaluation of the effects of the transgene on the phenotype. This topic has been the subject of numerous reviews (see Shuldiner, 1996). Factors that are important in the success of a transgenic animal include, amongst others, the strain of mouse from which it is derived, the level of expression of the transgene, the cell-specific expression of the transgene, the arrangement of the transgene. Because of the importance of mutations in Cu/Zn–SOD1 in some patients with FALS and neurofilamentous changes in tissue from ALS patients, transgenic mice have been produced which have mutations in these genes, or altered levels of expression of these genes (Table 3.6).

Cu/Zn–SOD1 mutations To evaluate the possible role of mutations in the Cu/Zn–SOD1 gene, transgenic mice have been constructed containing the mutant genes. One of the mutations selected was in exon 4

Table 3.6. *Mouse models with abnormal neurofilament accumulation*

Transgene	Neuronal populations affected	Axonal degeneration
Transgenic mice with motoneuron disease		
Human NF-H	Spinal motoneurons	Yes
(Collard *et al.*, 1995)	DRG neurons	No
MSV promotor/mouse NF-L	Spinal motoneurons	Yes
(Xu *et al.*, 1993)	DRG neurons	No
MSV promotor/mutant NF-L	Spinal motoneurons	Yes
(Lee *et al.*, 1994)	DRG neurons	No
SOD1 mutant hG93A	Prominent vacuoles in motoneurons	Yes
(Gurney *et al.*, 1994)	Spheroids in proximal motor axons	
SOD1 mutant hG37R	Vacuoles, some neurofilamentous inclusions	Yes
(Wong *et al.*, 1995)		
SOD1 mutant mG86R	Neuronal swellings	Yes
(Ripps *et al.*, 1995)		
Transgenic mice with no overt phenotypes		
Human NF-L	Thalamic neurons	?
	Cortical neurons	?
Human NF-M	Cortical neurons	?
	Forebrain neurons	?
MSV/mouse NF-M	Spinal motoneurons	No
	DRG neurons	No
Mouse NF-H-lacZ	Perikarya of CNS and PNS neurons	No
Mouse NF-H	Spinal motoneurons	No
	DRG neurons	

CNS, central nervous system; DRG, dorsal root ganglia; MSV, murine sarcoma virus; NF, neurofilaments; PNS, peripheral nervous system; SOD, superoxide dismutase.
Adapted from Julien (1997).

and consisted of a glycine to alanine substitution (Gly93Ala, G93A). The transgenic mouse line expressing the mutated Cu/Zn–SOD protein initially develops vacuolar degeneration of large anterior horn cells and subsequently anterior horn cell loss and atrophy with the deposition of neurofilamentous inclusions which resemble Lewy bodies (Dal Canto and Gurney, 1994). Posterior horns of the spinal cord remain unaffected, even in aged animals that have clinical and pathological features. Vacuolar changes appear to extend from the rough endoplasmic reticulum with swelling of this organelle. The Golgi apparatus is also disorganized and dilated. With increasing age and greater clinical involvement, intracytoplasmic vacuoles become more pronounced and tightly packed. Mitochondria become microvesiculated and vacuolar changes can be seen in the neuropil.

In mice which overexpress wild-type Cu/Zn–SOD1, neuropathological features are mild and consist of dendritic vacuolation with swelling of motor axons by accumulation of vacuoles and neurofilament bundles (Dal Canto and Gurney, 1994). The neuropathology of mice overexpressing mutant Cu/Zn–SOD1 bears some resemblance to the pathological changes seen in human ALS. Although vacuolar change is not a feature of human ALS, it is possible that vacuolar pathology might have occurred in humans at an early stage in the disease, before patients came to autopsy. In a few surviving neurons of animals with late stage disease, accumulations of tightly packed filaments are seen with a denser central portion. These hyalin inclusion bodies have some resemblance to Lewy bodies or the Lewy-like inclusions sometimes seen in ALS patients at autopsy. The pattern of involvement in the mutant Cu/Zn–SOD1 overexpressing mice also has some resemblance to the neuropathology seen following intrathecal administration of EAAs (Ikonomidou *et al.*, 1996).

The G37R mutants constitute several mouse lines having the substitution of arginine for glycine at codon 37 of Cu/Zn–SOD1 (Arg37Gly). Several of the G37R mouse lines express clinical features of motoneuron disease. Clinically, mice expressing higher levels of the mutant Cu/Zn–SOD1 protein activity in spinal cord have an earlier onset of motoneuron loss. Neuropathologically, affected mice develop bulbar and spinal motoneuron loss, with prominent vacuoles that are believed to include degenerating mitochondria.

Neurofilament gene transgenics As discussed above, transgenic mice which overexpress NF-H or NF-L develop abnormal neurofilamentous accumulations that are reminiscent of those that occur in ALS (Table 3.6). Among the notable features of these mice is the predominant involvement of motoneurons, suggesting that the selective vulnerability of this cell type is very high in the face of abnormal regulation of neurofilaments. The factors that could lead to abnormal neurofilament accumulation are listed in Table 3.3, and could include impaired phosphorylation of neurofilaments, or an impaired stoichiometry of different neurofilament subunits (Julien, 1997). For instance, a shift in the ratio of NF-H and NF-L subunits might be critical for neurofilament accumulation, rather than the absolute amounts of these subunits.

Paradoxically, accumulation of neurofilaments may give rise to no phenotypic changes whatsoever (Table 3.6). For instance, the NF-H-LacZ transgenic mouse is a recently derived strain in which the murine NF-H protein gene was replaced with a NF-H *E. coli* β-galactosidase (lacZ) gene (Eyer and Peterson, 1994). In this mouse, the expression of the fusion protein prevents the export of all classes of intermediate filaments from the nucleus and results in massively ballooned perikarya filled with filamentous aggregates. Motoneurons are particularly affected. Substantial hypophosphorylation of NF-H is apparent compared to control mice. However, clinically these mice are normal in spite of the dramatic vacuolization of spinal motoneurons (Eyer and Peterson, 1994). Other examples of transgenic mice with abnormal NF accumulation and no overt phenotype are listed in Table 3.6. The use of these transgenic models is undoubtedly one of the most promising techniques to explore the role of neurofilaments, Cu/Zn–SOD1, ageing and other factors in the development of motoneuron disease.

Summary

Clinically and neuropathologically, ALS can be broadly subdivided into different types depending on whether neuron losses are primarily of a lower motoneuron type (spinal muscular atrophy), or a combination of both upper and lower motoneuron loss. Isolated loss of descending tracts without motoneuron involvement (progressive lateral sclerosis) is generally believed to be a disorder distinct from ALS. Prominent bulbar involvement is a defining feature for the progressive bulbar palsy form of ALS.

Regardless of the form, ALS is characterized by variable losses of bulbar and spinal motoneurons with reductions in descending tract axons. The distribution of the cell loss is the defining feature of the illness. The distribution of neuronal involvement is relevant in terms of both the cell groups which are affected and those which are spared. Motoneuron loss is prominent in bulbar and spinal motoneurons, but rare in the sacral sphincteric motoneurons and in the nuclei of the extraocular muscles. In some patients, intraneuronal inclusions can be observed, including the relatively specific Bunina body, a $1–10\,\mu m$ cytoplasmic, eosinophilic inclusion, basophilic inclusions or, rarely, others. Often intracellular neurofilamentous accumulation is seen, which can occur in a generalized or focal manner within the neuron. Prominent, distended proximal segments can be ballooned to $20\,\mu m$ in diameter (spheroids). Many inclusions are ubiquitinated, although ubiquitin immunoreactivity is not specific for ALS. Occasional patients demonstrate chromatolysis. Loss of descending axons is variable but appears to involve corticospinal tracts in addition to other pathways. Rarely, cortical neuron loss, especially in the precentral gyrus, is sufficient to be seen on gross examination. In the peripheral nervous system, ventral horns are shrunken and a reduction in the numbers of large myelinated axons is seen. Neurogenic atrophy is apparent in muscle.

It is unresolved as to whether corticospinal tract loss precedes, follows, or is concurrent with the death of bulbar and spinal motoneurons. Current models suggest that upper and lower motoneuron loss proceeds independently. The mechanism by which the pathological changes arise in ALS is unknown. Neurofilamentous accumulation can occur in both patients with FALS and in some transgenic mice having mutations in the Cu/Zn–SOD1 gene. Mice having altered stoichiometry of neurofilament subunits also have neurofilamentous changes similar to those in ALS patients. However, some of these transgenic mice may have involvement of dorsal root ganglion neurons. It is possible that some of the pathological changes in ALS represent a continuum that arises as a consequence of impaired axonal transport.

4

Pathogenic mechanisms in ALS

Introduction

Despite the rapid proliferation of reports describing pathophysiological mechanisms in ALS, the cause of this disorder is still unknown. As for other diseases, it is important to distinguish between initiating factors for ALS (e.g. a genetic basis in familial disease), secondary effects induced by the disease (e.g. depletion of amino acid contents in brain and spinal cord) and effects produced in the late or terminal stages of ALS (e.g. agonal effects). Any review of the pathogenesis of ALS must also be mindful of the many promising leads in this area that have proved to be fruitless. Furthermore, the data reported in some studies related to ALS (for instance measurement of cerebrospinal fluid glutamate levels) are sometimes so inconsistent that it is impossible to draw firm conclusions.

Our view is that ALS is a heterogeneous disease in which a variety of relatively distinct initiating factors such as Cu/Zn–SOD1 mutations or abnormal glutamate metabolism lead to common clinical manifestations. The view that ALS is a multifactorial disease does not mean that different initiating factors cannot share similar pathophysiological mechanisms for motoneuron death. In fact, we expect that some, or perhaps all, of the initiating stimuli will trigger a common cascade of 'downstream' processes, ultimately resulting in neuronal dysfunction. For instance, it appears likely that mutations in the Cu/Zn–SOD1 gene are involved in some cases of FALS. This view is supported by recent work showing some relation between the specific mutation and the clinical course of the disease. However, it is also noteworthy that Cu/Zn–SOD1 mutations do not appear to be involved in most cases of FALS, or in sporadic ALS. Although the clinical course of FALS cases with Cu/Zn–SOD1 mutations may not be identical to that of cases without such mutations, the broad similarity in presentation suggests at least some shared pathophysiological

Table 4.1. *Subtypes of ALS*

Amyotrophy in the western Pacific (Guamanian ALS)
Familial ALS: autosomal dominant with and without Cu/Zn–SOD1
mutations
mechanisms of cell death
effects of aberrant Cu/Zn–SOD1
Sporadic ALS
involvement of cell surface receptors
excitotoxicity
neurotransmitter dysregulation
ionic channel dysregulation
increased intracellular Ca^{2+}
altered protein kinase activity
immunological mechanisms
growth factors
mitochondrial dysfunction

mechanisms are present. The nature of the common 'downstream' process that could be shared by a number of different initiating factors is unknown but could be mediated by aberrant regulation of protein kinases in ALS. This hypothesis is discussed further below. A case could also be made that sporadic ALS, young-onset disease, rapidly progressive disease and other presentations of ALS are distinct variations of a common clinical syndrome.

Epidemiological and biochemical data support the view that ALS is a multifactorial disease. For instance, there are at least three relatively distinct forms of ALS. These include: the epidemic form of ALS seen on the islands of Guam and Rota in the western Pacific, the familial form(s) of ALS (FALS) usually having autosomal dominant transmission, and the frequent, sporadic form of ALS. Table 4.1 indicates the three subtypes of ALS and the topics that are reviewed in this chapter.

Guamanian ALS

The high incidence of ALS in the Chamorro people of the Mariana Islands (Guam and Rota) has prompted numerous epidemiological investigations of the ALS–Parkinsonism–dementia complex of Guam (G-ALS), so called lytico–bodig disease. The clinical and pathological features of this condition are discussed in Chapters 1, 3 and 8, as are the many differences between this form of ALS and sporadic ALS. In the 1950s, the islands of Guam and Rota had prevalence and death rates of ALS more than 50 times higher than those in North America, but the incidence has declined over the past 15 years (Garruto and Yase, 1986). ALS patients from other high incidence areas in the Pacific were genetically, geographically and culturally different from the Guamanians, suggesting a local factor was independently responsible for the ALS in each of these high incidence areas. This observation prompted a search for an infectious, toxic or nutritional cause for G-ALS. In spite of considerable efforts to identify an infectious agent in G-ALS, none has been detected in more than two decades of intensive study (Gibbs and Gajdusek, 1982). Attention has been paid to other environmental factors as causative agents, such as low concentrations of magnesium and calcium and high levels of aluminium and iron in water and soil from high incidence foci. It has been hypothesized that patients in regions with a high incidence of ALS have a chronic nutritional deficiency of calcium, which leads to the development of secondary hyperparathyroidism, increased absorption of aluminium and the intraneuronal deposition of calcium and aluminium, leading to motoneuron death. This hypothesis has been supported by data showing that animals fed calcium-deficient diets develop abnormal intraneuronal accumulation of calcium (Yase and Ota, 1991). Rats fed a diet low in magnesium and calcium demonstrate motoneuron degeneration and some muscle atrophy (Garruto and Yase, 1986).

Nutritional studies have suggested that the consumption of the cycad nut (*Cycas circinalis*) could be a possible causative factor in G-ALS. More specifically, the compound BMAA has been implicated (Spencer *et al.*, 1987). This 'unusual amino acid' requires bicarbonate as a cofactor for its neurotoxicity in vitro. Some support for a toxic cause for G-ALS lies in its similarity to human lathyrism. Lathyrism is a neurodegenerative disease affecting corticospinal pathways that has been demonstrated to be associated with ingestion of chickling peas (*Lathyrus sativus*) containing the neurotoxin, BOAA (Roy, Spencer and Nunn, 1986). A well-described spastic paraplegia develops in humans after consumption of *Lathyrus* and feeding cynomologous monkeys a diet of *Lathyrus sativus* produces a spastic paralysis similar to human lathyrism (Roy *et al.*, 1986). However, while the likelihood of toxic environmental factors for G-ALS is high, the role of of cycad seeds is inconclusive (Duncan *et al.*, 1988). The cycad seed contains other toxins besides BMAA, including the carcinogen cycasin and its aglycone methylazoxymethanol (Spencer *et al.*, 1993). These other compounds have never been shown to lead to ALS. Furthermore, the presence of BMAA has not been detected in the plasma or cerebrospinal fluid of ALS patients with the sporadic disease (Perry *et al.*, 1990a).

Biochemically, brain amino acid contents in G-ALS and in the sporadic disease are different (Perry *et al.*, 1990a). Specifically, glutamate contents of the motor cortex in G-ALS are similar to controls and higher than in sporadic ALS. The high levels of taurine found in the cerebral cortex in sporadic ALS is not evident in brains from G-ALS patients.

Familial ALS

Familial ALS is an autosomal dominant disorder and occurs in approximately 5–10 per cent of ALS patients (Williams, 1991). In a few cases, an autosomal recessive mode of inheritance has been suggested. The evidence for this inheritance is weak except in juvenile-onset cases (Ben Hamida *et al.*, 1990). A recessive, adult-onset form of familial ALS has been described in families of Swedish and Finnish origin (Anderson *et al.*, 1996). It is not possible to distinguish patients with FALS from those with sporadic ALS on clinical grounds, although it has been claimed that as a group FALS patients may have an equivalent incidence in males and females, an earlier age of onset and more frequent disease onset in the legs than the sporadic disease. Pathologically, degeneration of posterior columns is considered by some neuropathologists to be a distinguishing feature of FALS, but even this feature may not discriminate between different forms of ALS (see Chapter 3). Studies of monozygotic twins have generally shown that when one of a twin pair develops FALS, the other will subsequently do so. The development of ALS in the later-affected twin can be variable – within 1–11 years (Williams, 1991) – suggesting that environmental or other factors are capable of modifying the genetic predisposition.

The application of molecular biology techniques to evaluate the genetic defects in FALS was pursued to understand this condition. The first step in this analysis consists in defining a chromosomal location for the disease gene. This is accomplished by 'linkage analysis'. Briefly, the co-inheritance of a given, established genetic marker and the disease gene is followed within a family. The probability that the inheritance of the marker and the disease gene could occur by chance is calculated, as is the probability that the disease gene and marker could recombine with a particular degree of linkage. The ratio of the odds for and against the particular degree of linkage is known as the logarithm of the odds, or lod score. A lod score of 3 or higher (odds of 1 in 1000) is arbitrarily used to indicate a significant likelihood of linkage. A lod score of -2 or lower indicates a significant probability that there is no linkage.

A large number of DNA markers have been used to screen for genetic linkage in ALS (Siddique *et al.*, 1991). Using these methods, Siddique and his colleagues found several moderately positive lod scores for markers on the long arm of chromosome 21 (Siddique *et al.*, 1991). These data also demonstrated genetic heterogeneity and indicated that at least two genetic subgroups of patients were present (some with the mutation on chromosome 21 and the other group having a different locus). Further analysis revealed tight genetic linkage between some cases of FALS and a gene on chromosome 21 which encodes a Cu/Zn–SOD1 (Rosen *et al.*, 1993; Siddique *et al.*, 1996). When DNA from 150 families with FALS was screened for mutations in the Cu/Zn–SOD1 gene, 11 different missense mutations were found in 13 different families (Rosen *et al.*, 1993). In the initial report, these mutations were found in exons 2 and 4 of Cu/Zn–SOD1. Later studies revealed that mutations were present in exons 1 and 5 as well (Deng *et al.*, 1993). The mutations in Cu/Zn–SOD1 appear to be specific for FALS and are not found in unrelated members of FALS pedigrees or normal controls (Rosen *et al.*, 1993). Currently, about 50 distinct mutations of the Cu/Zn–SOD1 gene have been described in FALS (Siddique *et al.*, 1996). These mutations occur in exons 1, 2, 4 and 5, but not in exon 3, for reasons which are unclear. With the exception of two splice junction mutations, a dinucleotide deletion and a premature stop codon, all other SOD mutations are missense (Siddique *et al.*, 1996). However, Cu/Zn–SOD1 mutations appear to account for only 15–20 per cent of FALS cases and are present only rarely in sporadic ALS, suggesting that FALS cases may not share identical pathophysiological mechanisms with sporadic ALS or even with other cases of FALS. Furthermore, some FALS cases are autosomal recessive rather than autosomal dominant.

The relation between the type of Cu/Zn–SOD1 mutation and the clinical expression is of interest. None of the mutations appears to influence the age of onset of the disorder; however, some mutations were associated with a more rapid progression (Juneja *et al.*, 1997). The Ala4Val mutation is among the most rapidly advancing, whereas Asp46Ala is slowly progressive (see Fig. 1.9). A recessive form of FALS occurring in Swedish and Finnish families has been linked with the Asp90Ala mutation and has a unique phenotype. The expression is characterized by slow progression and prominent upper motoneuron signs, initially in the legs and subsequently in the arms. Bulbar involvement is late and micturition is often abnormal. It is possible that the ethnic distribution of this syndrome is more widespread than described as the autosomal recessive pattern of transmission makes it likely that cases would not be recognized as being FALS.

Mechanisms underlying cell death in ALS

As is clear from the observations indicated above, it is highly likely that the causation of ALS is multifactorial. This is probably applicable both in terms of ALS having 'primary' and 'secondary' causes, as well as in different groups of ALS patients having relatively distinct primary causes for the disease (e.g. related to a unique Cu/Zn–SOD1 mutation). Although there are clinical differences between FALS patients having different genetic mutations and between patients with FALS and sporadic ALS, there is an impressive degree of clinical similarity. Until the time comes that specific genetic and biochemical abnormalities are identified, it is probably more reasonable to clarify the pathophysiological mechanisms underlying ALS, rather than hypothesize a single scheme. Furthermore, there are many limitations to our current knowledge of the pathophysiology of ALS, and consequently any attempt at a synthesis of various theories is fraught with difficulties and speculation. As a result, a fragmentary account of several of the currently favoured mechanisms of ALS is reviewed in light of our personal biases.

Effects of aberrant SOD in ALS

As a result of recent evidence that abnormalities in the Cu/Zn–SOD1 gene are present in some cases of FALS, considerable attention has been focused on the possible role of the SOD1 enzyme in ALS. Cu/Zn–SOD1 is one type of free-radical scavenging superoxide dismutase. In addition to the cytoplasmic Cu/Zn–SOD1, there is an intramitochondrial, manganese-containing SOD (Mn–SOD, SOD2) and an extracellular form of Cu/Zn–SOD (SOD3). These metaloenzymes are responsible for catalysing the dismutation of the superoxide ion (O^{2-}) to yield hydrogen peroxide (H_2O_2) and O_2. The removal of hydrogen peroxide is subsequently performed through the actions of glutathione peroxidase and catalase.

Several studies have shown that FALS patients with Cu/Zn–SOD1 mutations have reduced SOD activity in brain tissue, erythrocytes and lymphoblast cell lines compared to ALS patients (Bowling *et al.*, 1993; Deng *et al.*, 1993; Robberecht *et al.*, 1994). There is no reduction in Cu/Zn–SOD1 activity in FALS patients who do not have Cu/Zn–SOD1 mutations, or in patients with sporadic ALS. Immunocytochemical studies of Cu/Zn–SOD1 distribution in spinal cord have demonstrated Cu/Zn–SOD1 immunoreactivity, especially in substantia gelatinosa, interneurons and motoneurons (Pardo *et al.*, 1995). In motoneurons, Cu/Zn–SOD1 is apparent within the cytoplasm, both in the cell bodies and processes of these neurons. Axons and nerve terminals manifest considerable Cu/Zn–SOD1 immunoreactivity, suggesting that the enzyme may be transported anterogradely down the axon. In some cases, membrane-associated immunoreactivity is seen. Immunoreactivity for Cu/Zn–SOD1 is not restricted to spinal cord neurons; hippocampal CA3 and CA4 neurons also demonstrate substantial immunoreactivity for Cu/Zn–SOD. Generally, astrocytes and microglia do not demonstrate Cu/Zn–SOD1 immunoreactivity. These immunohistochemical studies have suggested that there are no correlations between the abundance of Cu/Zn–SOD1 immunoreactivity and the vulnerability of the neuronal types in ALS (Pardo *et al.*, 1995).

The effect of the Cu/Zn–SOD1 mutations in FALS is not understood. The SOD1 mutations are located in regions associated with enzyme dimerization or β barrel turns rather than at the catalytic site. Whether the mutation confers a novel 'gain of function', reduces 'wild-type' activity, enhances an existing toxic effect of SOD, or confers some other property to Cu/Zn–SOD1 is still a matter of much debate (Brown, 1995; 1996). The current consensus is that it is likely that the mutant SOD1 mutation represents a 'gain of function'. It may be more correct to say that the mutant SOD may amplify an unrecognized toxic effect of the normal (wild-type) SOD. Evidence that the Cu/Zn–SOD1 mutation confers a novel 'gain of function' includes the data summarized in Table 4.2.

Several hypotheses have been put forward to explain the gain of function of Cu/Zn–SOD1 observed with the FALS mutation. One hypothesis proposes that the mutant SOD1 potentiates the nitration of tyrosine residues by the peroxynitrite anion ($ONOO^-$) (Beckman *et al.*, 1993). Peroxynitrite is generated by the interaction of SOD with nitric oxide. Nitration of neurofilaments may result from elevated amounts of the peroxynitrite anion and this reaction, in turn, may interfere with motoneuron survival by disrupting the cytoskeleton as well as by interfering with axonal transport. Neurofilamentous change has been reported in one patient with a substitution mutation of Cu/Zn–SOD1 at Ile 113 (Rouleau *et al.*, 1996). An alternative suggestion is that the mutant Cu/Zn–SOD1 may catalyse the oxidation of substrates by H_2O_2 at a higher rate than the wild-type SOD (Wiedau-Pazos *et al.*, 1996). This

Table 4.2. *Evidence that Cu/Zn–SOD1 mutations produce a 'gain of function'*

Data that for some Cu/Zn–SOD1 mutations in FALS (e.g. D90A), the enzymatic activity of SOD is not reduced

Mice which overexpress mutant SOD1 develop a disorder that clinically and pathologically resembles human FALS (Gurney *et al.*, 1994; Brown, 1995) and that has features indicative of a toxic effect of the mutant protein

Yeast null mutants (not possessing Cu/Zn–SOD1) were rescued as efficiently by the mutant SOD as by the wild-type enzyme, indicating that the mutant enzyme possesses considerable enzyme activity (Rabizadeh *et al.*, 1995)

Mutant human Cu/Zn–SOD1 increased apoptosis in a neuronal culture model, whereas wild-type Cu/Zn–SOD1 inhibited cell death (Rabizadeh *et al.*, 1995)

---

latter view is supported by data showing that mutant Cu/Zn–SOD proteins seen in FALS produce a significant increase in the oxidation of several substrates. One explanation for the increased ability of mutant Cu/Zn–SOD to catalyse the oxidation of substrates may lie in the increased access to the active site in the mutant enzyme. Copper (Cu) ions are bound at each subunit of the active sites of Cu/Zn–SOD. These Cu ions appear to be critical for enzyme activity because greater extents of Cu metallization of both wild-type and mutant SOD will increase oxidation. Furthermore, Cu-chelating agents decrease the oxidation of substrates by mutant Cu/Zn–SOD (Wiedau-Pazos *et al.*, 1996). Wiedau-Pazos *et al.* (1966) have also shown that apoptosis of neural cell lines containing mutant Cu/Zn–SOD can be substantially reduced by Cu-chelating agents and that apoptosis does not occur with wild-type SOD. The observation that Cu-chelating substances inhibit apoptosis suggests that these compounds, although potentially toxic, should be studied in animal models of FALS.

In summary, mutations of the Cu/Zn–SOD1 gene have been closely linked with some cases of FALS, suggesting that the mutant Cu/Zn–SOD protein is responsible for some of the phenotypes of FALS. The SOD mutations appear to give rise to a novel, dominant, gain of function of SOD, probably related to altered oxidation of unknown cellular substrates. The gain of function may arise from a change in the morphology of the mutant Cu/Zn–SOD1 protein permitting greater access to the active site, leading to greater nitration or oxidizing ability compared to the wild-type Cu/Zn–SOD.

Sporadic ALS

Involvement of cell surface receptors in ALS

The vast majority of cases of ALS are not associated with a clear pattern of inheritance, but this does not preclude a genetic predisposition to ALS due to the operation of susceptibility genes. Although there have been a few case reports documenting Cu/Zn–SOD1 mutations in 'sporadic' ALS, some of these patients may have had an autosomal recessive pattern of inheritance. In the absence of evidence for Cu/Zn–SOD1 mutations, research in this area has been driven by a consideration of the pattern of the neuron loss in ALS. The specific pattern of neuronal involvement comprising motoneuron and corticospinal tract loss has lead to the hypothesis that the neuronal populations that are lost contain some unique characteristic that could render them susceptible to an insult and ultimately result in neuron death. Cellular receptors, including neurotransmitter or other receptors, as well as ionic channels are specific membrane-associated structures that could be the targets of a toxin or immune-mediated attack.

Excitotoxicity in ALS

The excitatory amino acid (EAA) receptors (also known as glutamate receptors) constitute an important group of neurotransmitter receptors that may be involved in ALS. Considerable recent evidence has indicated that exposing neurons to EAAs can lead to neuron death both in vitro and in vivo (Choi, 1988; Rothman, 1992). These findings are of considerable importance as glutamate and aspartate are EAAs and are probably the principal excitatory neurotransmitters of the corticospinal tract and of many cortical neurons. Thus, it is possible that excessive release of glutamate or impaired re-uptake of this neurotransmitter from synaptic clefts could lead to the death of postsynaptic neurons through an excitotoxic mechanism (Plaitakis, 1990). It has been well established that motoneurons possess NMDA, non-NMDA and metabotropic EAA receptors and therefore the actions of EAAs could be mediated through any or all of these pathways.

Broadly, six independent lines of evidence have been raised to implicate 'glutamatergic dysfunction', or excitotoxicity in ALS. These are listed in Table 4.3.

Table 4.3. *Evidence for 'glutamatergic dysfunction' in ALS*

An association between neurotoxin ingestion and the development of
   motor system disorders
Reports indicating elevated levels of EAAs in the cerebrospinal fluid and
   plasma of ALS patients
Observations of reduced contents of EAAs in spinal cord and brain tissue
   in ALS
Observations of impaired glutamate uptake in tissue from ALS patients
Autoradiographic data indicating altered binding of EAA receptors in
   ALS
Possible benefit of therapeutic agents that alter glutamate release

EAA, excitatory amino acid.

Intoxication with EAAs can lead to motor system loss

There are some precedents for the possibility that elevated concentrations
of EAAs can result in motoneuron and corticospinal tract loss. The
consumption of mussels containing the toxin domoic acid has been
linked to an encephalopathy associated with seizures, confusion and gaze
palsies (Teitlebaum *et al.*, 1990). Some of the patients who survive the
encephalopathic phase of this illness have electromyographic features of a
non-progressive motor neuronopathy. Neuropathological evaluation has
not shown motoneuron loss in brain stem or spinal cord. As discussed
above, the ingestion of chickling peas, containing the non-NMDA
receptor agonist BOAA, can lead to a neurological disorder. There has
also been the suspicion that G-ALS could be due to an excitatory amino
compound, BMAA. However, the weight of evidence suggests G-ALS is
caused by factors other than BMAA. As rare as these cases of EAA-
induced neurotoxicity are in humans, they do suggest that EAA-induced
mechanisms are at least possible in ALS.

Many animal studies using intrathecal or systemic administration of
EAAs or excitatory amino compounds have been performed. These
studies have shown that motoneurons and interneurons can be destroyed
by EAAs. However, neuropathological examination of treated animals
demonstrates prominent cell swelling, vacuolation and other features that
are dissimilar from those seen in patients with sporadic ALS but do
resemble the findings in transgenic mice with mutations in Cu/Zn–SOD1
(Ikonomidou *et al.*, 1996; see Chapter 3). The histological changes
observed in these studies may be different from those seen in patients
with ALS in that they reflect neuronal exposure to what may be a short

course of EAAs in high concentration. The effect of a more temporally prolonged, selective elevation of EAAs in a low or modest concentration at specific synaptic connections has not been determined.

Altered plasma and cerebrospinal fluid EAAs

To determine whether elevated concentrations of glutamate, aspartate or other EAAs could be associated with ALS, a number of investigators have measured EAA levels in the plasma or cerebrospinal fluid (CSF) of ALS patients and compared them to controls (see Table 4.4). The methods used in these studies have varied and this probably explains why the results are not entirely consistent. Nonetheless, it appears that in the majority of patients with ALS there are no significant differences in the levels of CSF glutamate and aspartate compared to controls. Some ALS patients do have values of CSF glutamate that are significantly higher than the mean control CSF level of this EAA. The significance of this observation is unclear. These high values could reflect the upper end of a normally distributed range of glutamate levels or might constitute an important subgroup of ALS patients. As indicated above, it is likely that ALS is a heterogeneous disorder and it is possible that patients with elevated levels of CSF EAAs could have a different disease mechanism than other patients. Potentially, these patients could have neuronal death produced by the elevated concentration of CSF EAAs. It is also possible that the variable levels of CSF glutamate reflect different stages of the disease. Early in the course of the disease, increased release of EAAs might predominate and account for samples with elevated levels of glutamate and aspartate. Later in the disease, as the neurotoxic effects of EAAs predominate, loss of the levels of EAAs might transpire. There is indirect evidence from electrophysiological studies to support this view and this topic is discussed further in Chapter 5. Studies that have also included measures of disease duration have not found a relation between CSF glutamate levels and the stage of disease (Perry *et al.*, 1990b).

It is not clear how CSF EAA levels relate to the synaptic concentrations of EAA in spinal cord and brain and this is a significant limitation of these studies. The CSF represents such a large pool of amino acids and other compounds that it is not evident that a localized increase of EAAs at the synapses of corticospinal tract neurons, or through impaired re-uptake, would modify CSF EAA levels appreciably. However, other studies of CSF from ALS patients have shown increased neurotoxicity for rat cortical neurons in culture. This toxicity is blocked by non-NMDA receptor antagonists but not by NMDA receptor antagonists (Couratier

Table 4.4. *Published reports on EAA levels in ALS patients*

Study	Number of MND patients	Number of controls	Plasma	CSF	Significant results in MND
1. Patten *et al.* (1978)	12	12	+	+	Increased serum tyrosine, total aromatic AA and total basic AA. Increased CSF total basic AA, lysine, essential AA and leucine
2. de Belleroche *et al.* (1984)	11	9	−	+	Increased isoleucine, glycine, alanine, phenyl-alanine and threonine
3. Plaitakis and Caroscio (1987)	22	81	+	−	Increased mean fasting plasma glutamate by approximately 100 per cent. Oral glutamate loading produced an increase in plasma gluta-mate and aspartate
4. Meier and Schott (1988)	5	17	−	+	No significant changes in the levels of 23 amino acids
5. Perry *et al.* (1990b)	Plasma 28	48	+	+	In plasma, increased mean levels of glutamic acid, glutamine, cystine, and decreased mean levels of threonine, GABA, methionine, phenyl-alanine and histidine.
	CSF 17	80			In CSF, increased mean levels of glutamine, alanine, GABA, isoleu-cine, leucine, trypto-phan, ethanolamine, lysine and arginine
6. Rothstein *et al.* (1991)	18	18	−	+	Mean CSF glutamate and aspartate increased by 100 to 200 per cent; 2–3 × increase in NAAG and NAA
7. Plaitakis *et al.* (1991)	84	46	+	−	Increased mean level of plasma glutamate by approximately 80 per cent. Greater in males and in patients with typical ALS

Continued overleaf

Table 4.4. (*cont.*)

Study	Number of MND patients	Number of controls	Plasma	CSF	Significant results in MND
8. Rothstein *et al.* (1991)	15	8	−	+	Increased mean levels of glutamate and aspartate in CSF
9. Iwasaki *et al.* (1992)	10	10	+	−	Increased mean levels of plasma aspartate, gluta-mate and glycine
10. Plaitakis and Constan-takakis (1993)	52	52	+	−	Increased mean plasma glutamate by approxi-mately 70 per cent
11. Lane *et al.* (1993)	Plasma 43 CSF 19	26 14	+	+	Glycine measured before and after an oral glycine load. No difference in baseline glycine level, but increased plasma level at 4 hours. CSF glycine increase at 2.5–4 hours
12. Camu *et al.* (1993)	Plasma 22 CSF 16	44 19	+	+	In plasma, decreased levels of alanine, methionine, leucine and thyrosine. In CSF, no differences in AA between ALS patients and controls
13. Blin *et al.* (1994)	10	10	−	+	No significant changes in CSF levels of 12 amino acids
14. Shaw *et al.* (1995)	37	35	+	+	In plasma, no significant changes. In CSF, ele-vated mean glutamate but heterogeneous, with 60 per cent of ALS patients in normal range

Modified from Shaw *et al.* (1995).
AA, amino acids; CSF, cerebrospinal fluid; GABA, γ-aminobutyric acid; MND, motoneuron disease; NAA, N-acetyl-aspartate; NAAG, N-acetyl-aspartyl-glutamate.

et al., 1993). Attempts to identify other possible excitotoxins in the plasma, CSF or nervous tissue from patients with sporadic ALS, such as quinolinic acid, cysteine, or BMAA, have so far been unrewarding (Perry *et al.*, 1990b; Krieger *et al.*, 1993a).

Tissue contents of EAAs

Contents of EAAs are reduced in brain and spinal cord tissue from ALS patients compared to controls (Perry, Hansen and Jones, 1987; Plaitakis, Constantakakis and Smith, 1988; Tsai *et al.*, 1991). Contents of N-acetyl aspartate (NAA) and N-acetyl aspartyl-glutamate (NAAG) are reduced in spinal cord (Plaitakis *et al.*, 1988; Tsai *et al.*, 1991) and possibly in cerebral cortex in ALS patients (Tsai *et al.*, 1991; Pioro *et al.*, 1994). These relatively consistent findings are important but may simply reflect the loss of neurons and synaptic terminals in brain cells, corticospinal tracts, interneurons and motoneurons. Reduced EAA contents are also observed in spinal cord ischaemia and following transection of the spinal cord. This makes it likely that the reductions in EAA contents could be a secondary effect of neuron loss and not specific for ALS.

Altered glutamate transport

A hypothetical mechanism for achieving excitotoxicity could be the failure of glutamate and aspartate uptake from synaptic sites because of impaired glutamate transporter function (Fig. 4.1). This mechanism has been postulated to occur for other disorders such as Huntington's disease (Perry and Hansen, 1990). Rothstein, Martin and Kuncl (1992) have reported a regional loss of high-affinity, Na^+-dependent transport in synaptosomes from spinal cord, motor and somatosensory cortex, but not from those regions of the nervous system usually spared in ALS (Rothstein *et al.*, 1992). The maximum velocity of transport of glutamate was decreased in ALS tissue compared to controls, but there was an unchanged affinity of the transporter for glutamate (Rothstein *et al.*, 1992). Using $[^3H]$-D-aspartate (ASP) binding as an autoradiographic marker for glutamate uptake sites, Shaw, Chinnery and Ince (1994a) demonstrated reduced binding in lumbar spinal cord from ALS patients compared to controls. The reduced binding was most apparent in the substantia gelatinosa and intermediate grey matter of spinal cord (Shaw *et al.*, 1994a). More recent studies by Rothstein and colleagues (1995) using immunoblotting and immunocytochemical analysis with antibodies to three distinct glutamate transporters, revealed a selective reduction in the levels of a glutamate transporter associated with astroglial cells (GLT-1 protein) in motor cortex and spinal cord tissue from ALS patients. Levels of a second type of glial glutamate transporter (GLAST) were normal, as were levels of the neuronal glutamate transporter EAAC1 (Rothstein *et al.*, 1995). A reduction in the amount of the GLT-1 transporter could

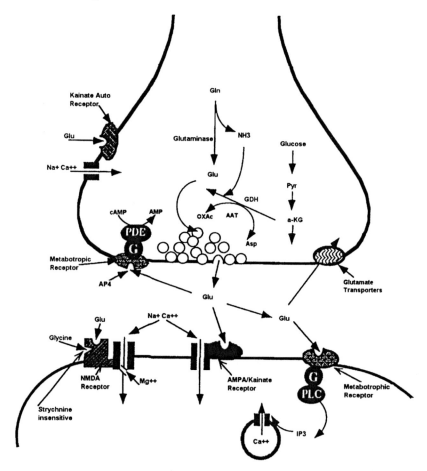

Figure 4.1. Schematic diagram showing the pathways involved with the metabolism of glutamate. The upper portion of the figure represents the synaptic terminal of the presynaptic neuron, and the lower portion represents the postsynaptic cell. Glutamate is released from vesicles (circles) into the synaptic cleft. It diffuses across the cleft, where it can activate receptors on the presynaptic and postsynaptic neurons. Among the receptor types activated are the metabotropic receptor, the AMPA/kainate receptor and the N-methyl-D aspartate (NMDA) receptor. Glutamate uptake from the synaptic cleft occurs by glutamate transporters found on the presynaptic and postsynaptic neurons, as well as on glial cells (not shown). Abbreviations: Gln, glutamine; Glu, glutamate; GDH, glutamate dehydrogenase; PDE, phosphodiesterase; Pyr, pyruvate; a-KG, α-ketoglutarate; OXAc, oxaloacetate; Asp, aspartate; G, G-protein; cAMP, cyclic AMP; PLC, phospholipase C; IP3, inositol-1,4,5-triphosphate; NH3, ammonia. (Adapted from Plaitakis, 1990.)

occur consequent to a change in the regulation of glial cells (see Chapter 3). Support for an impairment of glutamate re-uptake has been provided by Shaw *et al.* (1995), who found that the density of specific $[^3H]$-D-ASP binding was reduced to a greater degree in ALS patients with higher CSF glutamate levels. Thus, ALS patients with impaired glutamate transporters may have higher CSF glutamate levels.

Using organotypic rodent spinal cord sections, inhibition of glutamate transport produced degeneration of motoneurons and other neurons in culture. This toxicity was reduced by non-NMDA receptor antagonists, but not by NMDA receptor antagonists (Rothstein *et al.*, 1993). A puzzling aspect to these studies is that they do not clearly address why impairment of a glial EAA transporter would produce the relatively specific loss of corticospinal tract neurons and motoneurons. Furthermore, it remains to be determined whether the changes in transporter function occur secondary to altered synaptic and astroglial response as a reaction to neuron death, rather than as a primary event in ALS.

Alteration of EAA receptor binding

An alteration of EAA receptor binding has been reported in tissue from ALS patients obtained at post mortem. Some of the specific findings are listed in Table 4.5.

One of the difficulties in interpreting these findings is an inability to establish whether the results could occur as a consequence of selective neuron death. Furthermore, although up-regulation and down-regulation of receptors on surviving neurons have been suggested as a mechanism for the observation of altered EAA receptor binding, too little is known about the regulation of these receptors to provide a satisfactory explanation (Allaoua *et al.*, 1992).

Therapeutic trials

Evidence for the therapeutic benefit of drugs that produce EAA receptor blockade, or inhibit glutamate release (e.g. riluzole, see Chapter 7), provides indirect support for the belief that elevated levels of EAAs are relevant for ALS. The therapeutic efficacy of riluzole in some patients may relate to the observation that CSF glutamate levels are elevated in some patients with ALS (Shaw *et al.*, 1995). These issues are discussed further in Chapter 7.

Further substantiation for the involvement of EAA receptors in ALS would be provided by evidence that 'downstream' pathways, stimulated or inhibited by EAAs, would be involved. For instance, EAA receptor

Table 4.5. *Selected studies of EAA receptor binding in ALS*

EAA subtype and distribution	Effect of ALS on receptor binding
EAA (Kainate)	
Motor cortex: all layers	Increased binding in middle and deep premotor cortex, increased in superficial and deep regions of motor cortex (Shaw et al., 1994b)
Spinal cord: all laminae	Increased in substantia gelatinosa and intermediate grey (Shaw et al., 1994b)
EAA (AMPA)	
Motor cortex: all layers	No change (Shaw et al., 1994b)
Spinal cord: all laminae	Increased in substantia gelatinosa and intermediate grey (Shaw et al., 1994b)
	No change (Allaoua et al., 1992)
EAA (NMDA)	
Motor cortex: all layers, especially superficial	Slightly increased in deeper layers (Shaw et al., 1994b)
Spinal cord: all laminae, especially lamina II	Decreased in dorsal and ventral horn; ventral losses greater than dorsal (Allaoua et al., 1992)
	Decreased in dorsal and ventral horn; no change in receptor affinity (Krieger et al., 1993b)
	Decreased in ventral horns only: reduction correlates with motoneuron loss (Shaw et al., 1994b)

Modified from Krieger *et al.* (1996b). EAA, excitatory amino acid; AMPA, α-amino-3-hydroxy-5-methyl-1,4-isoxazole proprionic acid; NMDA, N-methyl-D-aspartate.

stimulation is known to affect many protein kinases (PKC, Ca^{2+}-calmodulin kinase II (CaMKII)) and proteases (e.g. calpains), although the temporal profiles of protein kinase and protease activation produced by EAA stimulation are poorly understood.

Involvement of neurotransmitter receptors in ALS

The finding of a selective depletion of a neurotransmitter (such as dopamine in PD), or an altered distribution of neurotransmitter receptors, has been influential in attempts to define a pattern of altered neurotransmitter function in ALS. As indicated above, there is consider-

Table 4.6. *Selected studies of neurotransmitter receptors in spinal cord and brain in ALS*

Neurotransmitter	Distribution	Effect in ALS
Substance P	Substantia gelatinosa, intermediolateral column, laminae IX, X	Reduced in ventral horn
Cholinergic (muscarinic)	All laminae, especially II, III and IX	Decreased in laminae IX (by 75 per cent), II, III, IV, VI, VII and VIII (by 50 per cent)
Benzodiazepine	All laminae, especially II, III and IX	Decreased in ventral horn
Glycinergic (strychnine-sensitive)	All laminae, especially II–III and IX	Decreased in VIII by (25 per cent) decreased in IX by (30 per cent)
Thyrotropin-releasing hormone	All laminae, especially II, IX	Decreased TRH binding in IX, no change in affinity
Serotonin	All laminae, especially II	Increased in lamina II and ventral laminae
β-Adrenergic	Homogeneous binding	No change
Opiate	Throughout grey, especially substantia gelatinosa	No change
Dopamine	Positron emission tomography: living patients (fluorodopa)	Reduced brain uptake, progressive fall in uptake with disease
Glutathione	All laminae, generalized	Generalized increase

Modified from Krieger *et al.* (1996b).
Unless otherwise noted, distribution refers to distribution within spinal cord.
References are listed in the text.

able circumstantial evidence for a role for EAA receptors in ALS. In a search for involvement of other neurotransmitter receptors in ALS a number of autoradiographic studies have been performed using brain and spinal cord tissue from ALS patients and controls. Results from some selected studies are shown on Table 4.6. In general, the reports listed in Table 4.6 have indicated reductions in binding to receptors for substance P (Dietl *et al.*, 1989), muscarinic cholinergic (Whitehouse *et al.*, 1983; Gillberg and Aquilonius, 1985; Manaker, Caine and Winokur, 1988; Berger *et al.*, 1992), benzodiazepine (Whitehouse *et al.*, 1983), strychnine-sensitive glycine (Whitehouse *et al.*, 1983), thyroid releasing hormone (Manaker *et al.*, 1985, 1988) and dopaminergic receptors (Takahashi *et al.*, 1993).

Most studies that have analysed both receptor numbers and affinity have indicated that the receptor number is reduced rather than there being a change in the receptor affinity (see Krieger *et al.*, 1996b). These observations are more consistent with the loss of receptors that could occur secondary to the death and disappearance of receptor-bearing neurons. As it is clear that motoneurons, interneurons and other neuronal classes are lost in ALS, it appears likely that the reduction in receptor binding is simply a result of neuron death and not the initiating factor for the disease. Several reports have been at variance with this general scheme. For instance, a higher concentration of serotonin receptors in lamina IX (the motoneuron pool) and other laminae is detected in ALS tissue compared to control (Manaker *et al.*, 1988). Binding studies of glutathione, a potential neurotransmitter candidate, have shown generalized increases in many spinal cord laminae in ALS (Lanius *et al.*, 1993, 1994). The significance of these binding studies is unclear, but it seems likely that receptor regulation is contributing to changes in receptor number (Krieger *et al.*, 1996b).

Involvement of other cellular receptors

In addition to neurotransmitter receptors, the surfaces of motoneurons, corticospinal tract neurons and other cells affected in ALS possess a large variety of cell surface receptors. It remains a tantalizing but unproven possibility that ALS may occur as a result of a direct interaction between a receptor and an injurious ligand, such as an antibody, neurotransmitter or neurotoxin. A number of studies have been undertaken to examine whether motoneurons possess distinct cell surface or intracelullar constituents. A number of candidate molecules have been reviewed (Hastings, 1992). To date, no well-characterized, motoneuron-specific proteins or genes have been identified. The MO-1 antigen is among the few molecules having a motoneuron-specific expression pattern (see Hastings, 1992). The structure of the protein which binds the MO-1 antibody is unknown. Several gene products are expressed in higher amounts in motoneurons than in other cells such as calcitonin gene-related peptide, agrin and peripherin (Hastings, 1992). However, the higher expression of these products in motoneurons may be correlated to some feature of these cells, such as their size, rather than to a cell-type-specific marker for motoneurons.

Involvement of ionic channels in ALS

As the activity of voltage-dependent ionic channels has profound effects on neuronal function and possibly viability, changes in the electrical properties of motoneurons have been evaluated in terms of the ionic channels operating under normal conditions (McLarnon, 1995) as well as in relation to disease. For instance, the duration of the afterpotential in slow α-motoneurons is subject to considerable control from some 'trophic' signal associated with the activity of the innervated muscle (Czeh *et al.*, 1978). Conversely, modulation of neuronal voltage-dependent ion channels can be produced by muscle. In co-cultured spinal cord neuron and muscle cell preparations, the presence of neurons produces a change in the conductance of the Ca^{2+}-dependent potassium channel in myotubes. Although involvement of ionic channels remains a possibility in ALS, the only channel type that has been extensively studied is the Ca^{2+} channel.

Ca^{2+} channels

With regard to possible initiating factors for ALS, considerable interest has developed as to the involvement of voltage-dependent Ca^{2+} channels. Several studies have supported a role for changes in the concentration of intracellular Ca^{2+} or flux through Ca^{2+} channels in ALS (Uchitel *et al.*, 1988; Delbono *et al.*, 1991; Smith *et al.*, 1993). Neurons express at least five types of Ca^{2+} channels, which have been classified by their electrophysiological and pharmacological properties as L, N, T, P/Q and R types. The results of biochemical and molecular cloning studies have shown that neuronal Ca^{2+} channels contain a complex of α, β and δ subunits (Birnbaumer *et al.*, 1994). Five types of cloned Ca^{2+} channel $α_1$ subunits ($α_{1A-E}$) are expressed in the central nervous system, each of which encodes an electrophysiologically and pharmacologically distinct type of Ca^{2+} channel. Structurally, each $α_1$ subunit consists of four homologous domains (I–IV) containing six to eight putative transmembrane regions and includes the pore region (SS1–SS2) and voltage-sensor (S4). While the $α_1$ subunits alone form functional Ca^{2+} channels, the biophysical properties of $α_1$ subunits can be modulated by co-expression with Ca^{2+} channel ancillary subunits. The major modulatory subunit appears to be the β subunit, which alters both the kinetic and voltage-dependent properties of the channel.

In ALS, increased Ca^{2+} influx may occur through specific Ca^{2+} channels. Initial studies by Appel and colleagues demonstrated that immunoglobulins (largely IgG) from the sera of ALS patients stimulated an increase in muscle miniature end-plate potential frequency in an in-vitro mouse muscle preparation, presumably by increasing Ca^{2+} influx into the presynaptic terminals of motoneurons, leading to increased quantal release of acetylcholine (Uchitel *et al.*, 1988). Later studies reported that IgG fractions from ALS patients bound to Ca^{2+} channels and reduced the amplitudes of the dihydropyridine-sensitive (L-type) currents of skeletal muscle (Delbono *et al.*, 1991; Smith *et al.*, 1992). Reports from the same group also indicated that ALS IgG will increase Ca^{2+} influx through P-type channels (Llinas *et al.*, 1993). These observations suggested that ALS sera had differing actions on various populations of Ca^{2+} channels. Potentially, the increased flux through P-type Ca^{2+} channels produced by ALS IgG is related to the augmentation of neurotransmitter release reported in the in-vitro mouse muscle preparation (Uchitel *et al.*, 1988). The net effect of these perturbations would probably be to increase the concentration of intracellular Ca^{2+} in the synaptic terminal. This view is supported by a recent study demonstrating that motor nerve terminals obtained from ALS patients at muscle biopsy had significantly higher Ca^{2+} values than disease controls (Siklos *et al.*, 1996). According to these studies, the effects of ALS IgGs appears to be twofold. First, ALS IgG can bind to Ca^{2+} channels (Smith *et al.*, 1992). Second, these IgGs are capable of modifying the physiological properties of the Ca^{2+} channels (Delbono *et al.*, 1991; Llinas *et al.*, 1993). A precedent for this type of action of ALS IgG exists in the disorder Lambert–Eaton syndrome, in which antibodies to Ca^{2+} channels bind to presynaptic channels, altering their function and resulting in impaired neuromuscular transmission (Lennon *et al.*, 1995).

Cell lines having some properties similar to those of motoneurons have been used to elucidate the pathogenesis of ALS. A report by Smith *et al.* (1994) demonstrates that one type of motoneuron clone, VSC 4.1, has reduced viability when incubated with ALS IgGs. The cytotoxicity associated with ALS IgGs was dependent on the extracellular Ca^{2+} concentration and could be blocked by pre-incubation of immunoglobulins with L-type Ca^{2+} channels or the purified α subunit of the L-type channel (Smith *et al.*, 1994). Selective blockers of N-type Ca^{2+} channels (ω-conotoxin) and P-type channels (Aga-IVA) attenuated cell death in this clonal line. Viability was not affected by incubation with an antagonist of L-type Ca^{2+} channels (nifedipine) or with Bay K8644 (an L-type channel activator). These data further substantiate the role of ALS IgG as enhancing various Ca^{2+} currents in neurons. A further report has claimed that the Ca^{2+}-induced cell death in this motoneuron cell line is due to apoptotic mechanisms (Alexianu *et al.*, 1994). Increased concentrations of intracellular Ca^{2+} appear to be the stimulus for neurotoxicity because expression of the calcium-binding protein calbindin-D_{28K} (CaBP) in these motoneuron hybrid cells reduces cytotoxicity due to IgGs from ALS sera (Alexianu *et al.*, 1994; Ho *et al.*, 1996).

One possible explanation for the selectivity of the Ca^{2+}-induced cytotoxicity in ALS could be the absence of Ca^{2+}-binding proteins from motoneurons and other susceptible cells. Thus, although ALS may be characterized by increased Ca^{2+} influx through N-type and P-type channels in many neurons in the neuraxis, most of these neurons possess sufficiently high levels of calcium-binding proteins effectively to buffer the increased Ca^{2+} influx and protect against Ca^{2+}-induced cytotoxicity. Several groups have recently provided support for the view that reduced calcium buffering could be present in ALS (Ince *et al.*, 1993; Reiner *et al.*, 1995; Elliott and Snider, 1996), with evidence that motoneuron populations which were lost early in ALS had lower levels of CaBP and parvalbumin (PV) immunoreactivity or mRNA than motoneurons lost later in the disease (Ince *et al.*, 1993; Elliott and Snider, 1996). Motoneuron hybrid cell lines which have lower levels of CaBP and PV have reduced viability following exposure to ALS IgG than other cell lines with higher amounts of CaBP and PV immunoreactivity (Alexianu *et al.*, 1994; Ho *et al.*, 1996). One limitation of these studies is that it is difficult to compare cell lines with regard to cell survival and conclude that the difference in viability is related to a single factor, such as the presence of CaBP or PV, as cell lines may differ in many respects from one another.

While Appel's model of IgG-induced changes in Ca^{2+} influx is of interest, several crucial issues remain to be addressed. First, the validity of the hypothesis remains to be tested by independent groups using sera isolated from larger numbers of both ALS patients and controls. Lennon and colleagues (1995) found antibodies to P-type or Q-type Ca^{2+} channels only in approximately 25 per cent of ALS patients. Antibodies to N-type Ca^{2+} channels were identified in around 15 per cent of patients with ALS. Drachman and coworkers have been unable to detect antibodies to either N-type or P-type Ca^{2+} channels in sera from sporadic ALS patients (Drachman *et al.*, 1995; Vincent and Drachman, 1996). A recent study by Arsac and coworkers showed that fewer than 10 per cent of patients with ALS had evidence for antibodies directed against N-type Ca^{2+} channels as measured using an immunoprecipitation technique (Arsac *et al.*, 1996). In contrast, about 60 per cent of patients with Eaton–Lambert syndrome had positive antibody titres. Enzyme-linked immunosorbent assays to N-type Ca^{2+} channels demonstrated immunoreactivity in only two of 25 serum samples from ALS patients. Immunoprecipitation assays of L-type Ca^{2+} channels did not demonstrate any positive ALS samples. These observations are at variance with the claims of Appel and colleagues that 75 per cent of patients with sporadic ALS have sera which react with L-type Ca^{2+} channels. Our view is that these data indicate that antibodies to Ca^{2+} channels are present in some patients with ALS. However, the frequency with which these antibodies are observed needs to be more precisely defined. Furthermore, the relation between these antibodies and the disease is unknown. The antibodies could be a byproduct of neuronal damage and unrelated to the course of the disease. The fact that ALS IgGs have been variously reported to interact with L-type and P/Q-type Ca^{2+} channels indicates that the exact molecular target of immunoglobulin binding remains to be precisely determined.

A further criticism of this work is that the evidence in favour of an immunological mechanism for ALS is controversial and limited (Drachman *et al.*, 1995; also see below). Furthermore, in the event that antibodies to Ca^{2+} channels were present and modulating the action of these channels in ALS, it is difficult to envisage a mechanism whereby they would selectively affect motoneurons and corticospinal tract pathways. Although Appel and colleagues have suggested that levels of Ca^{2+}-binding proteins might be relevant in this regard, this argument has little support. Studies examining the relation between levels of Ca^{2+}-binding proteins and the extent of excitotoxin-induced cell death have not yielded consistent results (see Abdel Hamid and Baimbridge, 1997). Although theoretically Ca^{2+}-buffering proteins could reduce the amplitude of a Ca^{2+} signal produced by an excitotoxic stimulus, the Ca^{2+}-buffering protein could also act as an intracellular source for Ca^{2+}, releasing this ion when intracellular free Ca^{2+} concentration returns towards normal. Thus, the dynamics of the Ca^{2+} entry system must be understood before this simplistic mechanism is accepted.

A possible alternative explanation for some of the results of Appel and coworkers is that ALS sera contains additional factors responsible for the false-positive binding studies. Nyormoi (1996) has suggested that ALS sera contain increased proteolytic activity which reduced the blockade of a monoclonal antibody to the α_1 subunit of a Ca^{2+} channel in a skeletal muscle preparation. Although this explanation may be true for one observation, it does not explain the results of other binding studies done by Appel and colleagues, or of neurophysiological experiments using ALS sera (Llinas *et al.*, 1993). An additional group has reported that ALS sera reduced the amplitude of Ca^{2+} current in cerebellar granule cells; however, this study only used serum samples from four ALS patients and a reduced current was seen only in three samples (Zhainazarov *et al.*, 1994). Furthermore, this study also reported that Ca^{2+} currents were modified by serum proteins in addition to IgGs.

In summary, although of considerable interest, evidence that ALS is due to antibodies directed to Ca^{2+} channels must be regarded with some scepticism until further substantiation of the numbers of ALS patients having antibodies to Ca^{2+} channels can be established. Also of importance will be to determine whether these antibodies have any physiological significance whatsoever.

Role of increased intracellular free Ca^{2+} concentration

Although the issue of whether antibodies to voltage-dependent Ca^{2+} channels are present in ALS has not been resolved, there are data indicating that the concentration of intracellular free Ca^{2+} is elevated in synaptic terminals from patients with ALS compared to disease controls (Siklos *et al.*, 1996). The increased intracellular Ca^{2+} might occur secondarily to a number of pathophysiological mechanisms. These include: (i) activation of EAA receptors, (ii) activation of voltage-dependent Ca^{2+} channels by antibodies, (iii) alteration of mitochondrial function (Beal, 1995), or (iv) low levels of Ca^{2+}-binding proteins. In the event that altered intracellular Ca^{2+} would occur in ALS, this ion could also influence free radical generation in neurons as Ca^{2+} is important at several points in free radical neurotoxicity. Specifically, increased intracellular free Ca^{2+} will increase the activity of a serine protease (calpain) which catalyses the formation of xanthine oxidase from xanthine dehydrogenase. Xanthine oxidase, in turn, is responsible for the production of superoxide anion, uric acid and H_2O_2. Raised intracellular free Ca^{2+} interacts with phospholipase A_2, which releases arachidonic acid and subsequently will elevate eicosanoids. Ca^{2+} also interacts with nitric oxide synthetase, leading to the production of nitric oxide which potentially can be toxic to neurons and motoneurons.

Altered protein kinase activity in ALS

Protein phosphorylation has been implicated in the control of many biological processes in the nervous system including neurotransmitter synthesis and release, control of ion channel conductance, as well as neuron differentiation. There is also strong evidence indicating that changes in protein kinase function are involved in some types of neuro-degenerative disease (see Krieger *et al.*, 1996a). The seemingly disparate mechanisms for producing neuronal loss in ALS, such as impaired function of Cu/Zn–SOD1 gene products, increased amounts of potentially excitotoxic EAAs, and disturbed transmembrane Ca^{2+} flux, may all be associated with changes in the activity and/or quantity of given protein kinases in ALS patients.

A study of the activity and amounts of PKC in cytosolic and membrane fractions from ALS and control tissue has shown that Ca^{2+}-dependent PKC activity was significantly increased in spinal cord tissue from ALS patients compared to controls (Lanius *et al.*, 1995). The increased activity appeared to be partially, but not completely, due to an increase in membrane protein. No statistically significant differences were apparent in motor and visual cortex, platelets and leucocytes between ALS patients and controls. Recent work on a cultured motoneuron cell line has demonstrated that increased PKC activity can be produced by raising the intracellular Ca^{2+} concentration. The augmented PKC activity may be produced by the phosphorylation of PKC itself (Hasham *et al.*, 1997). The mechanisms associated with the activation of PKC may be dependent on the level of intracellular Ca^{2+} achieved. When intracellular Ca^{2+} is only slightly elevated above control levels, PKC activation may be associated with translocation of PKC from the cytosol to the membrane. At higher levels of intracellular Ca^{2+}, phosphorylation of PKC may be important. It also appears that when intracellular Ca^{2+} concentrations are very high (> 400 nM), PKC may be proteolysed to yield protein kinase M (PKM), a constitutively active protein kinase. Whether raised intracellular Ca^{2+} concentration or stimulation by EAAs will result in a persistent elevation of PKC activity in motoneurons and spinal cord neurons over long time periods is presently unknown. There is evidence that stimulation of EAA receptors will result in a reduction of membrane-associated PKC activity. Protein kinase C has modulatory effects on the function of EAA receptors, as well as on voltage-dependent Ca^{2+} channels (see Krieger *et al.*, 1996a). Protein kinase C also has important stimulatory properties for 'down-stream' protein kinases. Because of its unique position in the cascade of protein kinases, it may serve as an important point of convergence for a number of distinct processes (Fig. 4.2). The role played by PKC is unclear. It is not known if the elevated PKC activity found in ALS tissue is simply a response to neuron death rather than a specific feature of the disease.

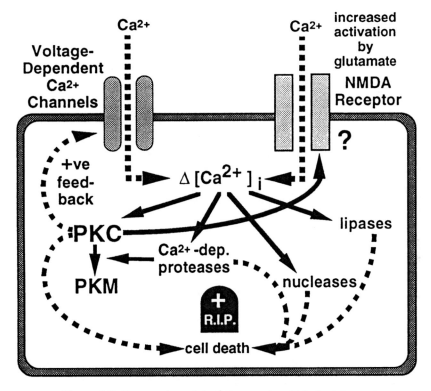

Figure 4.2. Proposed model of the events which lead to motoneuron death in ALS. Activation of excitatory amino acid receptors (or NMDA receptors) by glutamate results in increased intracellular Ca^{2+} levels and the activation of protein kinase C (PKC) and other enzymes. Protein kinase C can phosphorylate certain EAA receptor types as well as voltage-dependent Ca^{2+} channels, thus modifying the behaviour of these receptors. Elevated PKC may lead to cell death by activation of other protein kinases. Protein kinase C is proteolysed to protein kinase M (PKM) by the action of Ca^{2+}-dependent proteases.

Preliminary reports suggest that the activity of the lipid kinase phosphatidylinositol-3-hydroxy kinase is also increased in spinal cord tissue from ALS patients (Wagey *et al.*, 1996). This kinase is stimulated by several growth factors and also may stimulate certain isoforms of PKC.

The protein kinases are linked in a complex signal transduction network involving numerous protein kinases and protein phosphatases. Protein kinases are responsible for phosphorylating a number of important substrate molecules. Conversely, protein phosphatases act in an opposing manner to dephosphorylate substrates. Although our knowledge of the interaction between protein kinases is only rudimentary, several of the major signalling pathways have been identified. A few of the 'downstream kinases' in the signal transduction cascade are of considerable interest in view of their involvement in gene transcription and translation. Several important protein kinases, such as cyclin-dependent kinase 5, PKC, mitogen-activated protein kinase (MAPK), stress-activated kinases and glycogen synthase kinase 3, are capable of phosphorylating neurofilaments or other structural proteins, raising the possibility that they could be responsible for the aberrant phosphorylation of structural proteins that is observed in ALS tissue (see Chapter 3). For example, the in-vitro phosphorylation of the NF-L protein by either cyclic AMP-dependent protein kinase or PKC can block its polymerization, or cause disassembly of existing filaments. Protein phosphatases also regulate neurofilament phosphorylation. When cultured neurons are exposed to okadaic acid, which inhibits protein phosphatases PP2A and PP1, the fragmentation of neurofilaments is observed (see Julien, 1997). Although no direct evidence is available indicating an impairment of protein phosphatase activity in tissues from ALS patients, Wagey and colleagues (1997) have reported that protein phosphatase inhibitors have different effects on the binding of ligands to NMDA receptor channels in spinal cord tissue from ALS patients and controls. Direct measurement of protein phosphatase activities will be required to evaluate this observation.

Immunological mechanisms in ALS

Support for an immunological basis for ALS has been limited. To provide firm evidence that a disorder occurs through an autoimmune mechanism generally requires that several conditions be met. These conditions include: (i) the presence of antibodies directed to a suitable epitope, (ii) evidence that the antibody–antigen mediated-interaction can generate the appropriate physiological effect, (iii) the development of an immune-mediated animal model of the disease, (iv) evidence for passive transfer of the disorder, and (v) successful treatment of the disorder with immuno-suppressive medication or plasma exchange (Appel *et al.*, 1995). In ALS, the limited evidence in favour of an immunological mechanism includes the observation of raised titres of antibodies to several potentially important epitopes such as voltage-dependent Ca^{2+} channels or ganglio-sides in some patients with the disease. However, there is no clear support for the concept that the binding of an antibody in ALS patients leads to a pathophysiologically relevant response. Immune-mediated animal models of ALS are only a limited approximation of the disease in humans (Appel *et al.*, 1995). No passive transfer of the human disease has been demonstrated, and treatment of ALS patients with immunosuppressive medication has no clinical benefit. Thus, support for an immunological mechanism is not compelling. However, it is still possible that immunological mechanisms are involved in some aspects of the disease. Furthermore, although immune-mediated mechanisms may not be responsible for the initiation of ALS, they may be relevant for some features which occur later in the course of the disease. For instance, neuronal damage induced by a non-immunological mechanism could expose epitopes within neurons which could be a target for humoral responses and inflammatory changes.

The nature of the immunological mechanisms that may be involved in ALS has been reviewed (Antel and Cashman, 1995; Appel *et al.*, 1995; Drachman *et al.*, 1995). The neuropathological findings seen in ALS have been traditionally regarded as typical for a neurodegenerative disease without an inflammatory component. However, a number of recent studies have revealed features which are often seen in immune-mediated disorders. These features include:

1. deposition of immunoglobulin and complement in spinal cord and motor cortex of ALS patients (Appel *et al.*, 1995)
2. collections of T cells having restricted heterogeneity in spinal cord and motor cortex
3. the presence of macrophages, microglia and reactive glial cells in ALS tissue.

The deposition of immunoglobulins has been observed on motoneurons and cortical neurons in patients who died with ALS (Appel *et al.*, 1995). Potentially, immunoglobulins enter the motoneuron at the neuromuscular junction and are transported by retrograde axonal transport. The selective vulnerability of motoneurons for this process could arise because immunoglobulins gain access to the distal motor axon or synapse in the periphery.

Clinical features suggestive of an immune-mediated illness in ALS are few. Although it has been reported that ALS is associated with other autoimmune illnesses more commonly than expected, this effect is only slight (Antel and Cashman, 1995). Occasionally, monoclonal (or M) peaks are detected in the disease; however, these abnormalities are often seen in healthy, aged individuals. The nature of the epitopes that such antibodies would be directed to is unknown. Cerebrospinal fluid from patients with

ALS does not consistently show raised protein, altered cell counts or oligoclonal banding.

Reports of studies using tissue from patients with ALS and controls have been contradictory. Sera from patients with ALS have been reported to be toxic to neurons maintained in dissociated or organotypic tissue culture by some, but not all, investigators (see Antel and Cashman, 1995). For instance, Kiernan and Hudson (1993) found that sera from ALS patients frequently bound to spinal motoneurons but that sera from a similar proportion of control subjects would also bind. The cytotoxic effects of ALS serum may have an immunoglobulin-related component but passive transfer of the disease has not been achieved (Antel and Cashman, 1995). ALS sera have also been reported to inhibit terminal sprouting induced by botulinum toxin (Gurney et al., 1984). However, this has not been observed by other investigators (Donaghy and Duchen, 1986). Recent reports by Appel and colleagues have claimed that immunoglobulins from ALS patients are capable of binding several types of voltage-dependent Ca^{2+} channels (Appel et al., 1995). As described above, although antibodies to Ca^{2+} channels are found in the sera of some patients with ALS, this is probably not a frequent finding and the significance of these antibodies is unknown (Appel et al., 1995; Drachman et al., 1995; Vincent and Drachman, 1996).

Observations of patients demonstrating MMN with conduction block have revealed that some possess antibodies directed against components of peripheral myelin or the axonal membrane (Rowland, 1995). This disorder has been very influential in supporting the belief that there could be an immune-mediated process in ALS. In many cases of MMN with conduction block antibodies are directed to carbohydrate moieties which are present in gangliosides GM1 and GD1b of central and peripheral myelin. Antibodies to these gangliosides are found not only in MMN with conduction block but also in ALS, and it is likely that initial reports overestimated the prevalence with which these antibodies are observed in ALS patients (Drachman et al., 1995). Current estimates place the fraction of ALS patients with elevated levels of anti-GM1 or anti-GD1a antibodies, compared to controls, at around 25 per cent (Drachman et al., 1995). Elevated levels of these antibodies are often observed in autoimmune disorders and other neurological diseases. Drachman and colleagues (1995) have reported that fewer than 5 per cent of ALS patients have anti-GM1 or anti-GD1a antibody titres which are higher than those of patients with Guillain–Barré syndrome or MMN with conduction block. The spectrum of MMN with conduction block may overlap with ALS to the extent that there are patients with MMN who neither show conduction block nor possess anti-GM1 antibodies. Yet, as described in Chapter 2, there are clinical differences between MMN with conduction block and ALS, and clinical improvement may occur with the former.

Paraneoplastic syndromes arising in association with ALS could indicate an autoimmune mechanism. However, the relation between ALS and neoplasms is controversial (Rowland, 1995). Recent studies suggest that there may be a statistically significant increase in ALS among patients with lymphoproliferative disorders (e.g. lymphoma, multiple myeloma and macroglobulinemia) (Louis *et al.*, 1996), although this has been disputed (see Rowland, 1995). Anecdotal reports have described patients with lymphoproliferative disorders having ALS or 'ALS-like' symptoms and signs where the features of ALS improved following treatment of the lympoproliferative disorder (Rowland, 1995; Louis *et al.*, 1996). Louis and his colleagues estimate that the probable combined frequency of all forms of lymphoproliferative disease in patients with ALS is 2.5 per cent with an upper limit of 5 per cent (Louis *et al.*, 1996). Only two of 20 patients had some reversibility to their 'ALS-like' symptoms following immunosuppressive treatment. These results raise the possibility that the 'treatable' cases of ALS were actually motor neuropathies or MMN with conduction block.

Therapeutic efforts aimed at altering autoimmune activity in ALS using plasmaphaeresis, corticosteroids, cyclophosphamide, cyclosporine and total lymph node irradiation have not shown any benefit (Drachman *et al.*, 1995; Rowland, 1995). The failure to observe clinical improvement following immunotherapy does not disprove that the initiating factors were immunological in nature. However, the absence of improvement by these modalities is certainly not supportive of such a mechanism.

In summary, there is currently very little evidence in favour of autoimmunity in ALS. Antibodies to voltage-dependent Ca^{2+} channels or to gangliosides are detected in some patients. The significance of these antibodies is unclear. Rarely, minor neuropathological features suggestive of inflammation are seen. There is no support for a satisfactory immune-mediated animal model of ALS, passive transfer of the disorder, or beneficial effects of immunosuppressive treatment.

Involvement of growth factors or growth factor receptors in ALS

Studies of motoneurons and spinal cord neurons both in vivo and in vitro have clearly established that motoneurons require neurotrophic factors

Table 4.7. *Growth factors in motoneuron survival*

Neurotrophins
NGF
BDNF
NT-3
NT-4/5
Neuropoietic cytokines
INTERLEUKINS:
IL-1β, IL-2, IL-3, IL-4, IL-5
IL-7, IL-8, IL-9, IL-10
GP-130 RELATED FACTORS:
CNTF, LIF, IL-6, IL-11
TGF-β factors
TGF-β1, TGF-β2, TGF-β3
Other trophic factors
FGF
IGF
GDNF

NGF, nerve growth factor; BDNF, brain-derived growth factor; NT, neurotrophin; IL, interleukin; CNTF, ciliary neurotrophic factor; LIF, leukaemia inhibitory factor; TGF, transforming growth factor; FGF, fibroblast growth factor; IGF, insulin-like growth factor; GDNF, glial cell line-derived neurotrophic factor.

and other substances for survival, growth and phenotypic expression. Several recent reviews have addressed this issue (see Elliott and Snider, 1996). Several factors having possible trophic influence on motoneurons are indicated in Table 4.7. To be considered as a trophic factor, a substance should: (i) be available to motoneurons in vivo, (ii) have specific receptors to which it binds on motoneurons or other neurons, (iii) mimic the effect of the endogenous substance when applied exogenously, and (iv) when its supply is interrupted, result in neuronal dysfunction or cell death. Some of these conditions have been met for the factors listed below.

Neurotrophins

Neurotrophins constitute one of the best characterized families of neuro-trophic factors. These compounds are small, basic polypeptides that act at receptor tyrosine kinases of the tyrosine kinase receptor (Trk) family (e.g. TrkA, TrkB, TrkC), as well as at a low-affinity p75 receptor. Most neurotrophins except nerve growth factor (NGF) are capable of promot-ing the survival of embryonic rat motoneurons in culture (Henderson *et al.*, 1993). The reasons for differences in the neurotrophic activity of specific neurotrophins are unclear. The presence of a high-affinity receptor for a given neurotrophin is not sufficient to insure that a trophic effect is observed. This may occur because there are multiple isoforms of TrkB and TrkC, some of which lack the tyrosine kinase domain. Potentially, the presence of receptors without tyrosine kinase domains may reduce, or abolish, the ability of neurons containing the truncated receptors to respond to a specific neurotrophin.

Nerve growth factor Although NGF is among the most thoroughly studied of the neurotrophins, it does not appear to exert any trophic effects on motoneurons. Spinal motoneurons express NGF receptor mRNA and receptor protein. Autoradiographic studies demonstrate that motoneurons express NGF receptors during development and that NGF receptors are also present in the human spinal cord, both in patients with ALS and in controls.

Brain-derived neurotrophic factor Brain-derived neurotrophic factor is a neurotrophin having survival-promoting activity for motoneurons and other central nervous system neurons (Jones *et al.*, 1994). The administration of BDNF to chick embryos reduces the extent of programmed cell death in spinal motoneurons (Oppenheim *et al.*, 1992) and the application of BDNF to the nerves of postnatal animals is also capable of reducing motoneuron death due to nerve transection (Sendtner *et al.*, 1992).

Studies of the wobbler mouse (wr/wr), an autosomal recessive mutant having progressive motoneuron loss, have suggested that administration of BDNF will slow the progression of this motor system degeneration (Mitsumoto and Pioro, 1995). The survival-enhancing effect of BDNF appears to be synergistic with ciliary neurotrophic factor (CNTF). The co-administration of these two neurotrophic factors in wobbler mice is more than additive and arrests the decline in motor function temporarily (Mitsumoto and Pioro, 1995). As is discussed in Chapter 7, phase I and II clinical trials of BDNF have been completed in ALS patients. However, there does not appear to be any clinical benefit of BDNF when administered according to the protocols used (see Chapter 7).

Neurotrophin-3 Neurotrophin-3 also has trophic effects on motoneurons. Application of NT-3 to transected peripheral nerve results in greater motoneuron survival (Sendtner *et al.*, 1992). However, under some experimental conditions, the rescue of motoneurons is only temporary. Motorneurons possess receptors for NT-3 (TrkC) and this substance is synthesized by skeletal muscle. There are reports that NT-3 has neuro-trophic effects on corticospinal tract neurons. In ALS patients, spinal motoneurons have reduced NT-3-like immunoreactivity compared to controls, although there is no change in TrkC mRNA (Duberley *et al.*, 1997). No differences in NT-3-like immunoreactivity are seen in neurons of the motor cortex in ALS patients and controls. Whether the decrease in NT-3-like immunoreactivity in spinal motoneurons reflects decreased uptake, retrograde transport, or increased destruction is unknown.

Neurotrophin-4/5 Neurotrophin-4/5 (NT-4/5) acts on TrkB receptors which are present on spinal motoneurons. Local application of NT-4 is capable of preventing injury-induced death of facial motoneurons following nerve transection in neonatal rats. Choline acetyltransferase synthesis and motoneuron survival in vitro are supported by BDNF and NT-4 but are less efficiently promoted by NT-3 (Henderson *et al.*, 1993).

The importance of neurotrophins and their receptors has been clarified by the use of gene-targeted deletions ('knockout mice'). This has been accomplished for several neurotrophins that have trophic activity for motoneurons, as well as neurotrophin receptor tyrosine kinases (Elliott and Snider, 1996). Studies of knockout mice for BDNF and NT-3 have indicated that although these neurotrophins have prominent activity for motoneurons, the knockout mice themselves do not exhibit motoneuron loss except for some reduction in the numbers of γ motoneurons in NT-3 null mutants (see Elliott and Snider, 1996). Mice with knockout of the TrkB receptors do not demonstrate reduced motoneuron numbers, although this may not be the case in some TrkC null mutants (see Elliott and Snider, 1996).

Insulin growth factors

The biological activities of insulin and insulin-like growth factor-I (IGF-I) and IGF-II are mediated by specific, structurally related membrane receptors (Doré *et al.*, 1996). The actions of IGF-I, although mediated by the IGF-I receptor, may also involve stimulation of insulin and IGF-II receptors. Furthermore, the effects of IGF-I and IGF-II can be modified by a family of IGF-binding proteins. Considerable recent interest has been directed to IGF-I in ALS as this molecule potentiates motoneuron survival in culture (Ang *et al.*, 1992), as well as preventing programmed motoneuron death during normal development or following axotomy (Lewis *et al.*, 1993). In adult rodents, nerve sprouting can be induced by the subcutaneous administration of IGF-I (see Yuen and Mobley, 1996). Patients who died with ALS demonstrate increased IGF-I and IGF-II binding in spinal cord compared to controls, whereas insulin binding is unchanged (Doré *et al.*, 1996). The increased binding of IGF-I and IGF-II is generalized and not restricted to ventral grey matter or motoneurons and suggests that these receptors are up-regulated in ALS. The up-regulation of these IGF receptors could mean that they would respond to exogenously applied IGFs or endogenous sources, such as microglia or astrocytes. Therapeutic studies using this neurotrophic compound in ALS patients and animal models of ALS are described in Chapter 7.

Glial cell-derived neurotrophic factor

Purification of glial cell-derived neurotrophic factor (GDNF), originally characterized as a conditioned medium activity obtained from glial cell lines, has revealed it to be a member of the transforming growth factor-β (TGF-β) superfamily. The receptor for this factor is currently unknown. It is expressed in limb bud and cultured myotubes, suggesting that it may have a growth-promoting function prior to the establishment of neuro-muscular junctions. Schwann cells and type I astrocytes have mRNA for GDNF and may be the cell types which release this factor. GDNF is believed to bind to a surface receptor on motoneurons and to be transported in a retrograde manner. It has been reported to be a survival factor for purified rat spinal motoneurons in culture (Henderson *et al.*, 1994), for neonatal rat facial motoneurons following axotomy (Yan *et al.*, 1995), as well as for embryonic chicken motoneurons *in ovo* (Oppenheim *et al.*, 1995). Administration of GDNF to chick embryos rescues approximately 25 per cent of spinal motoneurons from programmed cell death and may have survival-promoting effects on sympathetic ganglion neurons (Oppenheim *et al.*, 1995), but not on dorsal root ganglion neurons or neurons in the nodose or ciliary ganglia. Embryonic chickens treated with GDNF after axotomy do not exhibit motoneuron loss. Therapeutic trials using this factor are described in Chapter 7.

Ciliary neurotrophic factor

Ciliary neurotrophic factor is one of a group of neuropoietic cytokines related to cholinergic differentiation factor (CDF), interleukin-6 (IL-6) and other cytokines. These proteins are predicted to have a common tertiary fold structure in spite of the absence of significant homologies in their amino acid sequences. Neuropoietic cytokines share signal-transducing elements including the gp130-related receptor and other subunits (Kishimoto *et al.*, 1994). The CNTF-related changes in phenotype may be mediated by the CNTF-α receptor. CNTF is expressed in Schwann cells and type I astrocytes and supports the survival of motoneurons and other neurons in vivo and in vitro. The evidence for this trophic support includes: (i) CNTF increases the survival of cultured motoneurons; (ii) CNTF administration to chick embryos in ovo decreases the extent of naturally occurring cell death; (iii) CNTF prevents the death of facial motoneurons following axotomy; (iv) CNTF induces terminal sprouting of motoneurons (Gurney *et al.*, 1992); (v) administration of CNTF to progressive motor neuronopathy mice (pmn/pmn) that have been subjected to facial nerve axotomy prevents the loss of motoneurons in the facial nucleus; and (vi) subcutaneous administration of CNTF retards disease progression in the wobbler mouse (wr/wr) (Mitsumoto and Pioro, 1995). As a consequence of the promising results of animal and culture studies, placebo-controlled trials of recombinant human CNTF were undertaken in patients with ALS. The results of these trials have been reported to be negative and are discussed in Chapter 7.

Fibroblast growth factors

Fibroblast growth factors (FGFs) are a family of polypeptide growth factors that have been established to enhance the survival and development of post-mitotic neurons, both in vivo and in vitro (see Gouin *et al.*, 1996). In-vitro studies have indicated that FGF-2 has survival-promoting activity for motoneurons (Gouin *et al.*, 1996) and increases levels of choline acetyltransferase of these neurons. The survival-promoting activity of FGF-2 in purified chicken embryonic motoneurons appears to be modest and may be potentiated by TGF-β, but not by GDNF. Cultured motoneurons express immunoreactivity for the FGF receptor and may also contain mRNA for the FGF receptor. The in-vivo sources for FGF that might support motoneuron development are unclear. The mRNAs for FGF-1 and FGF-2 are expressed in avian spinal cord and motoneurons at early developmental stages and are down-regulated later in life. Other members of the FGF family are expressed in muscle but not in spinal cord (Haub and Goldfarb, 1991). One potential source of these trophic factors could be motoneurons that have released endogenous FGF during the course of cell death.

Transforming growth factor-β

The transforming growth factor superfamily constitutes a family of ligands that activate a number of related receptors. TGF-β1 is absent from nerve and muscle but mRNA for TGF-β2 can be visualized in the ventral horns of embryonic mice. TGF-β3 has low levels of survival-promoting activity for embryonic chick motoneurons in culture, but can act synergistically with FGF-2 to permit increased survival (Gouin *et al.*, 1996).

In summary, the growth factor requirements of motoneurons and their central connections are clearly complex, with multiple neurotrophic substances involved, possibly showing developmental or injury-dependent regulation. It appears fairly clear that at least some members of the neurotrophin family provide neurotrophic support for motoneurons, including BDNF and NT-3. Whether alterations in these neurotrophins are involved in the pathogenesis of ALS is unknown. Even in the event that neurotrophins are unrelated to the pathogenesis of ALS, it is possible that administration of neurotrophins may still affect the clinical course of ALS. The fact that neurotrophins appear to aid some classes of neurons in their responses to oxidative stress, excitatory amino acids, axotomy and programmed cell death lends support to this idea. Although attention has hitherto been focused on the growth-promoting activities of neuro-trophins, it is also evident that a wide variety of substances will have neurotrophic activity. For instance, over a dozen known growth factors and extracts can influence motoneuron survival in chick embryos. It is prudent to bear in mind that molecules outside the major families of neurotrophic factors may be involved in cell death and development. For instance, the serine protease inhibitor protease nexin-1 rescues moto-neurons from naturally occurring and axotomy-induced cell death (Houenou *et al.*, 1995).

Summary

This chapter examines our fragmentary understanding of the patho-physiology of ALS. It appears clear that ALS results from the action of a number of distinct mechanisms. However, it is not clear whether these mechanisms ultimately trigger a common cascade of cellular events responsible for the neuronal dysfunction and death. There is an associa-tion between the presence of mutations in the Cu/Zn–SOD1 gene and the occurrence of familial ALS in some patients. In support of this association, it appears that there may be some relation between the specific mutation and the clinical phenotype of the affected ALS patient. The reason that Cu/Zn–SOD1 mutations lead to ALS is unknown, but is likely to be related to a novel 'gain of function' of the mutant protein. This novel function presumably relates to aberrant oxidation of substrates.

There has been considerable interest in a role for impaired EAA regulation in ALS, but the evidence for this is limited. Levels of EAAs are generally normal in the plasma and CSF of ALS patients, although some workers have questioned whether there exists a small subgroup of patients with elevated CSF glutamate, aspartate or other putative excitatory compounds. Several investigators have provided evidence for impaired glutamate re-uptake by specific transporters, but it remains to be seen whether this effect is causative of ALS or a consequence of the change in glial and neuronal functioning which accompanies ALS. The compound riluzole, which interferes with the release of EAAs at central synapses, does appear to have some modest beneficial effects. The observation of depressed contents of excitatory amino acids in nervous system tissue from ALS patients at autopsy is among the most consistent findings in the disease. However, these results are probably a consequence of the loss of neurons and corticospinal tract axons that occurs in ALS.

Immunological mechanisms, although of interest, have not had much experimental support. A few patients appear to have ALS-like conditions as a consequence of antibody-mediated effects, either from a lymphoproliferative disorder or, rarely, a remote malignancy. Anti-ganglioside antibodies are probably found as frequently in ALS as in other neurological disorders affecting the motoneuron. Although antibodies to voltage-dependent Ca^{2+} channels are found in some ALS patients, there is little evidence that they result in neuron death. Furthermore, treatment of patients with ALS using immunosuppression has been unrewarding.

Neurotrophic factors hold much promise for the treatment of ALS and other neurodegenerative disorders. However, there is little support for a primary abnormality in a neurotrophic factor as a cause of ALS. There is unquestionably a large number of neurotrophic factors, many of which have not been identified. It is thus difficult to be definite about this issue. Furthermore, it seems likely that many other compounds, not primarily regarded as trophic factors, may be beneficial in the maintenance of motoneuron survival and function.

In an attempt to find a point of convergence for a number of possible mechanisms for motoneuron dysfunction, several groups have focused on the possibility that impaired protein phosphorylation could arise from altered intracellular Ca^{2+} concentrations or EAA stimulation. In turn, activation of protein kinases, such as PKC, could lead to altered phosphorylation of neurofilaments and activate 'downstream' protein kinases, resulting in motoneuron death. Further study of these mechanisms is required.

5

The role of clinical neurophysiology in ALS

This chapter explores the role of clinical electrophysiology in ALS. The term EMG is used here generically to include various types of conduction studies and needle EMG. These procedures are of considerable aid in the diagnostic confirmation of ALS, and electrophysiological abnormalities have now been incorporated into the El Escorial criteria for ALS. Electromyography is also an aid in establishing the prognosis for an individual and for determining timely institution of, for example, BIPAP. Conduction studies are essential in the identification of some of the disorders that mimic ALS but which have a better natural history or are treatable. In addition, recent sophisticated physiological techniques have enhanced our understanding of the pathophysiology of ALS (Table 5.1).

Conduction studies in ALS

Motor and sensory nerve conduction studies are considered mandatory in all patients with suspected ALS. Motor conduction studies are the only means of detecting MMN with persistent conduction block (Bouche *et al.*, 1995; Trojaborg *et al.*, 1995; Parry 1996). MMN is now reasonably well characterized and, as discussed in Chapter 2, can closely mimic ALS. Its prognosis is considerably better than that of ALS, and when the disease is of recent onset and denervation of muscle has not occurred, the response to intravenous hyperimmune globulin (IVIg) may be quite dramatic (Bouche *et al.*, 1995; Parry, 1996).

It may be necessary to stimulate several nerves at multiple sites to demonstrate conduction block. The number of nerves required to be studied before concluding conduction block is absent is debatable, but three sites in each of three different nerves are probably the minimum. It is important that a sufficiently proximal stimulation site has been employed.

144

Table 5.1. *Role of electrophysiological studies in ALS*

Type of study	Application
Motor conduction studies	Rule out MMN with conduction block, CIDP
F-wave	A measure of motor unit loss; may be large in early spasticity, delayed or absent in MMN and CIDP
SNAP	Small or absent in Kennedy's syndrome
Needle EMG	Evidence of lower motoneuron disease in clinically normal limb or bulbar muscles
	Diaphragm to determine respiratory involvement
	Extent of denervation versus re-innervation
Motor unit estimates	Follow course of disease, track response to therapy
Transcranial magnetic stimulation	Assess function of central motor pathways
Peristimulus time histograms	Assess integrity of corticomotoneuron, track loss of corticomotoneurons

SNAP, sensory nerve action potential; EMG, electromyography; MMN, multifocal motor neuropathy; CIDP, chronic idiopathic demyelinating polyneuropathy.

Inadequate stimulus intensity may give a false impression of conduction block. When stimulating the nerve roots, the stimulus should be sufficient to induce movement in the unaffected limb. When this occurs, one can be confident that the stimulus was truly maximal. Conduction block is best defined as 'a combination of clinical paralysis or paresis occurring in association with the ability to stimulate the nerve and obtain visible muscle contraction distal to the block' (Kimura, 1997). One might add to this definition that there should be little, if any, wasting of the weak muscles and that if they are denervated, the amount of fibrillation should be limited. The site(s) at which conduction block occurs may be unusual; for example it may be detected in the distal forearm or, more commonly, proximal, usually rostral to Erb's point. Proximal conduction block is best demonstrated by nerve root stimulation using a monopolar needle electrode or a magnetic stimulator which easily excites the nerve roots percutaneously (Chokroverty and Chokroverty, 1992; Eisen, 1992). The conduction block in motor neuropathy is almost always very dramatic, with amplitude and/or area reductions after proximal stimulation of >80 per cent. Typically, the conduction block is not associated with conduction slowing (Fig. 5.1). In MMN, the physiological site of the

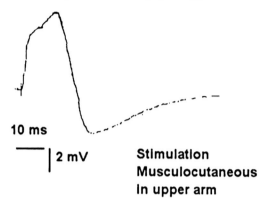

Stimulation
Musculocutaneous
in upper arm

10 ms

2 mV

Stimulation
Musculocutaneous
Erb's point

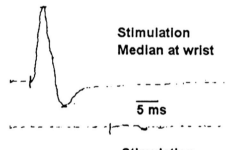

Stimulation
Median at wrist

5 ms

Stimulation
Median at Erb's point

Figure 5.1. Marked conduction block in multifocal motor neuropathy. In this patient (Chapter 2, Case report 2.5), the conduction block was proximal and could be documented after stimulation of the upper trunk of the brachial plexus at Erb's point (compare the top two traces), but also along the median nerve (compare the lower two traces). In both there is only a very small evoked response stimulating proximal to the block, representing a >90 per cent conduction block along both the median and musculocutaneous nerves.

Table 5.2. *Sites of physiological conduction block in 11 patients with multifocal motor neuropathy*

Upper limb nerves	Forearm	Arm	Proximal to axilla
Median	4	2	3
Ulnar	2		4
Radial		1	2
Musculocutaneous			2
Axillary		2	
Lower limb nerves	**Leg**		**Proximal to thigh**
Sciatic			1
Tibial	1		

With grateful thanks to our colleague Dr Gillian Gibson.

conduction block occurs most frequenty at sites along the nerve that are not typically prone to pressure (Table 5.2).

A modest reduction in amplitude or area of the CMAP (< 30 per cent) must be very cautiously interpreted. In the context of ALS, such a finding is much more likely simply to reflect physiological conduction block in motor fibres from phase cancellation (Kimura, 1997). This is not normally seen in motor conduction studies, but when there has been a significant loss of anterior horn cells there is a greater than normal variation in axonal conduction velocities and phase cancellation is more likely to occur. It is unclear whether MMN with conduction block is a specific entity or, more likely, one end of a spectrum of chronic dysimmune neuropathies, with CIDP being the prototype (Parry, 1996).

A demonstration of conduction block clearly implicates disease of the peripheral nerve, but it does not exclude the possible coexistence of central nervous system disease. Rowland (1994a) has argued that conduction block in peripheral motor nerves does not necessarily exclude ALS. Combined central and peripheral nervous system disease is certainly seen in other disorders, Guillain–Barré syndrome and MS to name just two. There has been a recent clinical–pathological description of a patient with motor neuronopathy and multifocal conduction block, who at autopsy had all the characteristic pathological features of ALS, as well as showing areas of focal demyelination in the peripheral nerves and extensively swollen anterior spinal nerve roots (Kinoshita *et al.*, 1997). The patient, a 64-year-old woman, developed slowly progressive left lower limb weakness and muscle wasting, without sensory complaints. Over the following two years, muscle weakness and wasting became widespread, involving the other leg and both arms. Tendon reflexes were brisk in the arms but hypoactive in the legs. Cranial nerves were normal throughout the course of the illness. Both median motor terminal latencies and the right tibial terminal motor latency were delayed and F-waves could not be obtained.

In classical ALS, routine motor and sensory conductions are essentially normal. However, in the terminal phases of disease, there may be modest slowing of motor conduction velocities resulting from the death of the faster conducting motor axons, but values of less than 15 per cent of age-matched control values are not encountered (Eisen and McComas, 1993). Sensory conduction velocities should be normal, and a significant reduction in the amplitude of SNAPs is worrisome in ALS, and another cause for such an abnormality must be sought. Small or absent SNAPs recorded in a patient with diffuse muscle weakness and wasting, including bulbar musculature, fasciculation and a 'neurogenic' EMG, strongly suggest X-linked recessive bulbospinal neuronopathy (Kennedy's syndrome) (Li *et al.*, 1995; Ferrante and Wilbourn, 1997). This possibility can be confirmed by DNA testing for the trinucleate repeats within exon 1 of the androgen receptor gene.

Needle EMG abnormalities in ALS

Characteristically, needle EMG in ALS shows fibrillation and/or positive sharp wave potentials, fasciculation potentials, and rapidly firing motor units producing an incomplete interference pattern. The MUPs are frequently complex and often unstable (Fig. 5.2). To support the diagnosis of ALS, these abnormalities must be seen in two to three extremities in a multimyotomal (multisegmental) distribution. Bulbar muscles are collectively equal to an extremity (Brooks, 1994). The extent of the abnormalities usually varies from myotome to myotome as well as with disease severity and duration. In general, the more spontaneous activity (fibrillation and/or positive sharp waves) that is present in a muscle, the more rapidly progressive is the disease. There is a very orderly pattern to normal MUAP recruitment. This was first described by Henneman *et al.* (1965) (Henneman size principle). Smaller motoneurons have a lower threshold and fire earlier than larger, higher threshold MUAPs. With increased contraction, the smaller motor units first increase their firing rate and then larger MUAPs are gradually recruited. Only at full force is interference complete. The frequency with which MUPs discharge varies with different muscles. On average, MUPs normally discharge at rates of 8–12 Hz.

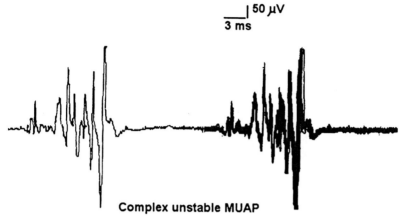

Figure 5.2. Complex, unstable motor unit action potential (MUAP) recorded from the tibials in ALS. The MUAP has at least seven easily recognized components, and superimposition of several traces of the same discharging MUAP (right part of the figure) shows that most of the components have increased jitter and are unstable (increased jiggle).

Facial muscles, including the tongue, discharge faster than distal limb muscles. Proximal limb muscles have the slowest rates of discharge. The firing frequency of the first-recruited motor unit divided by the number of other motor units that can be identified is called the recruitment ratio. Normally it is between three and five. Thus, if an indexed motor unit fires at a frequency of 16 Hz when four others can be identified, the recruitment ratio would be $16/4 = 4$. This measure is useful in the detection of early disease. When there is fallout of functioning motor units, as occurs in ALS, there are fewer units to achieve a given force-function. To compensate for this, the surviving motor units discharge at a higher frequency, but the interference at full force is reduced. This type of recruitment is referred to as reduced or incomplete recruitment or, more appropriately, discrete interference. The recruitment ratio is increased (>5) and values of between 15 and 20 are common in ALS (Eisen, 1994). For example, if an indexed MUAP had a discharge frequency of 22 Hz at a time when two other MUAPs could be identified (Fig. 5.3), the recruitment ratio would be $22/2 = 11$. This would suggest a mild loss of the number of functioning motor units. Recruitment ratios are also increased in association with acute reversible or chronic persistent conduction block without axonopathy, secondary to ischaemia and temporarily during recovery from local and general anaesthetics. Rapidly discharging motor units are also seen in upper motoneuron disorders. Therefore, in ALS, where there is combined

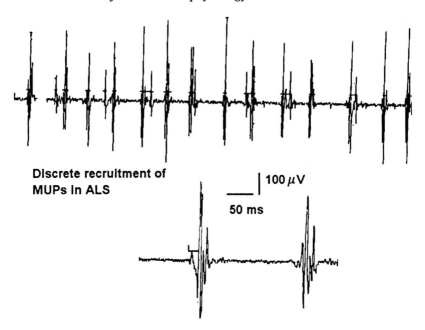

Figure 5.3. Discrete recruitment of motor units in ALS. The largest motor unit, which was the first to discharge, has a firing frequency of 22 Hz. The total sweep was 500 ms. Two other MUPs, a small one and a medium-sized one, were also discharging, giving a recruitment ratio of 22/2 = 11 (normal < 5). This suggests that there is a moderate loss of functioning motor units in the muscle motoneuron pool.

upper and lower motoneuron loss, increased motor unit firing frequency cannot be assumed to reflect loss of anterior horn cells.

None of the needle EMG abnormalities described above is specific for ALS, but in the context of the clinical picture, they are helpful in confirming a suspicion of the disorder and in assessing severity of the disease and a predictable rate of progression. EMG abnormalities are common in clinically unaffected limbs, and this can be used to confirm multisegmental disease. This is particularly helpful when the disease is of bulbar onset or when upper motoneuron features predominate and occur in the apparent absence of clinical lower motoneuron deficits. EMG abnormalities in different myotomes affecting two or more extremities strongly support the diagnosis of ALS. Muscle atrophy may not become obvious until > 30 per cent of the muscle's anterior horn cells have been lost (Wohlfart, 1957; McComas, 1987), and muscle strength may remain normal until more than 50 per cent of motor units are lost (McComas, 1987).

Certain abnormalities seen on needle EMG give a qualitative measure of disease progression. For example, a MUP with increased fibre density and increased 'jiggle' (instability) indicates there is ongoing re-innervation (see Fig. 5.2). It is at this stage of the disease that some therapeutic agents, such as neurotrophic factors, which may induce or encourage axonal sprouting, are most likely to be of benefit. However, motor units, which are enlarged through terminal nerve, or collateral sprouting in the course of re-innervation, may not always generate much force. This can be revealed by comparing the macro motor unit potential (macro-MUP) – the compound action potential derived from all the muscle fibres belonging to one motor unit (Stålberg, 1990) – with its twitch tension. Many large motor units generate low twitch tensions (Dengler *et al.*, 1990; Pouget *et al.*, 1994). Single fibre and macro-EMG abnormalities are more frequent in patients with prominent lower motoneuron findings, but most patients with predominant upper motoneuron findings will have increased fibre densities and instability of many motor units in clinically strong muscles (Stålberg, 1990).

Changes in the macro-EMG appear later than fibre density or jitter abnormalities (Stålberg and Sanders, 1984; Stålberg, 1986, 1990). The macro-EMG may be increased by a factor of 10 or more, indicating a good capacity for re-innervation. Slow disease progression is characterized by motor units with significantly increased fibre densities and relatively little jitter, and increased macro-EMG amplitudes. EMG recording of fibrillation potentials and/or positive sharp waves, which were not previously present, heralds a more rapidly progressive phase of the disease. Jitter in motor units becomes exaggerated while the increase in fibre density is less dramatic. The macro-EMG amplitude is normal or only slightly increased once the disease is in its terminal phases (Stålberg and Sanders, 1984). It may eventually become smaller than normal at a stage when the MUP is no longer capable of sending out sprouts to denervated muscle fibres.

Fasciculation in ALS

Fasciculations reflect the spontaneous, intermittent activation of some or all of the muscle fibres innervated through a single motor unit. They are seen clinically or recorded electrically in many diseases that involve the lower motoneuron. However, under these circumstances, fasciculations are seldom as diffuse or so prominent a feature as occurs in ALS (Lambert, 1969; Hjorth, Walsh and Willison, 1973; Eisen, 1995). Clinical and/or electrical fasciculation is considered essential for the diagnosis of ALS, and is often an early sign of disease. In most cases, both the patient and the physician note the fasciculation. As discussed in Chapter 2, fasciculations may pre-date other neurological deficits by many weeks or months. Fasciculations are readily recorded using surface electrodes (Howard and Murray, 1992). This type of recording should be employed before concluding that fasciculations are absent. Surface recording of fasciculation is facilitated by using a high gain (50–100 μV) and a narrow bandpass (500 Hz–5 kHz). The quantity and distribution of fasciculations seem to have little prognostic value. However, late in the disease, fasciculations are often less frequent. This is usually interpreted as indicating that there are too few remaining anterior horn cells that are capable of generating this activity, and presumes that fasciculations arise at or distal to the cell soma (Conradi, Grimby and Lundemo, 1982; Roth, 1984; Layzer, 1994). In a single experiment, Forster and Alpers (1946) cut the femoral nerve trunk in a patient with ALS. Within a few days the fasciculations evident in the quadriceps muscle became quiescent. This observation suggests that axonal death rather than sprouting may be relevant in the generation of fasciculations. Below is presented evidence to suggest that some fasciculations in ALS are generated proximal to the anterior horn cell.

There is a general perception that fasciculations associated with ALS cannot be differentiated from 'benign' fasciculations or those seen as part of the fasciculation–cramp syndrome (Trojaborg and Buchthal, 1965; Layzer, 1982). It is true that different types of fasciculation cannot be distinguished by their firing frequency; however, needle electrode recordings of fasciculations in ALS do, in our experience, have some characteristic features. They are often complex, with many fibre components which are unstable inducing increased jitter (Fig. 5.4). This type of potential clearly indicates a pathological process. When these large, complex fasciculations discharge, they often induce joint displacement, especially in muscles acting at wrist and finger joints (McComas, 1987).

Because fasciculations are so much a part of ALS, understanding their origin might give clues to some of the pathogenic mechanisms involved. The prevailing view is that fasciculations in ALS are generated anywhere between the anterior horn cell and the distal axon terminal. Using collision techniques, previous studies have clearly shown that some fasciculations in ALS arise in the distal axon or even the nerve terminals (Conradi *et al.*, 1982; Roth, 1984; Guiloff and Modarres-Sadeghi, 1992; Layzer, 1994). However, there is recent evidence suggesting that other

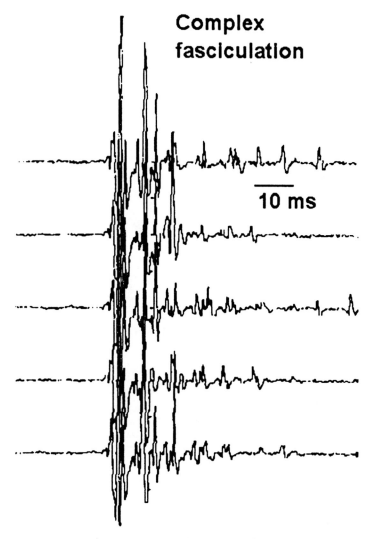

Figure 5.4. Complex fasciculation in ALS. This fasciculation, which was recorded from the quadriceps muscle, is very complex. Up to nine components can be recognized in some traces in this raster recording. Careful examination of it shows that some components drop out in some traces.

fasciculations in ALS are generated supraspinally (Kaji *et al.*, 1997). The evidence to support a supraspinal origin is:

1. Several subcomponents of a fasciculation may be seen consistently to 'drop out' when the same fasciculation potential is

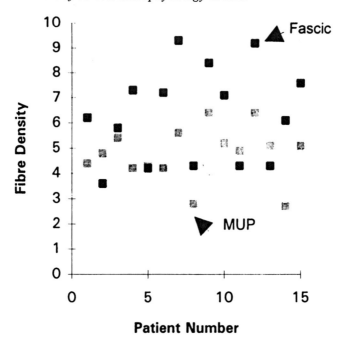

Figure 5.5. Comparison of fibre density of fasciculations and MUPs recorded at the same needle site in 15 patients with ALS. In each patient the fibre density of five motor unit potentials was measured. A small, light square represents the mean value. For the same 15 patients, fibre density of four to five fasciculation potentials was measured. The mean for each patient is represented by a larger black square. In each patient, both the motor unit potentials and the fasciculation potentials were recorded at the same needle site.

recorded sequentially. Careful analysis shows that the same subcomponents at other times can be recorded in isolation. This suggests that the fasciculation consists of two or more MUPs which at times discharge synchronously but which at other times discharge independently (Fig. 5.5).

2. Some of the subcomponents of complex fasciculations can be recorded during voluntary contraction, but voluntary contraction is never able to recruit MUPs that mirror a whole complex fasciculation, as might be the case if a synchronous, voluntary activation of MUPs had occurred. In fact, synchronous firing of voluntary activated MUPs does occur, but only rarely, and mostly in the intercostal and hand muscles (Datta, Farmer and Stephens, 1991).

3. Single-unit H-reflexes can be readily recorded with a single fibre needle electrode and they represent the discharge of a single anterior horn cell. In ALS, only 'simple' H-reflexes can be evoked at the same needle site as complex fasciculations can be recorded (Kaji, 1997).

4. The fibre density of fasciculations recorded at the same needle site as voluntary activated motor units is significantly different (Pant, Eisen and Stewart, 1992). The mean fibre density of 40 fasciculation potentials (pooled data recorded from different muscles in 15 patients) was 6.31 ± 4.2, which compared to a mean fibre density of 4.76 ± 2.9 for 60 voluntarily recruited motor units recorded at the same needle site as the fasciculation potentials. This difference is highly significant ($p < 0.001$) (Fig. 5.6). Thus, complex fasciculations can be recorded even when voluntary recruited motor units, recorded from the same muscle, at the same needle site, are of simpler morphology.

5. Transcranial magnetic stimulation can elicit the very same complex fasciculations that are spontaneously recorded (Fig. 5.7).

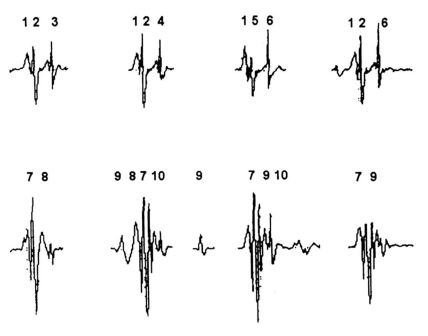

Figure 5.6. Fasciculations in ALS may reflect activity of two or more motor units.

Spontaneously discharging fasciculations

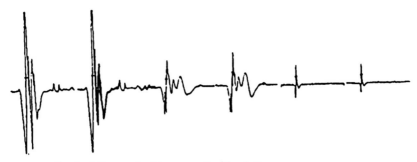

Fasciculation evoked by magnetic stimulation

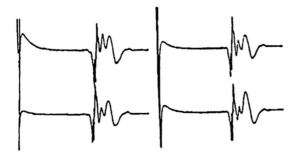

Figure 5.7. Spontaneous fasciculation also evoked by transcranial magnetic stimulation. Three different spontaneously occurring fasciculation potentials can be recognized in the top trace. In the lower two traces, the middle potential seen in the top trace was also evoked by transcranial magnetic stimulation of the motor cortex.

Taken together, the above observations, which have not been described in diseases other than ALS, suggest that in this disorder at least some fasciculations are of multi-unit origin, reflecting the synchronous discharge of two or more MUPs. The synchrony could occur at a spinal level or within the motor cortex as a result of the spontaneous firing of a parent corticomotoneuron. It is interesting that, over 30 years ago, Norris (1965) recorded fasciculations from muscles innervated by adjacent but different myotomes that discharged almost synchronously. Maybe some fasciculations in ALS are micro (single corticomotoneuronal) seizures. Certainly, as described below, there is abundant evidence pointing to a hyperexcitable motor cortex in ALS. Also, both lamotrigine and riluzole can dramatically reduce fasciculations. Both drugs have anticonvulsant properties (Eisen *et al.*, 1996).

Repetitive (or double) discharges of the same MUP are very common in ALS (Fig. 5.8). Repeat firing of the same motor unit may also reflect hyperexcitability of the anterior horn cell membrane and, as such, could be a fasciculation-related phenomenon. Repetitive discharges occur in several disorders but they are particularly frequent in ALS. They are rarely, if ever, recorded in progressive spinal muscular atrophies. The generator(s) of repetitively discharging MUPs is unknown. The interval between the first and second firing is variable but short, which suggests that they must originate at, or near, the cell soma. The increased frequency of double or repetitive discharges in ALS may be due to hyperexcitability of the cell membrane, possibly resulting from excess glutamatergic stimulation.

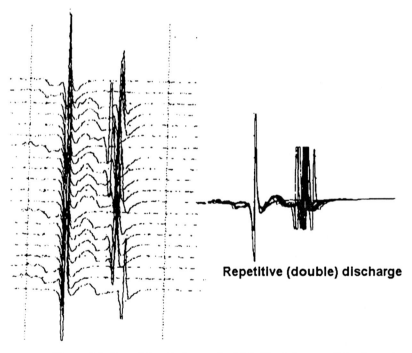

Repetitive (double) discharge

Figure 5.8. Repetitive discharges in ALS. The left part of the figure is a raster recording of a tibialis anterior motor unit. In most of the traces the same unit fires a second time. There is a variable interval between the first and second firing in sequential traces and this is seen as considerable jitter in the right part of the figure, which is a superimposition of the raster traces.

Examination of specific muscles in ALS

Needle EMG of specific muscles can have particular relevance for ALS because the anatomical distribution of involvement may allow one to conclude with greater confidence that the patient has ALS. Careful choice of the muscles for study limits the extent of discomfort to the patient. For example, abnormalities of the paraspinal muscles indicate that the lesion is at least as proximal as the ventral root. Unfortunately, needle EMG abnormalities of cervical and lumbar paraspinal muscles may be misleading since they may simply reflect changes associated with degenerative disc disease which commonly occurs in the age range of patients with ALS. Fibrillations can be recorded from the lumbosacral paraspinal muscles in about 15 per cent of asymptomatic, elderly subjects (Date *et al.*, 1996), but rarely to the extent that occurs in ALS. However, the thoracic spine is rarely subject to disc degeneration, and paraspinal muscles are easily examined in this region. Alternatively, the upper part of the rectus abdominus muscle can be examined. It is innervated through T8–T12 roots and is readily accessible.

Needle examination of the tongue and other bulbar muscles such as the masseter, facial muscles or sternomastoid, is particularly valuable when the clinical examination of these muscles appears to be normal. The tongue is most comfortably and efficiently needled from under the chin, introducing the needle electrode into the genioglossus muscle. The discharge rate of facial and tongue muscle MUPs is faster than that of limb muscles, and the increased firing frequency of the MUPs in them must be cautiously interpreted. However, other EMG abnormalities, including spontaneous activity, fasciculations and complex unstable MUPs, are all good indicators that the tongue is involved in the disease process. EMG abnormalities, especially the presence of fibrillation or positive sharp waves recorded in the chest wall muscles (intercostals) and the diaphragm, have important therapeutic and prognostic implications. As discussed in Chapter 7, timely institution of BIPAP greatly adds to patient's comfort and can significantly prolong life. Although a falling forced vital capacity (FVC) is a more conventional means of deciding when to implement BIPAP, this measure may be erroneously reduced when facial muscle weakness makes it difficult for the patient to form a tight seal around the spirometer tube. Serial oxygen saturation measurements usually remain normal until respiratory failure is imminent, so that they are a poor indicator of respiratory reserve in ALS.

The commonly held belief that needle EMG of the diaphragm is difficult and dangerous because of a potential risk of puncturing the lung, spleen, liver or other organs is unjustified (Bolton *et al.*, 1992). We routinely perform diaphragmatic EMG on most patients with ALS, and to

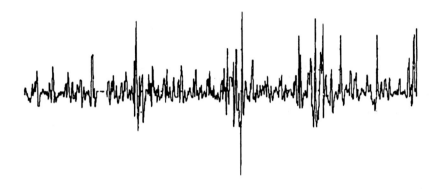

Needle EMG - Diaphragm
ALS

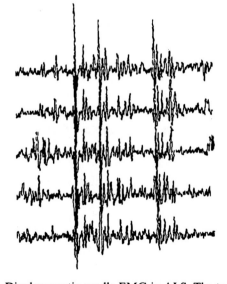

Figure 5.9. Diaphragmatic needle EMG in ALS. The top trace shows a few complex MUPs (the larger potentials) recorded during inspiration. The other activity is a mixture of fibrillations and some positive sharp waves, indicating the diaphragm is denervated. The lower traces are a raster recording of a complex repetitive discharge that also indicates denervation.

date have not experienced any untoward effects. A monopolar needle-recording electrode is inserted through the 8th–9th interspace at the anterior axillary line. Cartilaginous formation typical of those with ALS, especially in older subjects, may preclude introduction of the needle at lower intercostal interspaces. However, even at the 8th interspace, there is approximately 1.5 cm between the pleural reflection and the lower costal cartilage into which the diaphragm inserts. The needle tip should be pointed downwards, parallel with the rib cage. Some subjects experience a brief, sharp, pleuritic pain as the needle enters the diaphragm. MUPs in the intercostal muscles are recruited during expiration and are generally of much higher amplitude than those recorded from the diaphragm, which are largely recruited during inspiration (Fig. 5.9). Fibrillation, fasciculation and complex motor units are easily recognized in both muscles, indicating that they are subject to denervation or re-innervation (Chen *et al.*, 1997).

Motor unit estimates

One of the major pathophysiological correlates of ALS is progressive fall-out of anterior horn cells, and it would be valuable to measure the number of motor units innervating a muscle or myotome and the rate of their decline over the course of the disease. This approach has been helpful in following the natural history of disease and may play a role in monitoring future therapeutic trials. However, motor unit counting has problems and all physiological motor unit counting methods give estimates only. The procedure has been hampered by the lack of a 'gold standard', for even anatomical methods make the assumption that 50 per cent of large axons are sensory, but the actual number of motor units in a muscle is not known (McComas, 1991, 1994; Doherty *et al.*, 1995; Slawnych, Laszlo and Hershler, 1996; Daube, 1997). For this reason, the methods are best referred to as motor unit numerical estimates (MUNEs). Four methods have been developed. Each has its own distinct difficulties but there is reasonable agreement between them as to the estimates of the number of motor units that have been made in several different muscles. Three of the methods use nerve stimulation and recording of the compound muscle action potential; the fourth relies on voluntary EMG. The underlying principle for all methods is the same. The MUNE is determined by dividing amplitude or area of the CMAP by the average amplitude or area of a single MUAP. An erroneously large CMAP, usually due to phase addition from distant signals, will inflate the MUNE, and an erroneously small CMAP, usually due to phase cancellation, will reduce the MUNE. Similarly, an erroneously large MUAP will underestimate the MUNE and an erroneously small MUAP will overestimate it (Bromberg, 1993; Bromberg and Abrams, 1995).

The incremental response technique, which was first described by McComas *et al.* (1971) more than 25 years ago, is the easiest to perform, and is now fully computerized. Motor unit estimates derived using the computerized technique are more reproducible than was the case using the original manual method. The method assumes that small increments in stimulus intensity evoke an additional 'all or none' response reflecting the recruitment of an additional unit (Fig. 5.10). Variations on this method

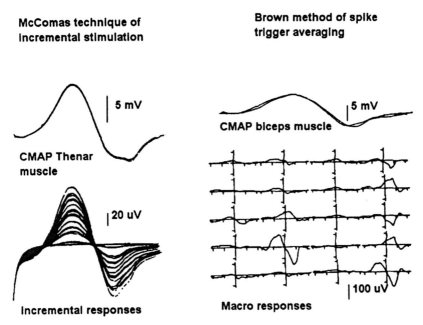

Figure 5.10. Motor unit counting. Two methods are shown. The left is the McComas method in which incremental stimulation (bottom traces) adds new 'all or nothing' components. The mean difference in these (about 25 µV) is divided into the maximum CMAP (about 12 mV), giving an estimate in this case of 480 units for the thenar muscle. On the right, the Brown method shows 20 macro responses obtained through spike trigger averaging (bottom traces). The mean macro amplitude is about 50 µV. This value is divided into the maximum CMAP, about 10 mV (top traces), giving a motor unit estimate for the biceps brachii of 200.

have included multiple point stimulation and stochastic activation (Doherty *et al.*, 1995; Wang and Delwaide, 1995; Slawnych *et al.*, 1996). It is questionable whether either adds much to the accuracy of the original method. The spike trigger averaging method developed by Brown and coworkers (Brown, Strong and Snow, 1988; W. F. Brown, 1994) involves voluntary activation of a single motor unit which is used to trigger a surface-recorded 'macro' potential of the same unit (Fig. 5.10). Window discriminators, which are available on most current EMG equipment, make it possible to record the macro potential triggered by different-sized motor units that are recruited during moderate voluntary muscle contraction. Both the incremental stimulation and spike-triggered averaging methods limit MUNE to the lower threshold, first-recruited motor units. Even though the spike-triggered averaging method is somewhat more complex than the incremental stimulation technique, we prefer it because it is more easily applied to proximal as well as to distal muscles. It also has the added advantage of being able simultaneously to record the complexity and stability of the activated MUAPs and the presence of fibrillations and positive sharp waves indicating denervation.

Even in the hands of those performing MUNEs regularly, the normal variation is large. For example, in the small hand muscles (thenar or hypothenar muscles), estimates range from 150 to over 350. Some of the variation is due to a true interindividual biological variation (McComas, 1994). However, the variation is much greater amongst different methods, and it is probably inappropriate to compare the results obtained from different methods. A given method, once mastered, has acceptable reproducibility and can be used to study the loss of motor units in ALS in a longitudinal manner. Motor unit estimates indicate that with normal ageing there is only a modest attrition of anterior horn cells up to about 60 years of age (Brown *et al.*, 1988; Dantes and McComas, 1991). In ALS, a significant reduction in the MUNE can be detected in clinically strong muscles, which becomes much more marked as the muscle weakens. This is one clue indicating the disease begins at some period before becoming clinically overt. As many as 80 per cent of functioning motor units in a muscle motoneuron pool can be lost without apparent clinical weakness (McComas, 1994; W. F. Brown, 1994). Once affected, approximately half the neurons in the motoneuron pool cease to function within six months, with a further 50 per cent becoming non-functional in the subsequent six-months (Dantes and McComas, 1991).

The upper motoneuron and use of magnetic stimulation in ALS

The corticomotoneuronal system

In mammals, several descending tracts converge on the spinal moto-neuron (SMN); their connections are largely polysynaptic. However, in humans, and to some extent in non-human primates, these tracts have been largely sacrificed at the expense of a greatly expanded corticomoto-neuronal system. This system originates from pyramidal cells in the primary motor cortex and is the only descending motor pathway making monosynaptic connections with the SMNs (Porter and Lemon, 1993). Glutamate is probably the sole excitatory transmitter subserving the corticomotoneuronal system (Shaw, 1993). The corticomotoneuronal system is the substrate for the diversity of human fractionated movements. These are almost unique to humans and are most evident for forearm and hand movements. They have resulted in our ability to perform an infinite variety of complex motor skills (Phillips, 1975; Palmer and Fetz, 1985; Humphrey, 1986). Using transcranial magnetic stimulation (TMS), it has been demonstrated that the amplitude of the MEP recorded from the first dorsal interosseus muscle is task dependent and that the amplitude is larger when the muscle is involved in more complex movements (Datta *et al.*, 1991; Flament *et al.*, 1993; Lemon, 1993). Fractionation of movement is evident in a wide selection of human motor skills including vocalization, which necessitates the combined activity of facial, laryngeal, chest wall and abdominal musculature. It seems that often the pattern of muscle involvement in ALS follows that which would be used in a fractionated movement. Each SMN receives input from many corticomotoneuronal cells, which form a cortical core facilitating a single SMN. Also, each corticomotoneuronal cell synapses with several to many anterior horn cells within a given muscle motoneuron pool as well as those of synergistic motoneuron pools (Jankowska, Patel and Tanaka, 1975; Edgley *et al.*, 1990; Palmer and Ashby, 1992a; Porter and Lemon, 1993; Eisen and Krieger, 1993). This arrangement would predict that, under some circum-stances, motor units are capable of synchronous activity, which has been shown to be true using cross-correlation analysis of multi-unit EMG in awake humans in hand and forearm muscles (Datta *et al.*, 1991; Bremnar, Baker and Stephens, 1991). As discussed above, this may be the basis of some of the complex fasciculations seen in ALS.

Disease of the corticomotoneuronal system is a major element of neuronal dysfunction in ALS, resulting in considerable clinical deficit. It has become possible to study the corticomotoneuronal system and the upper motoneuron physiologically by using TMS, and the remainder of this chapter is devoted to this particular topic. The remarkable discovery by Merton and Morton (1980) made it possible to stimulate the awake and intact human motor cortex. Initial experiments were performed using high-voltage, short-duration electrical stimuli applied to the scalp over-lying the motor cortex. This was tolerable but quite uncomfortable and not appropriate for routine clinical use. Electrical cortical stimulation excites the descending motor axons postsynaptically. It has been largely superseded by TMS, which activates the corticomotoneuronal system presynaptically through the apical dendrites of the corticomotoneurons. The local circuit cortical inhibitory interneurons are also activated. The current density induced by the magnetic coil is insufficient to directly excite descending motor tracts within the spinal cord. A rapidly changing magnetic field is generated which induces electric currents within the cortex (Eisen, 1992; Murray, 1993). Short-latency contractions are evoked in contralateral muscles, in keeping with a single synaptic connection (Barker *et al.*, 1985; Hess, Mills and Murray, 1987; Mills and Kohara, 1997). TMS is virtually free of discomfort. It also appears safe in both the short and long term (Barker *et al.*, 1985; Hess *et al.*, 1987; Day *et al.*, 1989; Eisen, 1992; Murray, 1993). Over the last decade, many thousands of individuals throughout the world have been subjected to TMS without adverse effects (Beric, 1993).

The corticomotoneuronal hypothesis of ALS

Anatomical and physiological studies in humans indicate that the corti-comotoneuronal system synapses with the motoneuron pools of all SMNs except those innervating the external ocular muscles and Onuf's nucleus, whose cell bodies supply innervation to the bladder wall (Gandevia and Rothwell, 1980; Gandevia and Plassman, 1988; Colebatch *et al.*, 1990; Iwatsubo *et al.*, 1990). These motor nuclei are almost invariably spared in ALS. This, and the absence of an animal model that truly mimics human ALS, led to the 'corticomotoneuronal hypothesis' of ALS. This hypo-thesis postulates that the disorder is primarily one of the corticomoto-neuron or its presynaptic terminal and secondarily affects lower motor and possibly other neurons (Eisen *et al.*, 1992, 1995). The idea that ALS might originate in the motor cortex was originally proposed by Charcot (Charcot, 1865; Charcot and Joffroy, 1869). There are arguments against the corticomotoneuronal hypothesis that postulate that the disease com-mences in the SMNs and spreads retrogradely to the upper motoneurons

(Chou and Norris, 1993). It is also possible that both the upper and lower motoneurons become involved independently of each other. For example, one hallmark of ALS is the accumulation of axonal spheroids in the lower motoneuron and conglomerates in the upper motoneurons. Chou *et al.* (1996) have performed experiments to suggest that these neurofilamentous accumulations result from the co-localization of peroxynitrite and superoxide which affect neurofilament assembly. These findings would support the idea that both cells are subjected to a common insult independently of each other. Kiernan and Hudson (1991) and, more recently, Pamphlett *et al.* (1995) studied the pathological correlates of upper and lower motoneuron demise and also concluded that both cells die independently of each other. However, autopsy material reflects end-stage disease and cannot be easily used to determine accurately the earliest structures that are involved in ALS (Eisen, 1995). Recently applied in-vivo techniques, including MRI (Cheung *et al.*, 1995), magnetic resonance spectroscopy (Pioro *et al.*, 1994), PET (Kew *et al.*, 1993), and neurophysiological studies involving corticospinal excitation of single motoneurons using TMS (Awiszus and Feistner, 1993, 1995; Mills, 1995; Eisen *et al.*, 1996, 1997; Nakajima *et al.*, 1996; Enterzari-Taher *et al.*, 1997; Mills and Kohara, 1997), have been used to study the corticomotoneuronal system in ALS. Each has lent support to the corticomotoneuronal hypothesis. It is also possible that inhibitory control of the corticomotoneuron, which is subject to modulation by several different classes of cortical interneurons, is impaired in ALS, and the following describes how it is possible to investigate this possibility.

Distinct types of inhibitory interneurons have been identified by their immunohistochemical reactivity to the calcium-binding proteins calbindin (CB), parvalbumin (PV) and calretinin (CR) (Celio, 1990; Baimbridge, Celio and Rogers, 1992; Conde *et al.*, 1994). The axon terminals of interneurons form symmetric inhibitory synapses on the dendritic shafts, somata and/or proximal axonal segment of the pyramidal neuron (corticomotoneuron) (Conde *et al.*, 1994). Those terminating exclusively on the corticomotoneuronal cell soma are called wide arbor neurons and they react for PV. They may be responsible for synchronizing events of the cell. Those which terminate on the apical dendrite are referred to as doublebouquet neurons, and they demonstrate immunoreactivity to CR and less frequently to CB. These interneurons modulate the response of pyramidal neurons to excitatory inputs. Neurons terminating on the initial axonal segment of the pyramidal cell are called chandelier neurons, and they immunoreact for PV and influence the probability of the cell firing

(DeFelipe and Jones, 1992; Conde *et al.*, 1994). These anatomical observations raise the possibility that ALS might be characterized by abnormal excitatory or inhibitory modulation of descending cortical volleys. Physiological studies that support this concept are described below.

Other arguments raised against the corticomotneuronal hypothesis included the problem of the PMA form of ALS and why motor stroke does not also cause lower motoneuron loss. As described in Chapter 2, most adult-onset PMA is hereditary and the responsible gene has been identified. It has nothing to do with ALS. Sporadic ALS beginning with lower motoneuron findings is common, but >85 per cent of patients develop upper motoneuron findings in a few weeks or months and if the lower motoneuron loss is severe, upper motoneuron findings may be difficult to detect. Some cases of lower motoneuron disease mimicking ALS turn out to have motor neuropathy with conduction block or hexosaminidase-β deficiency. The corticomotoneuronal hypothesis depends on intact, but not necessarily normal, corticomotoneurons that are excited by excess glutamate and/or similarly excite the anterior horn cell. This would not be possible in an acutely destructive process such as a stroke!

Central motor conduction in ALS

Early studies in patients with ALS employed electrical cortical stimulation (Hugon *et al.*, 1987). In many patients there was marked attenuation or absence of the MEP. Less frequently, the response was delayed in latency and there was modest prolongation of central motor conduction time – the time for the fastest conducting impulses to travel from the motor cortex to the cervical, or lumbar, spinal cord. The upper limits for these conduction times are 9 ms and 18.5 ms respectively. Abnormalities of central conduction were more frequent when MEPs were recorded from lower limb muscles (Ingram and Swash, 1987). Schriefer *et al.* (1989) studied 22 patients with ALS using TMS. The target muscle used was the hypothenar. There was a modest correlation between the extent of prolongation of central motor conduction time and hyper-reflexia of the limb, including brisk finger flexion, but not between central motor conduction time and impairments of fine finger movements or hypothenar muscle weakness. In some patients, abnormal MEPs were recorded even though there was no clinical abnormality of the limb under study. Subsequently, Eisen *et al.* (1990) performed TMS on 40 patients with ALS recording from the

Table 5.3. *Physiological evidence for hyperexcitability of the motor cortex in ALS*

Nature of fasciculations in ALS
Double (repetitive) discharges
Lowered cortical threshold to transcranial magnetic stimulation
Shortened cortical silent period
Failure of inhibition to paired stimulation
    Whole muscle recording
    Single unit recording

thenar, extensor digitorum communis and biceps muscles. In 12 patients with severe bulbar palsy and generalized hyper-reflexia, responses could not be elicited. In others, the main abnormality was a marked reduction in the MEP amplitude and MEP/CMAP ratio. This ratio is important because it takes into account any amplitude reduction of the MEP that may be due to lower motoneuron involvement. The latency to all three muscles was significantly prolonged, but only to a modest degree, as was central motor conduction time. More recent studies have shown that central conduction is generally either normal or modestly prolonged in ALS. This is not too surprising considering the disease results in axonal degeneration. There is one interesting exception; that is, the recently described Asp90Ala–SOD1 recessively inherited mutation, apparently restricted to patients whose origin is Finnish or Swedish. It is associated with a very slow central motor conduction time (Andersen *et al.*, 1996).

Excitability of the motor cortex in ALS

As is indicated in Table 5.3, a number of physiological observations have been made in ALS suggesting the motor cortex or its surrounds are hyperexcitable.

Cortical threshold, which is defined as the stimulus intensity required to evoke a motor response of $> 50 \mu V$ in three out of five trials (Hufnagel *et al.*, 1990), is a good measure of excitability of the underlying motor cortex. Normal values measure about 55 per cent with a $< \pm 5$ per cent side to side variation. The absolute value depends on the type of magnetic stimulator and coil that is used (Eisen *et al.*, 1992, 1993) and also on the patient's age. In infants, threshold is very high and frequently it is not possible to evoke a motor response by TMS before the age of 3–4 years. Normal threshold is not attained until about age 8 years or older (Eyre,

Miller and Ramesh, 1991). Even though cortical threshold is high, adult values for central motor conduction velocity are reached by age 4–5 years. This discrepancy implies that myelination of central motor tracts precedes maturation of synaptogenesis. The extent and age at which synaptogenesis nears completion account for the considerable variability in the acquisition of motor skills in humans.

Many patients with ALS have a normal or even surprisingly low cortical threshold (Caramia *et al.*, 1991; Eisen *et al.*, 1993a; Desiato and Caramia, 1997). Intuitively, this is an unexpected finding in a disease which is characterized by a loss of corticomotoneurons and axons. The explanation for this observation is not clear, but it is tempting to relate it to excessive stimulation by EAAs (see Chapter 4). Dysfunction of cortical inhibitory interneurons may also be important. Longitudinal studies suggest that the lowest cortical thresholds occur early in the course of ALS and that the thresholds increase with disease progression (Fig. 5.11). Eventually, threshold may become so high that it is no longer possible to elicit a MEP. Another measure of cortical excitability is the duration of the cortical silent period which characteristically follows a magnetic stimulus applied to the motor cortex during the voluntary activation of a target muscle. When recorded from hand muscles, the cortical silent period lasts about 120 ms (Fig. 5.12). The first 50 ms of this is due to peripheral inhibitory mechanisms, but supraspinal inhibitory mechanisms are responsible for the major part of the cortical silent period (Holmgren *et al.*, 1990; Cantello *et al.*, 1990; Fahr, Agostino and Hallett, 1991; Triggs *et al.*, 1992; Prout and Eisen, 1994). Thus far, studies measuring the cortical silent period in ALS have been limited and the results contradictory (Uozumi, Tsuji and Murai, 1991; Haug *et al.*, 1992; Prout and Eisen, 1994). The duration of the cortical silent period is dependent on the stimulus intensity and will lengthen with increasing stimulus intensity. The diversity of results reported may reflect different stimulus intensities that have been used. In normal subjects, the duration of the silent period increases by approximately 100 ms between perithreshold stimulation (the lowest stimulus able to elicit a clearly recognized cessation in the EMG activity) and maximum stimulation (the intensity at which there is no further change in the duration of the silent period). The same observation holds true for patients with ALS. Compared to age-matched controls, the cortical silent period is shortened in ALS (Uozumi *et al.*, 1991; Haug *et al.*, 1992; Prout and Eisen, 1994; Desiato and Caramia, 1997). The shortening, may be due to disordered cortical inhibitory interneurons (see below), excessive stimulation by EAAs, or to both mechanisms.

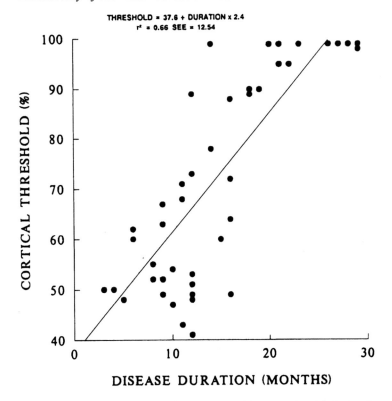

Figure 5.11. Cortical threshold to transcranial magnetic stimulation in ALS. There is a linear correlation between cortical threshold and disease duration ($r^2 = 0.66$). During the first year of disease, about half of the patients had a threshold to stimulation $\leqslant 55$ per cent. This increased with time and after about 18 months threshold in many was > 80 per cent. A threshold $= 100$ per cent means there was no response to maximum output of the stimulator. (From Eisen *et al.*, 1993a. Reproduced with permission.)

When transcranial double stimulation is applied to the normal motor cortex, so that the conditioning stimulus is subthreshold and the conditioning–test interval is very short (1–4 ms), there is marked attenuation of the test response. The suppression is due to local circuit cortical inhibitory mechanisms because responses to electrical brain stimulation, which stimulates postsynaptic structures, do not cause the same attenuation. Also the H-reflex is not attenuated. The same results were found in patients with spinal muscular atrophy (Yokota, Yoshino and Saito, 1996). However, in ALS the normal inhibition induced by a subthreshold conditioning stimulus is very much reduced. This, then, is another line of

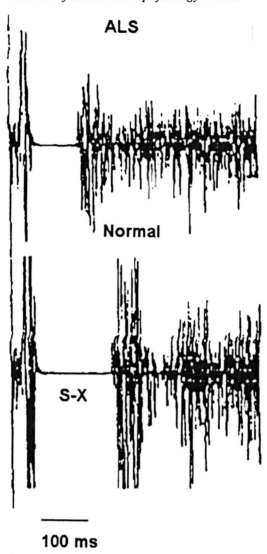

Figure 5.12. Cortical silent period. (See text.)

evidence pointing to a hyperexcitable motor cortex in ALS. Other recent
in-vivo studies using PET and functional MRI have also shown that the
motor cortex and its surrounds in ALS are overactivated. This presumably is due to loss of inhibitory mechanisms (Kew *et al.*, 1993; Abrahams
et al., 1996).

Table 5.4. *Conclusions derived from single unit studies using transcranial magnetic stimulation*

Age-dependent decline in the size of the EPSP
The size of the EPSP in ALS is frequently reduced
Normal or large EPSPs in ALS have an increased rise time
In ALS there is a dissociation between the cortical EPSP and the Ia afferent EPSP
Normally there is an inverse correlation between the macro-MUP and the size of the EPSP
In ALS there is no relation betwen the macro-MUP and the size of the cortical EPSP
A conditioning stimulus normally inhibits a test EPSP; this is modified in ALS

EPSP, excitatory postsynaptic potential; macro-MUP, macro-motor unit potential.

Single unit recordings in humans using TMS

If a motor unit is voluntarily recruited and at the same time random transcortical stimuli are applied to the motor cortex, the firing probability of the motor unit changes dramatically. This methodology has enabled inferences to be made about the physiology of single corticomotoneurons (Boniface, Mills and Schubert, 1991; Schubert and Mills, 1994; Awiszus and Feistner, 1993, 1995; Bawa and Lemon, 1993; Mills, 1995; Mills and Kohara 1997; Eisen *et al.*, 1997; Enterzari-Taher *et al.*, 1997; Nakajima *et al.*, 1997). Peristimulus time histograms (PSTHs) can be constructed that display changes in the firing of a single motor unit as a result of an intervening TMS (Fig. 5.13). Following a cortical stimulus, there may be two periods of excitation. The first has a short latency, occurring as early as 20 ms after the stimulus. This latency is in keeping with a fast-conducting, monosynaptic event. A later, much smaller and less consistent, period of excitation occurs at about 65 ms after the stimulus; its origin and significance are not clear (Boniface *et al.*, 1991; Bawa and Lemon, 1993). A later period of excitation is not seen in Figure 5.13.

PSTHs have shown abnormalities in ALS that suggest there is a supraspinal defect which is presynaptic to the SMN, possibly as rostral as the corticomotoneuron itself (Mills, 1995; Kohara *et al.*, 1996; Eisen *et al.*, 1996; Enterzari-Taher *et al.*, 1997; Nakajima *et al.*, 1997; Mills and Kohara, 1997; Eisen *et al.*, 1997). Using PSTHs, recent studies have led us

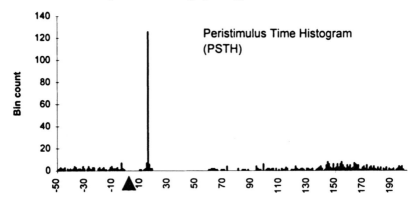

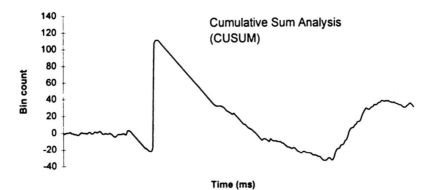

Figure 5.13. Normal PSTH describing how the firing of a single motor unit is altered by transcranial magnetic stimulation. *Top.* The x-axis represents time from − 50 ms to 200 ms. The total time has been divided into 250 × 1-ms bins. The magnetic stimuli are given at time 0 (arrow). The y-axis is the bin count and represents the number of times that the indexed motor unit fell into a particular bin. Prior to any stimulation (− 50 to 0 ms) the bin count is between 1 and 2. About 20 ms after the stimulation there is a large rise in the bin count, about 130 in the example shown. Immediately thereafter there is a period of absolute inhibition, with variable duration, but in this case it lasted about 30 ms. The prestimulus firing of the indexed unit is then resumed. *Bottom.* Cumulative sum analysis: this is another way of describing the same phenomenon as the top part of the figure. A downward deflection means inhibition and an upward deflection means excitation. Just before the large upward deflection there is a small negativity that is due to removal of the stimulus artifact. The second, much longer, negativity lasting about 70 ms is a true absolute and then relative physiological inhibition.

to several conclusions (Table 5.4; Eisen *et al.*, 1997). The findings, taken together, support the corticomotoneuronal hypothesis.

The essentials of the methodology involved in measuring the cortico-motoneuronal excitatory postsynaptic potentials (EPSPs) using PSTHs follow in some detail as some readers may wish to explore this rather elegant technology for themselves. Some background anatomy and physiology are necessary to better understand the methodology. A number of individual corticomotoneurons converge onto a single SMN; the actual number of corticomotoneurons varies with the muscle studied. The EPSP produced by the descending corticomotoneuronal volley represents a summation of all of the EPSPs of individual corticomoto-neurons converging onto a single SMN. The magnitude or amplitude of the EPSP reflects the number of corticomotoneurons that facilitate a given SMN (Fetz and Cheney, 1980; Ashby and Zilm, 1982a, 1982b; Fetz and Gustafsson, 1983; Mao *et al.*, 1984; Brouwer and Ashby, 1990). In humans and higher non-human primates, corticomotoneuronal projec-tions are strongest to the motoneurons innervating the hand and forearm muscles (wrist extensors and flexors), indicating a greater size and number of cortical projections to these muscles (Fetz and Cheney, 1980; Palmer and Ashby, 1992b; Porter and Lemon, 1993). These muscles have been used for most clinical studies.

Methodology for constructing PSTHs and measuring the corticomotoneuronal EPSP

Recordings are made using a disposable concentric needle electrode (Dantec 13R01, recording surface area = 0.07 mm^2). The bandpass is restricted (500 Hz to 10 kHz). An indexed motor unit is identified with a peak-to-peak amplitude > 500 μV and a rise time of < 50 μs. The subject should undergo a brief training period, learning to recruit a motor unit in isolation at a frequency of about 12 Hz. Constantly available audio-visual feedback is very helpful for this. A window discriminator is employed to help reduce contamination by other motor units that are usually recruited at the same time. In our experiments, a Dantec Magpro II is used to generate a brief, rapidly changing magnetic field to deliver stimuli to the contralateral motor cortex through a large, cup-shaped, round coil (MMC140) fixed over the head using a stand. The inducing current flows clockwise as viewed from above. The site of lowest stimulus intensity (threshold) capable of inducing a visible muscle contraction of the extensor digitorum communis (EDC) or the first dorsal interosseus (FDI) is located. This is usually 2 cm anterior and lateral to the vertex (Eisen *et al.*, 1996). The stimulus intensity is then reduced by 5 per cent, which is readily tolerable and it is unusual for the subject to feel any muscle contraction. Randomly generated TMSs (150–200) are delivered at intervals of 3–5 s. Specific software was written to collect the data on line and construct both PSTHs and a cumulative sum (CUSUM) analysis (Ellaway, 1978). Data are gathered into 1-ms bins over a 250-ms period, which includes 50 ms before the stimulus and 200 ms after the stimulus (see Fig. 5.13). The total number of consecutive bins with counts exceeding the mean prestimulus background by more than 2 standard deviations is used to measure the magnitude and rise time of the EPSP. An increase in motor unit firing probability can be also identified as an upward deviation in the CUSUM (see Fig. 5.13). The amplitude of the EPSP is estimated from the formula below (Ashby and Zilm, 1982a, 1982b; Mao *et al.*, 1984; Brouwer and Ashby, 1990; Eisen *et al.*, 1996). The total number of bins in the early peak with counts exceeding the mean prestimulus background by more than 2 SD is used to measure the magnitude and rise time of the composite corticomotoneuronal EPSP arising in the indexed motoneuron. The magnitude of the EPSP underlying the increase of firing probability (increased bin counts) can be estimated, assuming that the rise of the motoneuronal membrane potential to threshold (membrane trajectory) is linear and is normalized for the number of stimuli and mean interspike interval (Ashby and Zilm, 1982a, 1982b):

$$\text{Bin counts} = \frac{\text{number of stimuli} \times \text{EPSP amplitude (units)}}{\text{mean interspike interval (ms)}}$$

We converted the arbitrary 'units' used by Ashby and Zilm (1982a, 1982b) into mV, assuming an actual depth of the motoneuronal membrane from the resting (-65 mV) to threshold (-55 mV), that is 10 mV (Kandel and Schwartz, 1991).

$$\text{EPSP amplitude (mV)} = \frac{\text{bin counts} \times \text{mean interspike interval (ms)}}{\text{number of stimuli}} \times 10^{-1}$$

Normative data, age-related changes and abnormalities in ALS

Our initial studies were concerned with normative, age-related data and changes in the size of the EPSP, or primary peak after magnetic stimulation in patients with ALS (Fig. 5.13; Eisen *et al.*, 1996). Age was significantly correlated with the EPSP amplitude (Fig. 5.14, top). In patients with ALS, the mean EPSP amplitude was significantly reduced. Figure 5.14 (bottom), shows individual EPSP values for 84 ALS patients as a function of age. In most patients, the EPSP is small, and in about 10 per cent it could not be calculated because there was never a bin count that exceeded the prestimulus background + 2 SD. About 15 per cent of ALS

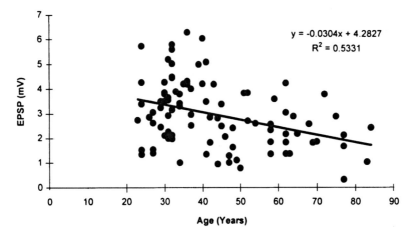

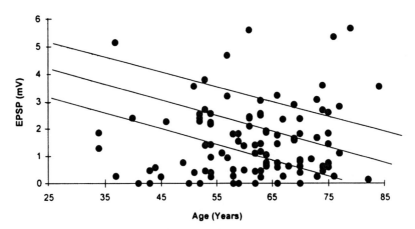

Figure 5.14. *Top.* Effects of age on the size of the EPSP. There is a positive linear correlation between age and EPSP magnitude ($r^2 = 0.533$, $n = 81$). The amplitude of the EPSP is a reflection of the number of corticomotoneurons innervating a single spinal motoneuron and the implication is that this number is reduced as one gets older. *Bottom.* EPSP values in 84 patients with ALS. Most of the EPSPs are of reduced amplitude but about one-third are normal and some (about 18 per cent) are larger than would have been predicted. See text for explanation.

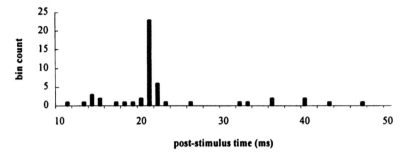

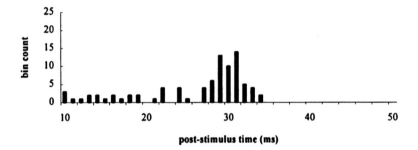

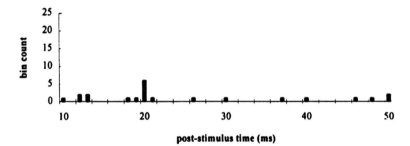

Figure 5.15. PSTH studies in ALS. Three examples are shown. *Top.* The EPSP is larger than predicted for age. There is a long rise time to the EPSP (6 bins are included). This is probably the result of dispersion in the descending corticomotoneuronal volley. *Middle.* The EPSP is much reduced in size, which is typical of ALS and reflects a loss of corticomotoneurons. *Bottom.* A primary peak could not be distinguished from the background, making it impossible to calculate an EPSP size.

patients have EPSPs that are larger than anticipated for their age, as is exemplified in Fig. 5.15 (top) in a 74-year-old man who had an EPSP of 3.59 mV. The predicted value would be 1.7 mV. Little is known about the extent and topography of the cerebral cortex that are subject to age-related neuronal attrition. In particular, there are no specific data regarding loss of human corticomotoneurons with ageing. Pathological studies do suggest an age-dependent reduction of pyramidal cells (but not specifically corticomotoneurons) ranging from 15 per cent to 40 per cent (Devaney and Johnson, 1980; Henderson, Tomlinson and Gibson, 1980; Mann, 1994). However, other studies conclude there is shrinkage of the perikaryon and dendritic arbor but little, if any, loss of cells (Terry, De Teresa and Hansen, 1987). Our data suggest that by 55 years of age, which is around the average age of onset of ALS, there is a substantial reduction in the EPSP. We believe that the size of the EPSP reflects the size of the corticomotoneuronal core converging on a single SMN. Corticomotoneuronal attrition probably subjects surviving neurons to greater metabolic demands and they become more susceptible to oxidative, excitotoxic or other stresses of the ageing neuron. Corticomotoneurons are amongst the largest neurons in the body, so they may be particularly susceptible to metabolic stress as they age and this may account for selective vulnerability of the corticomotoneuronal system in ALS. Additional loss of each neuron adds further stress to surviving ones. We are not suggesting that ALS is simply a disease of the ageing corticomotoneuron, although this concept was hypothesized many years ago in relation to the anterior horn cell by McComas (1977). More likely is that it is the product of age-related neuronal stress, the interplay of susceptibility genes, and environmental factors.

Methodological issues and interpretation of results in ALS

Although the PSTH paradigm is an elegant physiological means by which to study the descending motor cortical volley, there are several methodological concerns and assumptions that are made. These include:

1. The projecting corticomotoneurons that innervate one motor unit are widely dispersed over much of the motor cortex and it is assumed that the stimulus is sufficient to activate all of them. A low stimulus would result in an underestimation of the EPSP. A stronger stimulus cannot be used in the PSTH paradigm because it frequently evokes a complex response composed of more than one motor unit. The indexed unit would then be undertagged. This, too, will result in an underestimation of the EPSP.

2. It also has to be assumed that all of the fast-conducting anterior horn cells in a given motoneuron pool, which innervate a given muscle, receive similar convergent compound EPSPs. In our latest experiments we show that this assumption is not entirely

correct. In fact, there are variably sized EPSPs evoked from the same muscle motoneuron pool.

3. The formula used to estimate the amplitude of the EPSP assumes a rapid rise time and fairly large depolarization of the cell membrane. This assumption, although true for normal subjects, may not apply for all patients with ALS (Ashby and Zilm, 1982a, 1982b; Mao *et al.*, 1984; Brouwer and Ashby, 1990; Eisen *et al.*, 1996). However, since these types of experiments can only be done in limbs that are reasonably strong (MRC > 4), it can be assumed that most of the motor units are able to depolarize adequately.

4. The primary peak of the corticomotoneuronal EPSP (the large column in the PSTH shown in Fig. 5.13) consists of subpeaks and total estimates are based on the discharge probability of all these peaks. The number of bins, not counts per bin, included in this early period of excitation is referred to as the rise time of the EPSP. In normal individuals, the rise time of the EPSP can vary from 1 to 5 mV. Magnetic stimulation produces repetitive firing of corticomotoneurons, and some counts included in these consecutive bins are due to repeat waves of descending volleys. The total bin count used to estimate the compound EPSP may then include some repetitive activity of the same corticomotoneuron. This effect would result in overestimation of the amplitude of the EPSP and, as a result, of the corticomotoneuronal count.

Experiments described later suggest that in ALS repetitive firing is greater. More repetitive firing would increase the amplitude of the EPSP. Temporal dispersion may also be responsible for the greater rise time of the EPSP seen in ALS (Awiszus and Feistner 1993, 1995; Eisen *et al.*, 1996, 1997). There is a highly linear correlation between the rise time and amplitude of the EPSP in ALS (Nakajima *et al.*, 1996). A small-amplitude EPSP with a short rise time probably reflects a loss of corticomotoneurons supplying a given motoneuron (Fig. 5.16). The same abnormalities might result because of a problem at the presynaptic terminal. For example, axonal sprouts with poor safety factors may not all be able to sustain the descending volley. The anterior horn cell may also be abnormal and incapable of responding to the descending cortical volley. The large EPSPs with long rise times probably reflect a stage in the disease when there is corticomotoneuronal hyperexcitability, possibly induced by glutamate excess. This in turn could induce an increase in repetitive firing of the corticomotoneuron (Fig. 5.16).

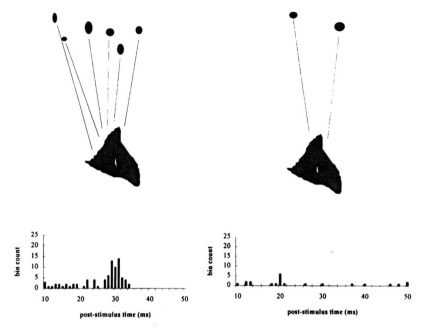

Figure 5.16. Temporal dispersion of descending corticomotoneuronal volley in ALS giving rise to a large EPSP. The cartoon on the left depicts a normal number of corticomotoneurons innervating a spinal motoneuron. However, they are diseased and their impulse traffic is dispersed, resulting in an EPSP of normal size but prolonged rise time. In the right cartoon, only two corticomotoneurons remain and the resulting EPSP is small.

Comparison between Ia afferent-driven and cortically driven EPSPs

It is tempting to interpret the changes that occur in the EPSP in ALS as being primarily due to disease or dysfunction of the corticomotoneuron itself or its presynaptic terminal acting on the SMN. Such a view would support the corticomotoneuronal hypothesis. However, a dysfunctional SMN could equally account for similar changes in the EPSP (i.e. reduced magnitude and increased rise time). In this next set of observations we show how this enigma can be solved, at least in part. It is possible to record a unitary EPSP from a motor unit by activation of peripheral Ia fibres in a way very similar to that described for evoking the cortical EPSP. This is done by giving a stimulus that is subthreshold for motor fibres to a peripheral nerve which then elicits a series of H-reflexes and a Ia afferent EPSP (Fig. 5.17). The Ia afferent EPSP, like the cortical EPSP, is

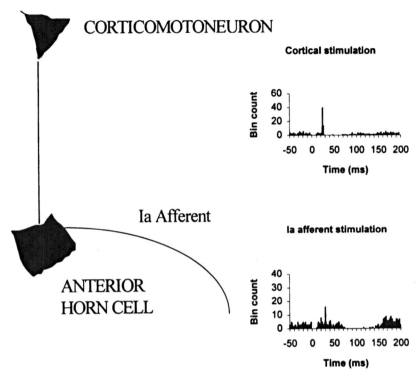

Figure 5.17. Ia afferent versus cortical EPSPs recorded from a first dorsal interosseus motor unit. The top EPSP was evoked by cortical stimulation and the lower one by stimulating the Ia afferent to the same spinal motoneuron. In this normal subject the cortical EPSP is larger than the Ia afferent EPSP.

excitatory and the transmitter is also glutamate. Presumably there is activation of the same spinal neuronal surface membrane. If the amplitude reduction in the cortical EPSP seen in many patients with ALS was secondary to corticomotoneuronal or presynaptic disease, then the Ia afferent EPSP should be normal, whereas if the anterior horn cell was responsible for the abnormalities, its EPSP would be reduced too. To investigate this possibility we compared a peripheral (Ia afferent) EPSP with a cortical EPSP evoked from the same motor unit. Postsynaptic events occurring in single motoneurons were derived from changes in the firing probability of single, voluntarily activated motor units in the FDI muscle during either electrical stimulation of the ipsilateral ulnar nerve or magnetic stimulation of the contralateral motor cortex. Transcutaneous electrical square-wave pulses of 1.0 ms duration elicited Ia afferent

NORMAL　　　　　　　　　　　　　　　　ALS

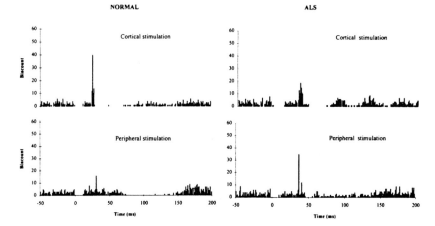

Figure 5.18. Cortical and Ia afferent EPSP in a normal subject and a patient with ALS. On the left, the upper EPSP was evoked by cortical stimulation and the lower one by peripheral Ia stimulation. Both were recorded from the same spinal motoneuron. The cortical EPSP is about 3.5 times the size of the peripheral EPSP. The right shows cortical (top) and peripheral (lower) EPSPs from a patient with ALS. The cortical EPSP is about one-third the size of the peripheral EPSP.

stimulation with the stimulus intensity adjusted to threshold for the motor unit under study. This paradigm is selective for the activation of the Ia afferents.

Following ulnar nerve stimulation of the Ia afferents, there was a period of increased firing probability of the motor unit, with an onset latency of around 30 ms (Fig. 5.18). Its latency correlated positively with the subject's height ($p < 0.001$), which would be in keeping with a mono-synaptic, afferent event such as an H-reflex. In normal subjects, the size of this primary peak is smaller in magnitude than the cortical EPSP recorded from the same motor unit. Thus, in normal subjects, the ratio of the amplitude of the EPSP in response to cortical stimulation to that of the EPSP in response to Ia afferent stimulation always exceeded 1.0 (Fig. 5.19). In contrast, in ALS, even when the cortical EPSP was small (mean value 0.71 ± 0.52 mV), the Ia afferent EPSP was of normal amplitude (mean value 2.09 ± 1.0 mV). This resulted in a cortical/Ia afferent EPSP ratio in ALS usually < 1.0 (Fig. 5.19). The reverse is the case for the soleus muscle unitary events (Mao *et al.*, 1984; Cope, Fetz and Matsumura, 1987). The difference probably reflects the very different functions of the two muscles. The FDI muscle, which was used to record the EPSP in this

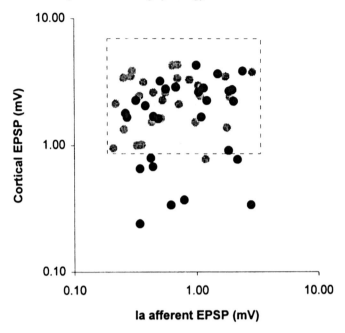

Figure 5.19. Scatterplot of Ia afferent versus cortical EPSPs in normal subjects (grey circles) and patients with ALS (black circles). The dotted square demarcates the boundaries for normal values. About a third of ALS values have cortical EPSPs that are reduced but whose peripheral Ia EPSPs are normal. This implies that the spinal motoneuron is capable of excitation and that the reduction in the cortical EPSP is due to loss or dysfunction of the corticomotoneuron.

series of experiments, is involved in a large repertoire of fractionated movements, necessitating large cortical facilitation. In contrast, the soleus is essentially involved in postural maintenance, for which it requires greater Ia afferent information but relatively little cortical demand, and the soleus has a much smaller composite corticomotoneuronal EPSP (about 0.6 mV) than does the FDI (2–3 mV) (Ashby *et al.*, 1987; Miles, Turker and Le, 1989; Mailis and Ashby, 1990). In most patients with ALS, the peripheral Ia EPSP is normal, even when the cortical EPSP is small or difficult to measure (Nakajima *et al.*, 1997). Both the cortical and the peripheral Ia projections terminate on the same anterior horn cell membrane and it is likely that distribution of NMDA receptors activated is the same in both cases. The observations of intact Ia afferent EPSPs in the face of altered corticomotoneuronal EPSPs then support the notion that in ALS spinal motor neurons frequently function normally even when the corticomotoneurons which innervate them are severely affected.

Comparison of the cortical EPSP and the macro-EMG in ALS

Early in ALS, the macro-EMG, which is a measure of the total motor unit territory, and the degree of collateral and terminal sprouting that is occurring are normal but, with progression of ALS, the macro-EMG enlarges. Subsequently, as the SMNs die and others can no longer efficiently sprout, the macro-EMG shrinks. The amplitude of the composite EPSP that we use is an estimate incorporating the total output of the SMN and varies with the product of the corticomotoneuronal synaptic current (input) and its own input resistance, given by Ohm's law (Ghez *et al.*, 1991):

$$E = IR$$

where E is the estimated amplitude of the composite EPSP, I is the corticomotoneuronal synaptic current, and R is the input resistance of the SMN. In keeping with the Henneman size principle (Henneman, Somien and Carpenter, 1965), SMNs that generate larger twitch tensions and larger motor unit potentials at the skin surface have a larger cell body; they also have a lower input resistance. As is shown in Fig. 5.20 (top), there is an inverse relation between the size of the macro-MUP and the EPSP amplitude so that MUPs with larger macro-MUPs have smaller composite EPSPs. This relationship is lost in ALS motor units. Although there are no available anatomical data, it is reasonable to assume that SMNs that have an enlarged motor unit territory and a larger macro-MUP amplitude also have an enlarged cell body, possibly in response to increased metabolic demands. The input resistance of such motor units should be decreased and this would tend to reduce the estimated amplitude of their composite EPSPs. However, in ALS, even those motoneurons with a large macro-MUP had large composite EPSPs and, conversely, most motoneurons that had a reduced composite EPSP did not have large macro-MUPs (Fig. 5.20, bottom). The findings indicate that in ALS, changes in the estimated amplitude of composite EPSPs must result from an abnormal synaptic current (input). A single cortical stimulus evokes repetitive, synchronous firing of corticomotoneurons. Kernell and Wu (1967) showed D-waves (direct) and I-waves (indirect) following the application of single electrical stimuli to the exposed motor cortex in the primate. The analogous responses have been demonstrated in

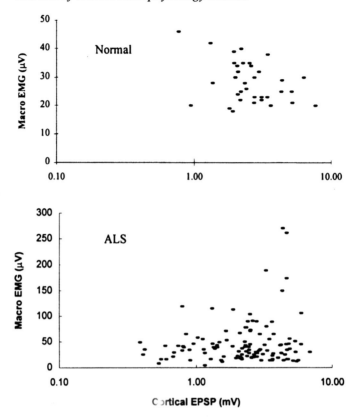

Figure 5.20. Correlation between the amplitudes of composite EPSPs and macro-MUPs in controls (*top*) and in patients with ALS (*bottom*). In normal subjects, the EPSP amplitude correlates inversely with the size of the macro-MUP. In ALS the correlation is not statistically significant, but in contrast to controls, the trend is towards a positive relationship. Grey points show EPSPs with a rise time equal to or greater than 6 ms. Both axes are logarithmic.

humans after transcranial electrical or magnetic stimulation (Day *et al.*, 1987; Amassian *et al.*, 1987). The trains of I-waves may last for 6.5–8.5 ms, and occasionally up to 10 ms, allowing the motoneuron to be depolarized. This duration is very similar to the prolonged EPSP rise time frequently seen in patients with ALS. We suggest that the prolonged rise time of ALS motor units which also have a larger EPSP results from excessive repetitive firing of the corticomotoneuron in response to a single brain stimulus. The cell could be rendered hyperexcitable because of chronic glutamate toxicity (Eisen, 1995).

Table 5.5. *Paired stimulation studies*

	Normals (n = 22)	ALS (n = 23)	Disease control (n = 15)
Age (years)	45.6 ± 15.9	62.5 ± 9.3*	53.7 ± 10
Stimulus intensity (%)	46.8 ± 9.5	48.8 ± 7.3	47.4 ± 10.5
Motor unit firing frequency (Hz)	78.7 ± 13.9	67.9 ± 11	81 ± 19.3
Onset latency 1st EPSP (ms)	19.5 ± 2.1	21.8 ± 2.5*	20 ± 2.4
Onset latency 2nd EPSP (ms)	22.2 ± 4	27.3 ± 6*	22.6 ± 5.1
Rise time 1st EPSP (ms)	3.7 ± 1.2	2.7 ± 1.2*	4.6 ± 2
Rise time 2nd EPSP (ms)	1.5 ± 1.09	4 ± 1.94*	2.3 ± 1.25
Amplitude 1st EPSP (mV)	3.26 ± 1.4	1.01 ± 0.7*	3.6 ± 1.4
Amplitude 2nd EPSP (mV)	0.48 ± 0.61	1.23 ± 0.69*	0.74 ± 0.38
Test conditioning EPSP ratio (%)	14.41 ± 15	131.6 ± 62.5*	26 ± 12.73

*A significant difference from normal at $p < 0.005$. EPSP, excitatory postsynaptic potential.

Paired stimulation studies and disordered inhibitory mechanisms in ALS

In the studies described thus far, we have shown that abnormalities of the cortical EPSP in ALS can be ascribed primarily to dysfunction of the corticomotoneuron or its presynaptic terminal. In the final set of experiments, using the PSTH paradigm, we examined the integrity of the motor cortical inhibitory interneurons. As alluded to earlier in this chapter, there is a growing body of evidence to indicate that the motor cortex in ALS is 'hyperexcitable'. This could result from excitation of the corticomotoneuron per se or from a loss of normally modulating inhibition. Inhibitory modulation of the corticomotoneuron occurs through local circuit inhibitory interneurons, which can be evaluated by delivering paired stimuli – a conditioning–test paradigm. The conditioning (first) stimulus will modify the response to the test (second) stimulus depending on the stimulus intensity used and the time between the two stimuli. In these experiments the conditioning–test interval was 30 ms and both stimuli were of the same threshold intensity. These characteristics are known to inhibit the test response.

Normal subjects

In the majority of normal subjects there is a very marked inhibition of the test EPSP (Table 5.5; Fig. 5.21). In many normal subjects there was no test

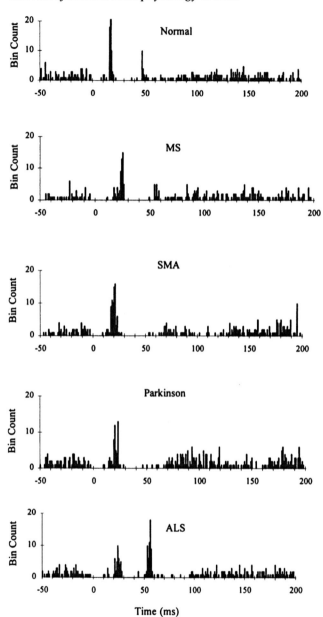

Figure 5.21. Paired stimulation studies. In each of the peristimulus time histograms a threshold-conditioning stimulus is given at time 0 ms. This is followed 30 ms later by a test stimulus of the same strength. In each example the conditioning stimulus produces a primary peak, the conditioning EPSP.   *Continued opposite*

Table 5.6. *Disease controls studied with paired stimulation*

Disease	Number of patients	Age (years)	Disease duration	Clinical findings
Multiple sclerosis	5	45–52	13–22	Spastic/hyper-reflexic
Benign fasciculation	2	45–46	1–1.5	Fasciculation
Kennedy's syndrome	1	43	2.5	Bulbospinal muscular atrophy, areflexia
Spinal muscular atrophy	1	65	4	Diffuse muscle atrophy
Parkinson's disease	1	67	10	Rigidity
Spondylotic myelopathy	1	75	3	Spastic paraparesis
Cerebral tumour	1	61	0.5	Spastic hemiparesis
Monomelic amyotrophy	1	38	20	Muscle atrophy

response and inhibition was complete. There was also a marked inhibition of the test EPSP in the disease control group, members of which had a variety of diseases but not ALS.

Patients with ALS

In most patients with ALS, the test EPSP was large, indicating failure of inhibitory mechanisms (Fig. 5.21). The majority had a conditioning–test EPSP ratio that exceeded 70 per cent. Disease controls (Table 5.6) do not show this abnormality. The mean conditioning–test EPSP ratio of the patients was about 10 times that of normal controls. Similar conclusions have been reached using a very short stimulus interval between the conditioning and test stimuli and recording from whole muscle rather than single motoneurons. The results of paired stimulation PSTHs in ALS patients suggest there is a failure of cortical inhibitory mechanisms (Yokota *et al.*, 1996; Enterzari-Taher *et al.*, 1997). We do not presently know if this is a primary event or occurs at the same time as disease of the corticomotoneurons. Interneurons release γ-aminobutyric acid (GABA)

Caption for Figure 5.21 (*cont.*)
The test stimulus induced a small test EPSP in the normal subject (top trace), and a large one in the patient with ALS (bottom trace), and none in the patients with multiple sclerosis (MS), spinal muscular atrophy (SMA) and Parkinson's disease. The large test EPSP in ALS indicates there is a failure of the normal inhibition typical of this paradigm and probably due to dysfunction of local circuit inhibitory interneurons.

onto the cortical pyramidal cells that include the corticomotoneurons. When $GABA_A$ receptors are activated, fast, inhibitory potentials are generated. In this way, GABAergic neurons regulate the amplitude and duration of EPSPs and, in the process, control the level of functional activation of NMDA receptors (McCormick, 1992; McCormick, Wang and Huguenard, 1993). Loss of GABAergic neurons could then result in chronic overactivity of the NMDA receptor.

As indicated earlier in this chapter, there are several lines of evidence indicating that the motor cortex of patients with ALS is hyperexcitable (see Table 5.2). This presumably reflects excessive drive of the output neuron which might be the result of overstimulation by excitotoxic amino acids or of a failure of inhibitory neurons, or both mechanisms. Local circuit cortical inhibitory interneurons are important in modulating the output of the corticomotoneuron. Those inhibitory neurons that immuno-react for parvalbumin and are responsible for controlling the firing frequency of the pyramidal neuron may be better able to sequester the excess calcium (Conde *et al.*, 1994). Those motoneurons that are typically affected in ALS do not express the calcium-binding proteins PV and CaBP (Ince *et al.*, 1993). Also, these motoneurons, unlike those innervating the eye muscles and bladder, which are generally spared in ALS, do not express the $GluR_2$ subunit of the AMPA receptor. The AMPA receptor has four protein subunits, $GluR_1$–$GluR_4$, and the expression of $GluR_2$ makes the AMPA receptor impermeable to calcium. It has been shown that there is a significant depletion of PV-immunoreactive GABAergic inhibitory interneurons in ALS motor cortex. This is independent of the severity of Betz cell loss (Nihei, McKee and Kowall, 1993; Snider, 1995; Reiner *et al.*, 1995). In normal brain stem, PV-containing neurons and interneurons are abundant in the oculomotor, trochlear and abducens nuclei, all of which are usually spared in ALS. In contrast, there are about one-third the number of PV-containing neurons and interneurons in the other brainstem motor nuclei (trigeminal, facial, ambiguus, and hypoglos-sal), and those which innervate skeletal muscle (Nihei *et al.*, 1992, 1993; Snider, 1995; Reiner *et al.*, 1995).

Summary

In recent years, conventional clinical electrophysiology (needle EMG and nerve conduction studies) has been complemented by newer, more sophisticated, electrophysiological approaches. Electrophysiology is important in ALS. It helps in the assessment of disease severity and rate of progression; it plays a role in evaluating the efficacy of therapeutic trials; and it has added insight into understanding the aetiopathogenesis of ALS. Currently, electrophysiology is the only means of confirming suspected ALS and is helpful in excluding some disorders that mimic ALS. Needle EMG identifies disease in clinically 'unaffected muscles', including bulbar musculature, confirms involvement of anterior horn cells, and can detect early involvement of respiratory muscles (intercostals and diaphragm). Conduction studies are imperative to rule out motor neuropathy with multifocal conduction block that may respond to therapy with immunosuppression or IVIg.

Various techniques employing TMS have demonstrated that the motor cortex in ALS is hyperexcitable. This may be secondary to excess release of excitatory amino transmitters, and glutamate is a likely candidate. Using PSTHs, it is possible to estimate the size of a unitary EPSP. This is a reflection of the number of corticomotoneurons innervating a single SMN. It is age dependent, and by 50 years of age as many as one-third of corticomotoneurons may be dead or non-functional. This may put added metabolic stress on the surviving corticomotoneurons. In ALS, the EPSP is often reduced in amplitude, but in about 20 per cent of patients it is normal or greater than predicted. These EPSPs are always associated with an increased rise time and there is a high correlation between the EPSP amplitude and rise time in ALS. Normal and large EPSPs in ALS are probably due to greater repetitive firing of the corticomotoneuron than normally occurs. When EPSPs evoked by cortical and peripheral Ia stimulation are compared in the same motor unit, the ratio of the cortical/Ia EPSP amplitude is normally > 1. In most patients with ALS it is < 1. This implies that the changes in ALS may be due to supraspinal mechanisms, probably involving the corticomotoneuron or its presynaptic terminal. The same conclusion can be drawn from a lack of any correlation between the macro-MUP and the EPSP recorded from the same motor unit.

Paired, threshold stimulation studies recording from whole muscle or in a PSTH paradigm induce marked inhibition of the test response. This is true of a wide variety of disease controls. Most patients with ALS demonstrate much less inhibition. This abnormality, which is further evidence of a hyperexcitable cortex in ALS, is probably due to dysfunction of local circuit cortical inhibitory interneurons.

6

The application of imaging techniques

Brain and spinal cord imaging has considerably extended our ability to understand the structure and function of the normal and disordered central nervous system. Data from imaging techniques can be obtained in living patients and permits an evaluation of a disease, not only at a given point in time, but over the progression of the disease. Some of the techniques reviewed in this chapter also have the potential to demonstrate an effect of drug therapy. Although, currently, these techniques are probably not sensitive enough to demonstrate a therapeutic response in an individual patient over time, it is possible that certain techniques may be capable of assessing changes due to therapy in a treatment group. This approach has been particularly powerful in disorders which are characterized by exacerbations and remissions, such as multiple sclerosis, where it has been possible to monitor changes in total cortical plaque load in response to treatment with β-interferon (Paty and Moore, 1997). Serial measurements using brain imaging will undoubtedly yield new insights, even in disorders marked by variable progression, such as ALS. To a large extent, imaging techniques can be thought of as an extension of pathological or biochemical measurements on brain tissue in situ.

The roles of imaging techniques in ALS are threefold. First, they are used to exclude causes of bulbar or limb weakness due to compressive lesions or other causes. Secondly, imaging techniques can identify abnormal signals that might be supportive of a diagnosis of ALS. Thirdly, MRI, PET, single photon emission computed spectroscopy (SPECT), functional MRI (FMRI) and functional ^{1}H-magnetic resonance spectroscopy (F^{1}H-MRS), in which the effects of activation are studied, are fast becoming important research tools in ALS. Each can help elucidate pathophysiological features of the disease.

190

Table 6.1. *Magnetic resonance imaging findings in ALS*

Cortical
   Signal loss in motor cortex
   Lobar atrophy
Subcortical
   Loss of white matter volume
   White matter signal change
Spinal cord
Corpus callosum changes
Tongue atrophy
Effects of ageing

Magnetic resonance imaging

Magnetic resonance imaging is a technique of tissue analysis in which radiowaves are applied in a magnetic field as a probe for the measurement and localization of the biochemical characteristics of a tissue. In practice, a strong, uniform magnetic field is applied to nervous system tissue leading to an alignment of atomic nuclei into one, two or more magnetic states. A pulse of radiofrequency waves of a frequency corresponding to the resonant frequency for hydrogen (in proton-based MRI) is used to stimulate protons into a higher energy state. Following the excitation pulse, protons 'relax' back to their original energy states, accompanied by the emission of radiowaves which are dependent on the structure and morphology of the tissue. Two tissue-specific relaxation constants can be identified, known as T1 and T2, and these constants allow for the characterization of the tissue analysed (e.g. white matter, grey matter, etc).

Based on what has been learned about ALS from neuropathological studies, one might anticipate that MRI would demonstrate: (i) neuronal loss in brain and spinal cord in the distribution of the corticomotoneuronal system as described in Chapter 3; (ii) Wallerian degeneration; (iii) demyelination; and (iv) an absence of inflammation. Our experience with cranial and spinal MRI in ALS has thus far proved disappointing because MRI scans have often been unremarkable, even in patients with advanced disease. However, we have sometimes seen abnormalities in ALS patients and many reports have described abnormalities detectable on MRI (Ishikawa *et al.*, 1993; Iwasaki *et al.*, 1994a; Kiernan and Hudson, 1994). These abnormalities are summarized in Table 6.1 and include altered signals in cortex, subcortical white matter, spinal cord and tongue.

Cortical lesions

Signal change can be seen in the brains of patients with ALS. The frequency of observation of these abnormalities depends on the extent of clinical involvement and probably on the pattern of neuronal loss (whether there is upper or lower motoneuron loss). The resolution of the MRI scanner, the scanning protocols used, and an awareness of the MRI changes that may occur in ALS also influence the frequency with which MRI abnormalities are seen. For example, using a 1.5 Tesla high-field strength MRI, three of seven patients with sporadic ALS had signal loss confined to the motor cortex on T2-weighted sequences. The abnormality was bilateral and extended from the vertex to the centrum semiovale. These abnormalities were not seen on T1-weighted and proton density images (Ishikawa *et al.*, 1993). However, one of the seven patients studied also had symmetrically increased signal intensity on T2-weighted images along the pyramidal tract, extending between the internal capsule to the cerebral peduncles. The authors did not see similar MRI findings in a cohort of 70 age-matched patients having a variety of neurological diseases. It is not clear whether the radiologists were blinded to the diagnosis of ALS in these patients. However, the MRI abnormalities could not be correlated with the clinical features in individual patients, and the number of ALS patients examined was small. The reduced cortical signal was attributed to a high cortical iron content, but this claim was not supported by substantiating evidence (Ishikawa *et al.*, 1993). Paradoxically, decreased signal intensity has also been reported in ALS (Oba *et al.*, 1992). The significance of the hypointensity of motor cortex on T2-weighted images is controversial. Iwasaki *et al.* (1994a) claim that similar changes may occur in older patients, with and without neurological disease, who do not have ALS. This prompted a re-evaluation of all cases of low-intensity signals at their institution. The authors found that hypointensity was seen in patients with several types of neurological disease, including AD, PD and other disorders, but not in 20 ALS patients. As a result of their study, Iwasaki and colleagues (1994a) conclude that the altered cortical intensity is an age-related phenomenon and not a specific finding for ALS. We agree with this interpretation.

To evaluate the extent of frontal lobe atrophy in ALS, Kiernan and Hudson (1994) used a 1.5 Tesla magnet to image T2-weighted sequences in 11 patients. Cortical surface area was determined from T2-weighted scans. Even though there was no significant change in the frontal lobe cortical surface area of patients with ALS compared to controls, there was a significant reduction in the anterior frontal lobe white matter area. In other brain areas, including the corpus callosum, the precentral gyri and parietal lobes of ALS patients, the white matter area estimates showed no difference compared to 49 age-matched controls. This study also attempted to correlate reductions in the volume of brain regions to the patterns of paresis. The only positive correlation was between the extent of bulbar dysfunction in ALS and a reduction in anterior frontal lobe area. A significant correlation between limb function and the amount of white matter in the anterior frontal lobes and precentral gyri was seen only in PLS and not in ALS (Kiernan and Hudson, 1994). It was suggested that the reduction in frontal white matter area resulted from a loss of afferent fibres to the anterior frontal cortex. Potentially, these fibres could originate from the thalamus and corticocortical connections. The limited change in the area of the motor cortex on MRI scans is not too surprising given the modest loss of cortical tissue in ALS which rarely results in detectable atrophy at post-mortem examination (see Chapter 3). The loss of corticocortical and descending corticomotoneuronal fibres in ALS is generally insufficient to alter the cortical area in a significant, reproducible way to produce changes on MRI in a small cohort of ALS patients. As described later, ^{1}H-MRS is considerably more sensitive than conventional MRI in detecting neuronal loss. It is possible that MRI studies in ALS patients with dementia will have reductions in cortical areas, compared to controls, but this has not been studied systematically.

Subcortical white matter changes

The first reports of MRI findings in patients with ALS described symmetrical areas of increased signal that extended from the cortex through the corona radiata and posterior limb of the internal capsule to the cerebral peduncles and into the pontine tegmentum (Goodkin, Rowley and Olney, 1988). In one report of five ALS patients, two had symmetrically positioned focal areas of increased signal intensity on T2-weighted scans in the subcortical regions indicated above. The two patients demonstrating these findings were young and their clinical course was rapid. A third patient had symmetrically placed regions of increased signal intensity either in or near the posterior limb of the internal capsule. Two other patients had normal MRI scans. The white matter changes were interpreted to reflect tract degeneration with demyelination, as is seen pathologically in ALS patients (Goodkin *et al.*, 1988). Sales Luís and colleagues (1990) studied MRI scans from 20 ALS patients and in eight there was increased signal in the centrum semiovale, corona radiata, internal capsule, cerebral peduncles, pons and medulla. As in other studies, the authors did not find any relationship between the presence of MRI abnormalities and the disease duration or the type of clinical deficits. Scans were obtained from four patients with progressive bulbar palsy and in three patients the scans were abnormal. Two of these patients had hyperintense lesions in periventricular regions and subcortical areas. Eleven healthy control subjects were also studied; in all controls the MRI was essentially normal except for small, discrete, bright spots located in the periventricular white matter in seven subjects (Sales Luís *et al.*, 1990). Similarly, Iwasaki and colleagues (1992a) studied 10 ALS patients using MRI on a 1.5T scanner. Four of the 10 patients had asymmetrical focal areas of increased signal on T2-weighted sequences. The MRI changes were limited to white matter in these patients. Udaka *et al.* (1992) found focal high signal regions in the posterior limb of the internal capsule and cerebral peduncles in four of 21 patients with ALS. No abnormalities were seen in the medullary pyramids in these patients. Figure 6.1 shows symmetrically increased signal (arrows) in the white matter at multiple levels in an ALS patient. A more recent report described high signal changes bilaterally in regions corresponding to the pyramidal tract in four of 13 ALS patients (Terao *et al.*, 1995). The lateralization of these high signal changes did not necessarily correspond to the clinical signs. The ALS patients who had abnormal white matter signals on cranial MRI also had abnormal, high signal change in T2-weighted sequences in the spinal cord. However, some patients with no evidence of demonstrable signal change in the brain did have abnormal findings in the spinal cord (Terao *et al.*, 1995).

In a retrospective review of 17 ALS patients, Cheung *et al.* (1995) identified sharp, well-defined symmetrical lesions, which were best seen around the internal capsule on T2-weighted sequences. These abnormalities in the corticospinal tracts were better visualized with proton-density-weighted images than with T2-weighted sequences. Low signal was also identified in six of eight patients in which proton density sequences were used. Several factors correlated with the visualization of corticospinal tract abnormalities on MRI. These included extension of the abnormal white matter signal intensity to motor cortex and increased signal intensity of the corticospinal tract (Cheung *et al.*, 1995). The MRI abnormalities correlated best in patients having a typical or rapid clinical evolution of the disease.

In summary, focal regions of increased signal intensity are seen in deep white matter, possibly in as many as 40 per cent of ALS patients (Sales

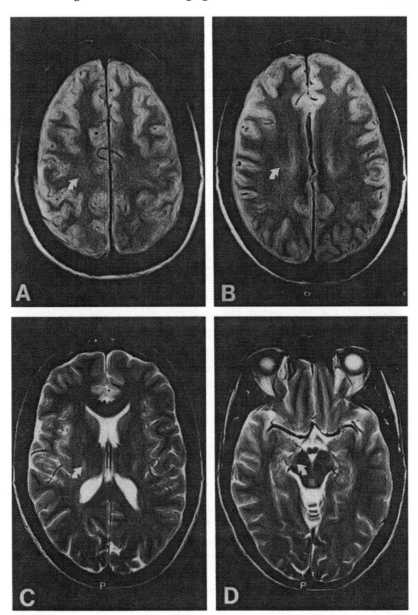

Figure 6.1. MRI scans of a patient with ALS. Four axial views are shown: (A) at the upper end of the centrum semiovale, (B) in the centrum semiovale, (C) at the level of the internal capsule, and (D) at the level of the mesencephalon. Scans in (A) and (B) are proton density weighted (long TR, short TE), those in (C) and (D) are T2 weighted (long TR, long TE). Symmetrically increased signal can be seen at multiple levels in the white matter (arrows). Arrows indicate densities on one side only.

Luís *et al.*, 1990; Iwasaki *et al.*, 1992). These findings correlate reasonably well with neuropathological studies which typically demonstrate cortico-spinal tract loss and demyelination in 30–90 per cent of patients (Brownell *et al.*, 1970). Increased signal intensity in the posterior internal capsules, especially when bilateral and symmetric, is a frequent finding in healthy controls, particularly in T2-weighted images. This observation has been attributed to the less dense myelination of axons of the parieto-pontine tract than in adjacent fibres. However, a distinguishing feature between normal and abnormal signals may depend on the regional extent of the abnormal signal. In cases where signal changes are more extensive, tract loss is more likely (Martí-Fàbregas and Pujol, 1992). Use of proton density sequences is more sensitive than T2-weighted sequences for evaluation of white matter changes.

Spinal cord

Although spinal cord atrophy is sometimes seen at autopsy in ALS patients, it is not usually detected on MRI. However, some patients do have sufficient tract loss for an abnormal signal to be detected. Several reports have described bilateral, symmetrical degeneration of the cortico-spinal tracts within the spinal cord with high signal noted on axial T1-weighted and T2-weighted sequences. Axial images of the spinal cord may show flattening of the ventral and lateral aspects, especially in the cervical segments. This gives rise to an appearance that has been likened to an inverted horseshoe (Friedman and Tartaglino, 1993). However, sagittal T1-weighted and T2-weighted images of the cord are typically normal (Thorpe *et al.*, 1996). Occasionally, it is possible to detect mild hyper-intensity of the anterior corticospinal tracts in the ventral white matter. The basis for this is unknown, but it is probably due to myelin loss and gliosis. It has been claimed that there is a correlation between the extent of clinical 'upper motoneuron' involvement and the selective hyperintensity of corticospinal tracts, whereas 'lower motoneuron' deficit is reflected by focal spinal cord atrophy with signal attenuation. Often the abnormal signal is situated symmetrically in the lateral aspect of the spinal cord. Signal change in the lateral columns can also be seen in thoracic spinal cord (Thorpe *et al.*, 1996).

Correlations between the MRI observations and post-mortem findings have been obtained in several patients (Terao *et al.*, 1995). In two patients whose MRI demonstrated high signal intensity in the cervical spinal cord, post-mortem examination showed atrophy of the ventral roots with a severe loss of ventral horn cells. Pallor was also seen in a localized region of the dorsolateral columns where severe axon loss, macrophage infiltration and oedema were present. The pathological changes appeared to give rise to the abnormal signal on MRI. Nine of 13 patients had abnormal signals in the dorsolateral columns on axial T2-weighted sequences and it was concluded that spinal MRI was more sensitive than cranial MRI for the detection of ALS lesions, especially those having 'upper motoneuron' type clinical features. Three of the 13 patients in this study exhibited only 'lower motoneuron' findings clinically, yet MRI demonstrated signal change within the spinal portion of the corticospinal tracts (Terao *et al.*, 1995).

ALS with Parkinson's disease and/or dementia

Only a limited number of studies have addressed MRI findings associated with cognitive decline in ALS. It has been claimed that between 3.5 per cent and 5 per cent of patients with sporadic ALS have significant cognitive impairment (see Chapters 2 and 7; Hudson, 1991b). This low incidence may hinder the accumulation of a cohort large enough for study. To evaluate involvement of cerebral regions outside primary motor cortex and its connections, Yamauchi and colleagues (1995) studied the area of the corpus callosum in 25 patients with ALS and a similar number of age-matched control subjects. They found that as a group, ALS patients had a significantly reduced callosal/skull ratio where atrophy was especially prominent in the anterior aspect of the corpus callosum. Those patients with cognitive decline or psychiatric symptoms had more substantial atrophy. The reduction in callosal area was attributed to a widespread decrease in corticocortical connections in ALS. The authors also point out that the large pyramidal neurons in layer 3 that are involved in ALS include a significant fraction which contribute projections to corpus callosum (Yamauchi *et al.*, 1995). A MRI and SPECT study by Abe and coworkers (1993) did not report specific MRI findings in ALS patients related to cognitive impairment. In contrast, SPECT was useful in delineating neuronal degeneration (Abe *et al.*, 1993). In cases of ALS associated with Parkinsonian features, signal hypointensity has been seen in the putamen and subcortical U-fibres.

Tongue

MRI imaging of the tongue in ALS patients has revealed radiographic evidence of atrophy, which can be more sensitive than clinical measures.

In a study of 16 ALS patients (Cha and Patten, 1989), major abnormalities of the size, shape and structure of the tongue were apparent in 14 patients, whereas these findings were not apparent in controls. The authors assumed that decreased tongue size, abnormal internal signals and the altered shape of the tongue in ALS were due to lower motoneuron disease, whereas the abnormal position of the tongue was attributable to upper motoneuron involvement.

Effects of ageing

An important consideration with MRI interpretation is age-related change. Age-related changes are important in two ways. First, they must be identified to establish whether a given MRI finding is abnormal or merely a normal variant. Secondly, a description of these changes permits an understanding of the normal ageing process of nervous tissue. This topic will be considered here only in relation to ALS. In general, MRI changes with ageing relate to: (i) altered volumes of the cerebral hemispheres, including cerebral atrophy and ventricular enlargement, and (ii) focal regions of signal change, usually in the white matter and basal ganglia.

Several studies have evaluated cortical and subcortical areas with advancing age and gender differences. The studies of Kiernan and Hudson (1994) have indicated that the mean area of the parietal lobes at the level of the superior aspect of the corpus callosum was greater in males than females, but that no other gender difference was apparent in the frontal or precentral region area. The region of the anterior frontal lobe was found to decrease with age, but no changes were apparent in the precentral gyri or parietal lobes between the ages of 30 and 80 (Kiernan and Hudson, 1994). These observation are of interest with regard to speculation that 'premature ageing' may be relevant to the development of ALS (see Chapter 7). Focal signal change in the posterior internal capsule has been noted to vary with age (Mirowitz *et al.*, 1989).

Magnetic resonance spectroscopy

Magnetic resonance spectroscopy (MRS) is a technique that permits the biochemical characterization of tissue by obtaining spectra of metabolites containing nuclei sensitive to magnetic resonance. It is the only technique currently available that can non-invasively analyse the chemical components of the brain. Most studies of normal and abnormal brain have used proton-MRS (^{1}H-MRS), which can measure brain metabolites with concentrations exceeding 1 mmol/l. Typically, long echo time ^{1}H-MRS provides spectral information on the methyl resonances of N-acetyl acetate (NA), choline (Cho) containing compounds, creatine (Cr), phosphocreatine (PCr) and, when elevated, lactate. Short echo time sequences can be used to detect additional resonances. The concentration of N-acetyl-aspartate (NAA) as measured by ^{1}H-MRS provides an index of the viability of the neuronal pool in the brain area measured. Several groups have used this index to evaluate changes in neurons of the motor cortex in ALS patients. Pioro and colleagues (1994) have employed ^{1}H-MRS to analyse levels of N-acetyl groups, such as NAA and N-acetyl-aspartyl glutamate (NAAG) in a number of cortical areas in ALS. These authors found that in ALS patients with definite upper motoneuron signs, the ratio of the N-acetyl to creatine spectra was significantly decreased ($p < 0.001$) in the primary motor cortex compared to normal controls (Fig. 6.2). In patients with probable upper motoneuron signs (PUMNS), the NA/Cr ratio was also reduced but to a lesser degree and at a lower level of significance ($p < 0.05$ compared to $p < 0.001$ for the ALS group).

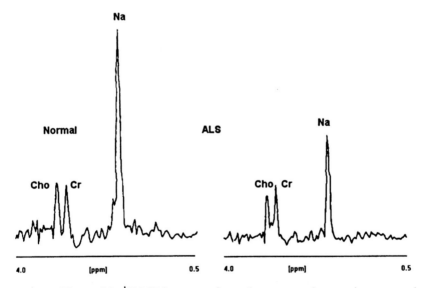

Figure 6.2. ^{1}H-MRS spectra from the precentral gyrus in a control subject (left) and an ALS patient (right). The size of the N-acetyl (Na) component, which is a measure of neuronal integrity, is reduced in the ALS patient. In order to minimize background 'noise', the signal is usually expressed as the Na/Cr ratio. This ratio is also reduced in the ALS patient. (Modified from Pioro *et al.*, 1994.)

In patients who had only lower motoneuron signs (PSMA), the NA/Cr ratio was not significantly different from normal (Fig. 6.3; Pioro *et al.*, 1994). Patients with ALS also had a reduced NA/Cr ratio in primary sensory cortex, superior parietal gyrus and the posterior premotor region (Pioro *et al.*, 1994).

Some of the results described by Pioro *et al.* (1994) are similar to those reported by Jones and colleagues (1995). Jones *et al.* (1995) found reduced levels of NAA in motor cortex from patients with ALS compared to controls. Although ALS patients and controls were not well matched for age, the NAA to Cr/PCr ratio and the NAA to Cho ratio were reduced in ALS. More recent studies by Gredal *et al.* (1997) have examined ^{1}H-MRS spectra in motor cortex and cerebellum from seven patients with ALS, three subjects with PSMA and eight controls. They found that concentrations of NAA were decreased only in those ALS patients with both upper and lower motoneuron signs. No differences were detected between Cho and Cr/PCr concentrations in brain or cerebellum between ALS patients

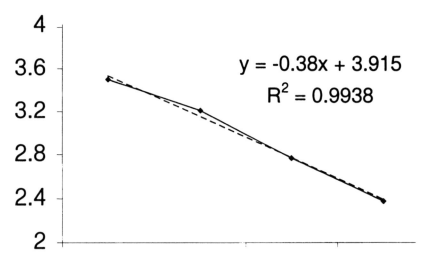

$$y = -0.38x + 3.915$$
$$R^2 = 0.9938$$

Normal PSMA PUMNS ALS

Figure 6.3. Relationship between the Na/Cr ratio and upper moto-neuron features in normal subjects and ALS patients with definite upper motoneuron signs (ALS), probable upper motoneuron signs (PUMNS) or only lower motoneuron signs (PSMA). The interrupted line is the cal-culated regression line and is highly significant ($r^2 = 0.99$). The data are taken from the literature (Pioro *et al.*, 1994; Gredal *et al.*, 1997) and suggest that the Na/Cr ratio is related to the extent of upper moto-neuron involvement in ALS patients.

and controls. These data confirm the observations of Pioro and colleagues (1994), as well as those of Jones *et al.* (1995), that NAA is reduced in motor cortex in patients with ALS. This reduction in NAA is seen in patients with upper motoneuron involvement and probably reflects a loss of neurons in motor cortex. This finding would be expected based on data from neuropathological studies (see Chapter 3). The ability to analyse ^{1}H-MRS signals from small brain volumes has allowed measurement of the NA/Cr ratio in the pons and upper medulla. The mean NA/Cr ratio is reduced in the brain stem of ALS patients compared to controls, presumably reflecting a loss of neurons in the cranial motor nuclei (Cwik *et al.*, 1997).

The compounds NAA and NAAG are believed to be confined to neurons and are not present in glial cells. Thus, the reduction in NA groups can be attributed to neuronal loss. The relation between the NA/Cr ratio and the clinical presentation of disease is of interest. Figure 6.3 shows Na/Cr ratios for controls (Normal), patients with PSMA having only lower motoneuron involvement, patients with PUMNS, and those with definite ALS. There is a good correlation between the fall in the NA/Cr ratio and the extent of presumptive involvement of cerebral cortex. However, it remains to be seen if this reduction in the NA/Cr ratio is due to neuronal loss. It is not yet clear if a reduced NA/Cr ratio is only seen in situations in which there is an actual loss of neurons or whether it can also occur if the neurons are living but dysfunctional. It seems that the changes detected by ^{1}H-MRS are greater than would be anticipated by the modest loss of neurons in the motor cortex generally found at autopsy (see Chapter 3). It would be helpful to correlate post-mortem brain concentrations of NAA with the ^{1}H-MRS NA spectra measured in-vivo. However, it appears that the correlation is poor. In autopsied spinal cord tissue, the levels of NAA measured by high-performance liquid chromatography are substantially reduced in ALS patients compared to controls, but this is not the case in the frontal or motor cortex (Tsai *et al.*, 1991). ^{1}H-MRS of the spinal cord is not feasible at present, and therefore comparison to NAA and NAAG levels measured in spinal cord tissue at autopsy cannot yet be made. The concentrations of NAA and NAAG obtained from ^{1}H-MRS measurements and those determined using liquid chromatography may differ as a single spectral peak in MRS may reflect protons from more than one chemical, which may cause erroneous interpretation in the identification of spectral peaks in ^{1}H-MRS (Knight *et al.*, 1996). The discrepancy between in-vivo and post-mortem analysis may also indicate a greater sensitivity of the in-vivo technique (Pioro *et al.*, 1994).

Despite these uncertainties, ^{1}H-MRS may provide a sensitive means of detecting or confirming upper motoneuron involvement in ALS. In ALS patients who have definite or probable upper motoneuron signs, there may also be a significant reduction of the NA/Cr ratio in the primary sensory cortex (Pioro *et al.*, 1994; Jones *et al.*, 1995; Shibasaki, 1997) and in the cerebellum (Gredal *et al.*, 1997). This suggests that reductions in NAA and NAAG occur in a widespread distribution in the brains of patients with ALS. There are other lines of evidence, including abnormalities of somatosensory evoked potentials and changes seen with PET and SPECT, which indicate that the somatosensory cortex is involved in ALS. ^{1}H-MRS may also prove to be a useful tool for the longitudinal evaluation of ALS patients, especially patients receiving therapy designed to alter intracellular concentrations of glutamate, aspartate, NAA and NAAG. Serial measurements of the motor cortex using ^{1}H-MRS may prove to be an objective measure of the progression of ALS, as well as an aid in determining a response to drug therapy.

SPECT scanning

Single photon emission computed tomography can be used to assess cerebral blood flow as well as cortical metabolic activity. A flow tracer, typically N-isopropyl-p-^{123}I-amphetamine (^{123}I-IMP), is tagged with a radionuclide, which readily crosses the blood–brain barrier and is distributed proportionally to the regional cerebral blood flow (rCBF). The uptake is imaged by CT and depends on the rCBF and other characteristics of the perfused tissue. SPECT has parallels with PET, but lacks its spatial resolution. Ludolph and colleagues (1989) performed SPECT scanning on 17 ALS patients, all of whom showed decreased cortical fixation of N-isopropyl-p-^{123}I-amphetamine (^{123}I-IMP) in brain. The pattern of reduced fixation could be categorized into several distinct groups. The first consisted of global impairments of IMP fixation; a second group had reduction in rCBF, especially in the frontotemporal regions; and a third group had findings which were combinations of the other two groups, having a generalized reduction of CBF, but which was most prominent in the frontotemporal regions. The changes in fixation could not be clearly related to the clinical features of the disease, or to the age of the patient, but patients with ALS of longer duration had more profound impairment of ^{123}I-IMP fixation. The most striking observation of this study was the impressive reduction of rCBF to frontotemporal structures. Although the resolution of this technique is limited, the findings are comparable to those acquired with [^{18}F] 2-fluoro-2-deoxy-D-glucose (FDG) PET scans, which demonstrate widespread hypoperfusion (except for cerebellum, which is relatively normal). Differentiating the reduced CBF in ALS from dementing disorders can be difficult (Ludolph *et al.*, 1989).

The abnormalities described in these earlier SPECT studies have been confirmed by several other groups using either SPECT or PET (Ludolph *et al.*, 1992; Tanaka *et al.*, 1993; Abrahams *et al.*, 1996). About a third of the patients who have reduced flow in the frontotemporal regions of the cortex are overtly demented; the dementia is usually mild. Patients with normal SPECT scans are almost never demented. Ludolph and colleagues (1992) correlated regional cerebral glucose utilization measured by high-resolution PET with neuropsychological testing in 18 ALS patients. All the patients had upper and lower motoneuron signs. Compared to controls, glucose utilization was significantly reduced in the frontal lobes of the patients, and the degree of reduction correlated well with disturbances in psychological testing. In a more recent study, Abrahams *et al.* (1996) measured rCBF using PET specifically to explore frontal lobe dysfunction in ALS (see Chapters 2 and 8). Comparison of rCBF with an activation paradigm of executive frontal lobe function (verbal fluency) was compared with word generation and word repetition in ALS patients with and without cognitive impairment, as well as in normal, age-matched controls. The patients who were cognitively impaired had significantly impaired rCBF to activation in cortical and subcortical regions including the dorsolateral prefrontal cortex, lateral premotor cortex, medial prefrontal and premotor cortices and insular cortex. Although the literature on SPECT scanning in ALS is not extensive, it does not appear that SPECT is either sufficiently sensitive or specific to recommend as a diagnostic test for ALS. In patients with ALS and dementia, SPECT scanning may have some diagnostic value, but the specificity of the SPECT findings for ALS remains to be determined. A recent evaluation of regional SPECT scanning using the radionuclide technetium-99m hexamethylpropylene amine (99m Tc–Hm PAO) in patients with AD has concluded that this technique lacks sensitivity for the diagnosis of this disease (Mattman *et al.*, 1997).

Positron emission tomography

Positron emission tomography is an imaging technique permitting the analysis of the metabolic activity or blood flow in a given tissue volume in vivo. PET has become an important tool to probe the metabolic status of

Verbal Fluency Activation

Left Hemisphere

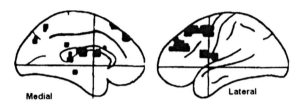

Medial   Lateral

Right Hemisphere

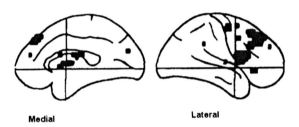

Medial   Lateral

Joystick Movement R hand

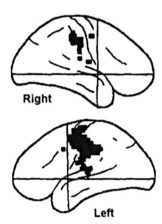

Right

Left

Figure 6.4. Measurement of regional cerebral blood flow (rCBF) using $H_2{}^{15}O$ PET in an activation paradigm. The dark areas in the pictures are regions of the brain displaying significant differences from normal in rCBF with activation (p < 0.001). The top four pictures show the effect of executive frontal lobe function (verbal fluency) in non-demented ALS patients who had impaired word generation.   *Continued opposite*

brain structures using FDG and other ligands. The methodology and technical aspects used for these studies have been reviewed recently (Snow, 1994). Early studies in ALS using FDG and PET demonstrated reduced cerebral metabolic rates for glucose in many cortical and subcortical regions in ALS patients having upper motoneuron findings. These regions included frontal, temporal, parietal and occipital cortical areas, as well as caudate, putamen, thalamus and pons (Dalakas *et al.*, 1987). PET studies in these ALS patients were compared to seven patients who had only lower motoneuron findings, three patients with post-poliomyelitis syndrome, and four patients with PSMA. The PET scans in these other patient groups were normal, suggesting that the reduction in cortical metabolism in the patients with ALS was not simply secondary to disuse. This study also indicated that disturbed cortical metabolism in ALS occurs largely in patients with clinical evidence of upper motoneuron disease.

The widespread abnormalities of cerebral metabolism seen with PET scanning in ALS patients (Dalakas *et al.*, 1987) have been confirmed in more recent studies. These studies have found significant reductions in all areas of cortex, including primary sensorimotor cortex, lateral premotor cortex, the supplementary motor area, the anterior cingulate cortex, the paracentral lobule and the partietal cortex, compared to age-matched controls (Kew *et al.*, 1993). The abnormalities in rCBF are probably partially attributable to neuronal loss in cortex and, specifically, nerve fibre degeneration in sensorimotor and premotor cortices. Involvement of the supplementary motor area, paracentral lobule and parietal lobe is believed to reflect either neuron loss in these areas or a reduction of corticocortical afferents to these brain regions (Kew *et al.*, 1993). Changes in rCBF have also been measured while patients and controls performed stereotyped or freely selected movements of the right hand. Under resting conditions, there was a significantly reduced rCBF in several brain regions

---

Caption for Figure 6.4 (*cont.*)
There is significantly reduced rCBF activation in the frontal and prefrontal cortices and other cortical and subcortical regions of the brain. The lower two pictures show significantly increased rCBF in ALS patients in response to hand movement using a joystick. The main changes are in the contralateral premotor and supplementary motor and sensorimotor cortices. It is possible that a loss of inhibitory interneurons resulting in relative excitation of the cortex that surrounds the motor cortex accounts for some of the changes. (Modified from Kew *et al.*, 1994; and Abrahams *et al.*, 1996.)

in ALS patients. Surprisingly, the movement-associated changes in rCBF were significantly larger in ALS patients than in controls. These changes were evident in the contralateral sensorimotor cortex, the premotor cortex and the parietal association cortex (Fig. 6.4). Elevated rCBF was also apparent in the contralateral insula and ipsilateral anterior cingulate cortex. The increased blood flow observed with the activation protocols was originally interpreted as an expansion of cortical regions related to the control of the upper limb, possibly due to an opening up of previously 'silent' neural pathways. However, other recent PET studies and electrophysiological data suggest that in ALS there is a reduction of cortical inhibition. This hypothesis may best explain the increased activity-induced metabolic changes seen with PET scanning (Eisen *et al.*, 1997; Shibasaki, 1997; Desiato and Caramia, 1997). In a subsequent study, Kew and colleagues (1994) compared rCBF in ALS patients having both upper and lower motoneuron signs with those who had only lower motoneuron signs, as well as with normal controls. At rest, the patients with ALS having both upper and lower motoneuron involvement showed reduced rCBF in the primary sensorimotor cortex. These reductions in rCBF were not seen in patients with only lower motoneuron signs, or in controls. In ALS patients with upper motoneuron signs, activation (movement of a joystick with the right hand) increased rCBF in the hand and arm area of the sensorimotor cortex bilaterally, the face area of the contralateral sensorimotor cortex, as well as the contralateral premotor and supplementary motor cortices. The findings of reduced rCBF at rest with abnormal bilateral activation and altered somatotopy during movement in ALS patients with upper motoneuron signs were thought to reflect a loss of pyramidal neurons (Kew *et al.*, 1994). However, it is possible that a loss of inhibitory interneurons accounts for some of the changes. The abnormal activation of the perisylvian areas during limb movement, which was seen in patients both with and without upper motoneuron findings, suggests a non-specific recruitment of accessory sensorimotor areas in response to limb weakness.

There have also been PET studies using 6-fluorodopa designed to study subclinical lesions in the nigrostriatal dopaminergic pathways. The issues of overlap between ALS and PD and between ALS and AD are discussed in Chapter 8. Takahashi *et al.* (1993) found a significant, progressive fall in 6-fluorodopa uptake in 16 patients with ALS that correlated with the time from diagnosis. In three patients who had ALS for longer than 10 years, there was an absolute reduction in dopaminergic function. Przedborski *et al.* (1996) used 6-fluorodopa PET to assess dopaminergic function in 14 patients with FALS. Seven of these patients had mutations of the CuZn–SOD1 gene. CuZn–SOD1 is present in large amounts in nigrostriatal dopaminergic neurons, raising the possibility that FALS patients having a mutation of this gene could have subclinical nigrostriatal dysfunction. Striatal/occipital ratios of fluorodopa uptake for the caudate and the putamen were calculated. The fluorodopa uptake ratio for the caudate did not differ between FALS patients with or without mutations in the CuZn–SOD1 gene, or in age-matched controls. However, putamenal uptake was significantly reduced in the FALS patients who did not have CuZn–SOD1 mutations. This may indicate that mutations of the CuZn–SOD1 gene are less cytotoxic to dopaminergic neurons than to motoneurons.

Summary

Conventional radiological techniques such as standard X-rays or CT scanning have provided little information in ALS. These studies are useful to exclude other causes for clinical signs suggestive of ALS. MRI may show symmetric or asymmetric lesions along the descending white matter pathways such as the pyramidal tract. However, the specificity of these lesions is uncertain and they are demonstrated in fewer than 40 per cent of patients. The extent to which they correlate with upper motoneuron findings remains to be determined. ^{1}H-MRS can be used as an in-vivo marker of neuronal loss. In particular, the NA/Cr ratio is markedly reduced in ALS patients with upper motoneuron signs and may be slightly reduced in patients with only lower motoneuron abnormalities. Recent ^{1}H-MRS studies have detected neuronal loss in the brain stem, but it is not currently possible to explore the spinal cord using this technique. When this does becomes possible, it will be an excellent method for comparing the relative rate of loss of upper and lower motoneurons in ALS. ^{1}H-MRS is potentially useful for monitoring a response to therapy by detecting a change in the rate of neuronal loss, but at present individual patient variation is considerable, making it necessary to study patient groups. SPECT and PET have been useful research tools in ALS. They have demonstrated that the disease clearly affects cortical areas beyond the motor cortex. Prefrontal and frontotemporal abnormalities seen on SPECT or PET are frequently associated with impaired neuropsychological testing, suggesting that cognitive impairment in ALS may be more frequent than bedside examination would indicate. PET studies used in an activation paradigm show a paradoxical increase in rCBF involving orbitofrontal, prefrontal and supplementary motor cortices. At rest, rCBF is reduced in the motor cortex. The increase in rCBF with activation suggests that there is a disinhibition of the motor cortex, a phenomenon also detectable using transcranial magnetic stimulation. This disinhibition of cortex could arise as a consequence of a loss of inhibitory interneurons. Although of limited assistance at present, imaging studies provide in-vivo measures of physiological and biochemical aspects of brain activity and will undoubtedly yield new insights. For instance, the findings suggestive of cortical disinhibition described above lend support to the view that cortical control is greatly altered in ALS patients. This can be viewed as evidence for the corticomotoneuronal hypothesis of ALS that is described more fully in Chapter 5.

7

ALS therapy, therapeutic trials, and neuroprotection

As discussed in Chapter 4, the pathogenesis of ALS is multifactorial and includes the interaction of one, or more likely several, susceptibility genes, undetermined environmental factors and cellular ageing mechanisms (Eisen and Krieger, 1993; Eisen, 1995). There is no clear indication when the disease begins, but the symptomatic disease is preceded by an incubation period of unknown length. Duration of symptoms is also quite variable, although disease starting in younger patients runs a significantly longer course (Eisen *et al.*, 1993c). These variables, which are not well understood, have added to the difficulty in assessing treatment which in the past resulted in a degree of therapeutic nihilism. This view is certainly being replaced by growing optimism as several therapeutic strategies based on known or suspected aetiopathogenic mechanisms are being translated into an abundance of therapeutic trials. Given our present knowledge of the aetiopathogenesis of ALS, it seems doubtful that a single, specific compound will be capable of arresting further neuronal loss and promoting regeneration. It is to be expected that the greatest therapeutic success will derive from a combination of substances that are aimed at different aspects of the disorder. This approach is routinely used in cancer therapy. Polytherapies might include neuroprotective agents, strategies directed to combat the terminal cascade of events in ALS, and symptomatic measures. Some of these approaches are summarized in Table 7.1. There are other treatment strategies detailed in this chapter, which, although based on rational concepts, have been only marginally helpful, of no benefit, or whose role is unknown.

As discussed in Chapter 1, there is evidence suggesting that the incidence of ALS and other neurodegenerative disorders is increasing (Lillienfeld *et al.*, 1989; Brooks, 1996). If this proves correct, it implies that environmental factors may have an important triggering function for ALS, and

Table 7.1. *Therapeutic strategies in ALS*

Approach	Comments
Symptomatic	
Bimodal passive airway pressure	Timing and indications still to be determined
Percutaneous endoscopically placed gastrostomy	Timing and indications still to be determined
Mucolytic agents	Mucomyst 1–2 cc twice daily
	Radiation to the submandibular gland
Antidepressants	
Hypnotics	
Aids for daily living	
Neuroprotection	
Vitamin E	400–800 i.u. daily; neuronal protection not proven
Selegiline	5–10 mg daily; patch and liposomal delivery may be more effective
N-acetyl cysteine	50 mg/kg per day; difficult to administer; rescues cells exposed to oxidative stress
Dehydroepiandrosterone	200 mg daily; effectiveness not proven; has growth factor properties
Antiglutamate medications	
Riluzole	100 mg daily; approved for ALS; mode of action uncertain; effectiveness marginal
Lamotrigine	200–400 mg daily; value in ALS unproven; modulates presynaptic release
Branched chain amino acids	L-leucine, L-isoleucine, L-valine; enhance oxidation of glutamate
Gabapentin	800 mg daily; further trials needed; modulates brain glutamate dehydrogenase
Dextromethorphan	7 mg/kg per day; further trials needed; non-competitive glutamate receptor antagonist
Neurotrophic factors	
Insulin-like growth factor-1 (IGF-1, myotrophin)	0.05–0.1 mg/kg per day; slows rate of decline of Appel score, survival and forced vital capacity

continued efforts are needed to identify and eliminate such factors. This chapter reviews current therapies in ALS, how the nature of therapeutic trials has changed, and what might be anticipated in the future.

Trial design – placebo controls in ALS

Approval of the glutamate antagonist riluzole (Rilutek) as the first specific medication for use in ALS exemplifies how a large therapeutic trial can have a major impact on a disease, even though the drug itself has only marginal benefit. Riluzole has been shown to prolong life expectancy in ALS by a few weeks (Bensimon *et al.*, 1994; Lacomblez *et al.*, 1996; Miller *et al.*, 1996a). It has been approved in many countries and is the first drug designated for the treatment of ALS. However, the greatest benefit of the riluzole trial may be that it brought together an international group of neurologists with an interest in ALS. These investigators have established an International Consortium for ALS Clinical Trials, which has been developed under the auspices of the World Federation of Neurology (WFN) Research Subcommittee on Motor Neuron Diseases. The consortium has considered strategies for instituting clinical trials using combination therapy. Two such trials are underway at the time of writing, one using insulin-like growth factor (IGF-1) and riluzole, the other using SR57746A (Sanofi Recherche), which is an oral neurotrophic–neuroprotective agent with riluzole. The outcomes are awaited with interest. It is likely that most combination trials for the foreseeable future will include riluzole and/or IGF-1 (myotrophin) as they are the only approved therapies for ALS. Additionally, the riluzole trial and the many other trials planned or presently underway have had a major impact on the overall care of patients with ALS. New ALS clinics have been established, few of which had previously existed, and the quality of care of ALS patients is improving and becoming more uniform throughout much of the world. Public awareness of the disease has increased considerably.

The difficulties of placebo-controlled trials in ALS

Now that Rilutek has been approved for use in ALS, and IGF-1 is currently under an expanded access programme, true placebo-controlled trials in ALS are becoming difficult to implement, and some may consider them unethical. Furthermore, the Internet has resulted in a substantial information service being made available to patients, families and physicians. Patients are thus well informed about clinical trials that are proceeding, medications that may be of some value in ALS, and anecdotal therapies without proven benefit. This creates problems in the design of placebo-controlled trials. Many ALS patients are taking vitamin E, even though it does not cross the blood–brain barrier. Mega doses of vitamin E have not proven beneficial in ALS (Zech and Telford, 1943). Other prescription medications used by ALS patients include selegiline (Deprenyl), gabapentin (Neurontin) and lamotrigine (Lamictal). These medications are used in the treatment of PD and epilepsy, respectively, but may have some benefit in ALS. This uncontrolled polytherapy is difficult to monitor but is less likely to occur if the patient is offered an approved medication as a placebo.

One way of avoiding randomized, placebo-controlled trials is to use historical controls (Munsat, 1996). This necessitates monitoring disease progression prior to starting the trial drug (wash-in period) for two to three months. Alternatively, but less accurately, one can compare the patient's course with that of a previously studied large patient population. This has the advantage that 50 per cent fewer patients are required than for traditional placebo-controlled trials. To be successful, trials using historical controls assume the following: (i) the natural history of the disease is defined with reproducible accuracy; (ii) the progression of the disease is reasonably linear; (iii) the disease is uniformly progressive to death; (iv) the assessment instrument is reliable, valid and reproducible; and (v) the same measurement techniques can be used reliably across different centres. None of these assumptions holds entirely true for ALS; nevertheless, there does seem to be a role for natural history-controlled trials in phase II studies.

Designing clinical trials for ALS

Prior to 1940, there were no organized therapeutic trials in ALS and the use of placebo-controlled trials was unusual until the early 1970s. During the subsequent 20 years, parallel or cross-over placebo-controlled trials became more sophisticated. The conclusions of some previous studies may have to be re-examined in the light of imprecise definitions of ALS, diagnostic criteria and small sample sizes. An internationally accepted definition of ALS has only recently been formulated (Brooks, 1994; Munsat, 1995). This should aid in recruiting a homogeneous patient population, which is essential for the performance of good therapeutic trials. Because of the rapid and progressive nature of ALS cross-over trials, which compare equal, back-to-back periods of time (usually three to six months) on and off the trial drug in the same patient, they are best suited to phase II exploratory or screening trials. Sample size of past trials was frequently too small to reject a null hypothesis. It can be anticipated that most interventions in ALS will have a small benefit which will not be detected if the sample size is too small. The smallest sample size able to detect a significant but marginal benefit has been calculated to be about 120 patients (Munsat, 1995).

Table 7.2. *Common endpoints used in ALS trials*

Death, tracheotomy or use of continuous bimodal passive airway pressure (23/24 hours)
ALS Functional Rating Scale (ALSFRS)
Norris Scale: combines functional, observational and measured items
Appel ALS Rating Scale: includes pulmonary function testing and manual muscle testing
Vital capacity: usually forced vital capacity; slow vital capacity (VC) also used
Tufts Quantitative Neuromuscular Exam: measures standardized isometric muscle contraction
Sickness impact profile: assesses quality of life

Clear primary and secondary endpoints are vital to the success of trials. In recent years, as a better understanding of the natural history of ALS has unfolded, this aspect of trial design has greatly improved. Common primary and secondary endpoints are shown in Table 7.2.

Of the endpoints shown in Table 7.2, the TQNE is the most complex, using computerized measurement of isometric muscle contraction in arm, leg and bulbar muscles (Andres, Finison and Conlon, 1988). The measurements obtained from different limb muscles are combined to form a limb megascore that is applied into a grand megascore. Over most of the course of ALS, megascores decline linearly. This has been interpreted as reflecting a linear progression in the course of ALS (Munsat *et al.*, 1988). Other measurement scales suggest that, preterminally, the rate of progression of ALS increases. Although there is a large degree of objectivity in the TQNE, it requires special equipment such as a frame on to which the strain gauges for measuring isometric muscle strength are attached. It takes time to become familiar and consistent with measurement of the TQNE. Intra-individual rater variability is small and statistically acceptable, but inter-rater variability is large. This variability in inter-rater assessment is a major limitation in the use of TQNE for multicentre trials (Miller *et al.*, 1996c). TQNE is also time consuming, and needs considerable patient co-operation and motivation, which may vary from assessment to assessment. It has now become apparent that in addition to measurement of motor function, a secondary endpoint must include an assessment of quality of life. The issue became evident as a result of the riluzole trial in which this medication was found to extend life without measured concomitant improvement of well-being. The most commonly

Table 7.3. *The Sickness Impact Profile*

Ambulation
Mobility
Communication
Alertness behaviour
Social interaction
Sleep and rest
Eating
Emotional behaviour
Body care and movement
Home management
Recreations and pastimes
Work

---

employed quality-of-life measure is the Sickness Impact Profile (SIP), which looks at the 12 different categories listed in Table 7.3.

The SIP questionnaire is completed by the patient, usually at home. It is not ideal. It takes about 45 minutes to complete and patients who can no longer write have to be aided by a family member or other care-giver. This can result in a biased view or misinterpretation of how the patient really wants to answer some of the questions. There is clearly a need to devise a simpler profile which the patient can complete without having to rely on others.

Several recent trials have used death (or the requirement for tracheotomy) as an endpoint (Eisen *et al.*, 1993b; Bensimon *et al.*, 1994; Lacomblez *et al.*, 1996), and other ongoing trials will use it as a primary endpoint. This definitive endpoint allows for the accurate comparison of survival curves between drug and placebo. However, trials using death as an endpoint need to run over a long period, usually 18 months or more (approximately half the length of the natural course of the disease) in order to obtain sufficient information to construct a statistically sound survival curve. Also, patients with bulbar onset usually succumb to respiratory failure earlier, giving a false impression of shorter disease duration, which may not truly reflect the course of the disease. The cost of clinical trials has escalated as trial design has become more sophisticated and trials involve large numbers of patients at multiple centres, sometimes for many months. This translates into a significant increase in the cost of the drug when approved and results in reluctance of health care agencies to cover the added financial burden. It would be very helpful if future trials were to include a measure of anticipated cost–effectiveness into the outcome, as well as the usual primary and secondary endpoints. The Research Subcommittee of the WFN on Motor Neuron Diseases (1995) has recently discussed some of these aspects.

Neuroprotective therapy

The use of neuroprotective strategies in ALS has considerable appeal. However, there are inherent problems with this approach, such as the identification of neuroprotective agents, the choice of patients and the timing of therapy. The lack of a specific biochemical marker for sporadic and most types of familial ALS precludes preclinical identification of those who are at risk. It is very likely that the true onset of the disease predates development of clinical deficits by months, or maybe years, which could provide a 'therapeutic window' for the use of neuroprotective compounds to prevent the final cascade of events invariably leading to death. The data in Figure 1.1 (see Chapter 1) show that onset of this incubation period is not known. The data in Figure 1.3 (see Chapter 1) suggest that there may be a progressive failure of natural protective mechanisms starting around the age of 45 years, and this might be the time to commence protective therapy. There is now evidence that both excitotoxicity and free-radical accumulation with oxidative stress play important roles in neuron death in ALS (Eisen *et al.*, 1995). Evidence has also accumulated that may implicate iron deposition as a result of free radicals in the pathogenesis of the neurodegenerative disorders. This raises the possibility of periodic iron chelation as a therapeutic approach. Metal-induced oxidant stress damages fundamental biological mechanisms, initiating mitochondrial dysfunction, excitotoxicity and increased cytosolic free calcium, leading to cell death (Cohen and Werner, 1994; Olanow and Arendash, 1994). Free radicals are normally neutralized by efficient systems in the body that include antioxidant enzymes (SOD, catalase and glutathione peroxidase) and nutrient-derived antioxidants such as vitamin E, vitamin C, carotenes, flavonoids, glutathione, uric acid and taurine (Sardesai, 1995). Therefore, any or all of these antioxidants, or their precursors, might be useful protective agents. Protein carbonyl formation, which is thought to reflect free-radical damage to proteins (Sohal *et al.*, 1994), is significantly increased in the motor cortex in both sporadic ALS and familial ALS (FALS) (Bowling *et al.*, 1993; Robberecht *et al.*, 1994). This process, too, might be negated by antioxidants. Several medications with antioxidant properties are now available. They are considered below.

Vitamin E (DL-alpha-tocopherol)

Supplemental vitamin E taken in doses of 400 iu or greater is currently consumed by a sizeable part of the population over the age of 45 years. Vitamin E acts as a natural antioxidant and has free-radical scavenging properties (Duval and Poelman, 1995). Its antioxidant properties are enhanced by the addition of other antioxidants including vitamin C, beta-carotene and flavonoids (Tonstad, 1995). Recent evidence indicates that vitamin E is protective against heart disease (Bellizzi et al., 1994; Singh et al., 1994; Tonstad, 1995). Also, experimental studies suggest that high levels of vitamin E in tissues prior to injury are essential for biological efficacy in repair, and that its administration after injury is often ineffective, supporting the protective nature of vitamin E (Vatassery, 1992). Re-examination of the use of vitamin E for the treatment of ALS is underway. It did not prevent the progression of disease in the baseball player Lou Gehrig, but it may be that there are subpopulations with ALS that do respond to vitamin E (Reider and Paulson, 1997). Alpha-tocopherol and its oxidized form α-tocopherol quinone are significantly reduced in the cerebrospinal fluid of patients with ALS (Hideo et al., 1996). This suggests that there may be a role for vitamin E supplementation. Presumably, vitamin E needs access to neurons to have an effect, and unfortunately very little vitamin E crosses the blood–brain barrier after oral administration. Therefore, before it will have any protective effect on central nervous system structures, a delivery system that allows it to cross the blood–brain barrier is needed.

L-Deprenyl (Selegiline)

Deprenyl is a selective monoamine oxidase-B (MOA-B) inhibitor. Evidence indicates that it is not effective in the long-term treatment of PD but that it can protect dopaminergic neurons against 1-methyl-4-phenyl-1,2,3,6-tetrahydropyridine (MPTP) toxicity. These effects may not simply reflect its MOA inhibition, but may relate to a unique antioxidant property of Deprenyl (Wu et al., 1994). Deprenyl significantly increases superoxide dismutase and catalase activity (Kitani et al., 1994); both enzymes are essential for the normal neutralization of free radicals. Deprenyl delays the development of disability in patients with early PD who are not on anti-PD medication. This is probably the result of its neuroprotective antioxidant properties (Olanow, 1993).

MOA-B is markedly increased in post-mortem ALS spinal cord, specifically in regions of neuronal degeneration (motoneuron laminae and corticospinal tracts) and white matter of the cortex (Aquilonius *et al.*, 1992; Josson *et al.*, 1994). This makes Deprenyl a rational therapeutic consideration in ALS. Deprenyl has also been shown to exert trophic effects on spinal motoneurons and significantly enhances neurite outgrowth (Iwasaki *et al.*, 1994b). Thus far, only one small negative crossover study in 10 ALS patients who received Deprenyl 10 mg per day has been reported (Josson *et al.*, 1994). Larger studies are warranted, and Deprenyl should certainly be considered as a potentially useful component in a combination therapy. The failure to demonstrate efficacy may indicate that well-tolerated doses of 5–10 mg per day are inadequate to produce sufficient concentrations of the drug in the brain. Patch and liposomal administration are two possible solutions being investigated to overcome this. Both appear to increase drug concentration in target neurons by manyfold. A small, phase II trial of patch deprenyl in PD in presently underway.

N-acetyl cysteine

N-acetyl cysteine (NAC) is a precursor of glutathione, which is one of the most important natural intracellular antioxidant defence mechanisms. Chronic inhibition of superoxide dismutase activity in organotypic spinal cord cultures induces apoptotic degeneration of spinal motoneurons occurring over several weeks and this apoptosis can be entirely prevented by NAC (Rothstein *et al.*, 1994). NAC also partially rescues cultured neurons exposed to oxidative stress (Colton *et al.*, 1995) and has the additional properties of enhancing the contractile function of isolated diaphragm and inhibiting muscle fatigue in humans who are pretreated with NAC (Khawli and Reid, 1994; Reid *et al.*, 1994). There has been one recent, randomized, placebo-controlled trial in ALS using NAC. The medication was administered by subcutaneous infusion (50 mg/kg body weight per day) and 12-month survival was used as the primary endpoint measure. The study population comprised 35 patients and 30 placebo controls (Louwerse *et al.*, 1995). The power analysis of the sample size indicates that the number of patients used was too small and the results indeterminate, so that further trials with NAC are warranted. The medication is safe but difficult to administer and the infusion site can become quite sore.

Dehydroepiandrosterone

Considerable amounts of steroids ('neurosteroids') accumulate in the mammalian brain. They are metabolized from peripheral steroid hormones but are also synthesized de novo in brain glial cells (Lanthier and Patwardhan, 1986; Beaulieu, 1991). Two in particular – pregnenolone (3β-hydroxy-5-pregnen-20-one) and DHEA (3β-hydroxy-5-androsten-17-one) – have been identified in the brain in unconjugated and sulphated forms (DHEAS) (Mathur *et al.*, 1993). DHEA and DHEAS are found in uniform concentrations throughout all brain regions (Regelson, Kalimi and Loria, 1990; Regelson and Kalimi, 1994). There is minimal circadian cyclical activity, especially of DHEAS, and intra-assay and interassay coefficients of variation are small, so that reliable measurements can be made at any time. Serum concentrations of DHEA and DHEAS demonstrate a marked age-dependent decrease such that, by age 65 years, production of these hormones is approximately 10 to 20 per cent of that at age 20 years (Bird *et al.*, 1978; Birkenhager-Gillesse, Derksen and Lagaay, 1994). Although men have substantially higher serum concentrations of DHEA and DHEAS than women, the rate of decline of DHEAS with ageing is more rapid in men. There is a more significant reduction in DHEAS concentrations in men with ALS compared to age-matched controls. This is not the case in women with ALS.

Amongst other properties, DHEA has a trophic role in the maintenance of neurons. Less effective concentrations of DHEA are probably deleterious to neuronal survival, and this may be one explanation for the higher incidence of ALS in men compared to women (see Chapter 1; Eisen *et al.*, 1995). DHEA or its sulphate is possibly protective in a number of diverse non-neurological conditions such as systemic lupus erythematosus, myocardial disease and diabetes. It remains to be seen if they have neuroprotective properties. However, these neurosteroids are involved in maturation and ageing of the nervous system and may exert important trophic effects on neurons (Birkenhager-Gillesse *et al.*, 1994). DHEA and DHEAS can maintain the integrity and growth of isolated 14-day-old mouse embryonic brain tissue (Kalimi and Regelson, 1990), and induce inhibition of neurons associated with an increase of neurofilament and glial fibrillary acidic protein. They also enhance NMDA-gated currents whilst at the same time inhibiting the inhibitory glycinergic and $GABA_A$ amino acids (Kalimi and Regelson, 1990; Friess *et al.*, 1995). Recent studies indicate that serum DHEA levels are uniformly lower in men with AD compared to age-matched controls (Nasman *et al.*, 1991; Ebeling and

Koivisto, 1994), and DHEA (or DHEAS) has been shown to improve memory in rodents, as assessed by the speed at which animals find their way through a maze (Flood, Smith and Roberts, 1988; Mayo *et al.*, 1993).

An open label, phase I and II pilot study using oral DHEA, 200 mg daily, is being investigated for the treatment of ALS at our clinic. At the time of writing, survival curves are not significantly different between non-treated patients, or between treated patients and those on riluzole who are in an open label, extended treatment programme.

Glutamate excitotoxicity and antiglutamate therapy

Glutamate is an important excitatory neurotransmitter in the mammalian central nervous system. Receptors for glutamate are ubiquitous throughout the neocortex and glutamate excitotoxicity has been implicated in a variety of acute and chronic neurological disorders (Shaw, 1993; Zeman *et al.*, 1994; Leigh, 1994; Lipton and Rosenberg, 1994; Plaitakis, Fesdijan and Sashidharan, 1996; Rothstein, 1996a, 1996b). Patients with ALS have been reported to have increased plasma levels of glutamate, abnormal clearance of orally administered glutamate loads, and reduced glutamate contents (e.g. concentrations/mg wet weight) throughout the central nervous system (Plaitakis *et al.*, 1996). Extracellular glutamate concentrations are tightly regulated through high-affinity, sodium-dependent glutamate transporters. Three glutamate transporters, labelled GLT1, EAAC1 and GLAST, have been identified and have been shown to act specifically on neurons, astroglia and both neurons and astroglia, respectively (Rothstein *et al.*, 1992, 1995). In ALS, there is a variable loss of the transporter GLT1, which localizes to astroglia; a 20–40 per cent loss of EAAC1, which localizes mainly to the large cortical pyramidal neurons (presumably many are corticomotoneurons); but there are no abnormalities of GLAST, which is localized to neurons and astroglia in the cerebellum (Rothstein *et al.*, 1995). Reduced glutamate transporter presumably translates into increased glutamate contents within the brain. The therapeutic implication arising from these findings is the need for targeted therapy able to enhance the reduced glutamate transporter activity in ALS.

In the human spinal cord the distribution and density of glutamate transporter sites, measured by quantitative autoradiography, show highest levels in the substantia gelatinosa and central grey matter (Shaw *et al.*, 1994a). In ALS, binding density for these putative glutamate transporter ligands is reduced. The reduction in binding is more evident in the lumbar as compared to the cervical spinal cord and is not seen in PMA or other neurological disorders (Shaw *et al.*, 1994). Ways to counteract the deleterious effects of excess glutamate release include: (i) modulate presynaptic glutamatergic production; (ii) enhance glutamate transport; (iii) modify glutamate receptor activity; and (iv) protect neurons from glutamate-induced intracellular processes (Plaitakis *et al.*, 1996).

Glutamate antagonism could be used therapeutically in ALS, but it requires caution. Antagonism sufficient to protect neurons from degeneration might be dangerous, especially in the later stages of the disease when very few neurons remain. Glutamate reduction in this situation could compromise vital functions such as respiration. Baroreceptor control uses glutamate as its transmitter and, although there is no firm supporting evidence, failure of this reflex might underlie some of the anecdotal reports of unexpected, sudden death in patients with ALS whilst they are receiving either lamotrigine or riluzole. Another inherent problem in the use of glutamate antagonists is the difficulty in making accurate and easy measurements of glutamate concentrations in human tissues which would allow the administration of appropriate drug doses during the course of disease. Concentrations of ALS serum and cerebrospinal fluid are variable because of changing concentrations as the disease progresses, heterogeneity of disease progression or heterogeneity of the disease itself. In any event, there is a need to develop methodology for serial glutamate measurements to titrate optimal dose regimes of riluzole and other glutamate antagonists. Until this can be achieved, it is probably best to administer riluzole early in the disease and curtail or stop it later, especially in the face of impending respiratory failure. The glutamate receptors are complex, and selective inhibition of one or more components, while allowing normal function to proceed through others, would be the ideal for which to aim (see Chapter 4).

Modulation of presynaptic glutamatergic mechanisms

Lamotrigine (3,5-diamino-6 (2,3 dichlorophenyl)-1,2,4-triazine) is a phenyltriazine compound, initially developed as an anticonvulsant. It is thought to inhibit the synaptic release of glutamate through its blockade of voltage-gated sodium channels (Brodie, 1992). A single, placebo-controlled trial in 67 patients with ALS using an oral dose of 100 mg daily did not demonstrate a difference in survival between treated and untreated patients (Eisen *et al.*, 1993b). About a third of the treated patients noted a lessening of fasciculations. This effect was not quantified, but we have also observed that patients treated with riluzole and Gabapentin report a decrease in fasciculations. This effect suggests that the frequency of fasciculations in ALS may have some glutamate dependence. The lessening of fasciculations with disease progression may relate to reductions in glutamate concentrations near spinal neurons. The 100 mg dose of lamotrigine used in this study, the only reported trial of lamotrigine in ALS to date, was probably too small; 400 mg is routinely given in the treatment of epilepsy, and further trials using 200–400 mg doses in a larger study are warranted before it can be concluded that lamotrigine is not beneficial in ALS.

Riluzole (amino-2-trifluoromethoxy-6-benzothiazine), like lamotrigine, was also originally developed as an antiepileptic drug, but was not as effective as lamotrigine. As well as inhibiting glutamate release, it also blocks voltage-dependent sodium channels, antagonizes NMDA-evoked entry of calcium, and can affect the uptake of GABA (Hebert *et al.*, 1994; Hubert *et al.*, 1994; Mantz *et al.*, 1994). However, its mode of action as a glutamate antagonist is poorly understood. Riluzole is the only drug thus far that has been approved for the treatment of ALS in some European and Asian countries as well as in the USA. It has not been approved in Canada and Australia. Riluzole appears to extend the survival of ALS patients on average for a few weeks and is not associated with improved well-being, improved quality of life or improved muscle strength (Lacomblez *et al.*, 1996; Miller *et al.*, 1996a). In an initial phase II study from France, which involved 155 ALS patients (Bensimon *et al.*, 1994), riluzole given in a dose of 100 mg daily was found to extend median survival by a mean of 90 days compared to placebo. The treatment effect was most marked with patients who had a bulbar onset. This remains an unexplained finding (Rowland, 1994b) but was not seen in the larger multinational trial that involved 959 patients, 301 of whom were treated with riluzole. In both studies, the difference between the treated and the placebo Kaplan–Meier survival curves lost significance with time: at about 12 to 15 months, the survival difference was no longer significant. Unfortunately, the large, multinational riluzole trial was terminated before it became clear whether or not the curves would meet (Fig. 7.1). The loss of significance at 12–15 months might simply reflect that the disease had progressed to a point beyond that at which riluzole could have an effect. Failure of sustained significance has also been interpreted as being due to reduced power because of too few surviving patients remaining toward the end of the trials. However, the loss of significance

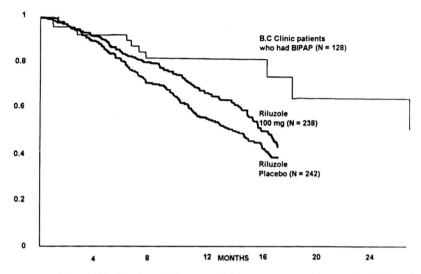

Figure 7.1. Kaplan–Meier survival curves comparing survival of ALS patients taking riluzole 100 mg daily, placebo, or riluzole and BIPAP. The riluzole data were supplied by Rhone-Poulenc-Rorer Inc., which sponsored the worldwide multicentre dose-ranging, placebo-controlled riluzole trial. The use of BIPAP in our clinic has increased and there are presently no 'standards' for its institution. Also, not all of the 128 patients who had BIPAP had riluzole. These variables make statistical comparison difficult. However, use of BIPAP is apparently favourable in terms of survival.

could reflect a deleterious effect of the drug later in the disease. There is, in fact, experimental evidence to support this. Transgenic mice having mutations in the SOD1 gene were given riluzole in much higher relative doses than were used in the human studies. Benefit was significant but also limited to the early and mid-terms of the induced disease (Gurney, 1996, unpublished). There is a dose-dependent effect of riluzole: 50 mg is not effective but 100 mg and 200 mg doses show similar efficacy. The 100 mg dose is less likely to induce side-effects, the commonest of which include nausea, dizziness, neurasthenia and a rise in liver function tests without overt liver disease, and this is the recommended dose for treating ALS.

Non-NMDA receptor-mediated neurotoxicity

The receptor for AMPA is a subtype of the ionotropic glutamate receptor of the non-NMDA type selectively gated by AMPA. It mediates neuronal damage in adult and infant brains, and BOAA, an AMPA agonist, is a candidate agent for neurolathyrism. When AMPA is continuously infused intrathecally for seven days into adult rats, it induces a dose-dependent, delayed-onset motor neurological deficit associated with damage to anterior horn cells (Nakamura, Kamakura and Kwak, 1994). This effect can be antagonized by concomitant administration of a non-NMDA receptor antagonist, but not by a NMDA receptor antagonist. Support for involvement of non-NMDA receptors in ALS comes from results of autoradiographic measurements of the density and distribution of AMPA and kainate receptors in human motor cortex and spinal cord (Shaw *et al.*, 1994b). Compared to normal controls, there is increased binding of kainate but not AMPA in the deep layers of the motor cortex of ALS patients. Both receptor subtypes show increased binding in the spinal cord of ALS patients compared to controls, but this seems to be restricted entirely to patients with combined upper and lower motoneuron features. There has been considerable research into AMPA antagonists in recent years, but there are currently no suitable AMPA antagonists available for human studies. However, such medications are likely to be important in ALS and several may become available for phase II studies in the near future.

Therapeutic agents that may act on glutamate metabolism
Branched-chain amino acids

Glutamate is metabolized partly by the enzyme glutamate dehydrogenase (GDH) that interconverts glutamate and α-ketoglutarate. GDH can be activated in vitro by the branched-chain amino acids (BCAAs) L-leucine and, to a lesser extent, L-isoleucine (Yielding and Tomkins, 1961). These BCAAs enhance glutamate oxidation by brain synaptosomes (Erecinska and Nelson, 1990). They are readily absorbed after oral administration; however, there is competitive transport in the intestine between different BCAAs such that intake of one BCAA decreases plasma and cerebrospinal fluid concentrations of the others. This can be prevented if L-leucine, L-isoleucine and L-valine are administered together – an approach that has been employed in several therapeutic trials (Plaitakis *et al.*, 1988b; Testa *et al.*, 1989; Plaitakis *et al.*, 1992; Beghi, 1993; Steiner, 1994; Tandan *et al.*, 1996). Some of these studies showed a trend in favour of the treatment group but none reached a statistically significant level. In all but one trial the sample size was small (Steiner, 1994). The most recent study (Tandan *et al.*, 1996) is the best validated: 31 patients received BCAA as a mixture of 12 g of L-leucine, 8 g of L-isoleucine and 6.4 g of L-valine powder daily for six months. Another 32 patients received L-threonine (4 g daily) and pyridoxal phosphate (160 mg daily), which is a cofactor in the conversion of L-threonine to glycine by the enzyme threonine aldolase. This study, which measured a variety of endpoints, showed no beneficial effect of either BCAA or L-threonine compared to controls. There was, in fact, a greater loss of pulmonary function in both treatment groups, which may have been due to an adverse effect of these amino acids.

Gabapentin (Neurontin)

This drug, which has been used successfully in the treatment of epilepsy, is a BCAA homologue and is stero-similar to L-leucine (Taylor, 1994). It is a potent inhibitor of branched-chain aminotransferase and, like L-leucine, it modulates brain GDH activities, but is concentrated in astrocytes to a greater extent than L-leucine. Branched-chain amino acids can serve as precursors for glutamate, and it has been postulated that Gabapentin could decrease the synthesis of glutamate (Taylor, 1994). Unfortunately, to achieve therapeutic levels which can significantly antagonize glutamate synthesis, the doses of Gabapentin required are toxic and cannot be tolerated. However, smaller concentrations of Gabapentin can sensitize GDH to stimulate L-leucine, which in turn enhances glutamate oxidation by brain synaptosomes (Plaitakis et al., 1996). This suggests that combination therapy with Gabapentin and BCAAs may have merit, and this combination is worthy of a therapeutic trial.

A recent placebo-controlled trial used Gabapentin alone, at a dose of 800 mg daily for six months in 152 patients. The primary endpoint was the slope of the arm megascore of maximum voluntary isometric strength (Miller et al., 1996b). The megascore was a summation of eight arm muscles standardized against a reference ALS population. Vital capacity was used as a secondary endpoint. Differences between treated and control groups did not reach significance, but there was a trend in favour of the treated group, suggesting that further studies with a larger sample and a longer trial period are needed.

Agents acting on glutamate receptors

Dextromethorphan is a sigma opioid agonist and a selective, non-competitive antagonist of the NMDA subtype of glutamate receptor. It is a component of most cough medication. In-vitro experiments have demonstrated the ability of dextromethorphan to antagonize NMDA-induced and glutamate-induced excitotoxicity in both central and peripheral motoneurons (Church, Lodge and Berry, 1985; Choi, Peters and Viseskul, 1987). Asmark *et al.* (1993) treated a small group of patients with ALS in a placebo-controlled, cross-over trial in which 150 mg/day of dextromethorphan was administered orally for 12 weeks. No benefit was noted. High-dose therapy (about 7 mg/kg per day) has been shown to be tolerable and phase II and III trials using larger doses are underway (Hollander *et al.*, 1994).

Therapy with immunosuppressants

There are some arguments to support a role for disordered immunity as a possible mechanism in the death and degeneration of motoneurons in ALS (Appel *et al.*, 1993, 1995). This need not imply that disordered immunity is the primary cause of ALS, but that immune mechanisms may play an important role in the ultimate demise of the involved neurons. The presence of other autoimmune disorders in ALS patients, such as paraproteinaemias and lymphomas, the presence of lymphocytes and activated macrophages in ALS spinal cord, IgG within ALS motoneurons and antibodies against calcium channels are all circumstantial evidence for an autoimmune process in the disorder (Appel *et al.*, 1995). However, many of the features typical of a conventional autoimmune disorder are lacking (Drachman *et al.*, 1995). For example, there is no inflammatory infiltrate, and cytokine levels, such as interleukin-6, are normal, indicating that there is no tissue response to inflammation. The course of ALS has not been significantly altered by treatment with a variety of immuno-therapies including steroids, cyclophosphamide, cyclosporin, plasma-phaeresis and total lymphoid irradiation (Drachman *et al.*, 1994). However, the approaches used to date have not been targeted. Targeted therapy directed against relevant peptide epitopes, as, for example, the calcium channel antibodies seen in a large number of patients with ALS (Appel *et al.*, 1995) or the T-cell receptors with which they may interact, might show an effect.

Aspirin and other non-steroidal anti-inflammatory drugs

Several years ago it was observed that there is a remarkable proliferation of activated microglia expressing high levels of major histocompatibility complex glycoproteins (especially HLA-DR) in the brains of patients dying of neurodegenerative diseases (McGeer and McGeer, 1994; McGeer, Rogers and McGeer, 1994). This led to the postulate that there was an autodestructive inflammatory process perpetuating neuronal damage and demise once it had commenced. This hypothesis provided a rationale for treatment with anti-inflammatory medications. It is likely that AD and PD share some pathogenic aspects. Observations that there is a reduced risk of developing AD and that the rate of disease progression is slower in patients that have been previously treated with non-steroidal anti-inflammatory drugs (NSAIDs) including aspirin, encourages their use in ALS (Breitner *et al.*, 1994; Rich *et al.*, 1995; Andersen *et al.*, 1995). A six-month, double-blind, placebo-controlled study of 100–150 mg/day of indomethacin lessened the rate of cognitive decline in patients with mild to moderately severe AD when compared to placebo controls (Rogers *et al.*, 1993). It is not known if aspirin or chronic use of other NSAIDs confers a similar protection in ALS. This effect would be more difficult to substantiate in ALS than in AD, which has an incidence that is approximately 200 times that of ALS. Nevertheless, given the overall safety of aspirin and its proven value in cardiovascular and cerebrovascular disease, it would be a reasonable medication to try as a potential neuroprotective agent in ALS.

Neurotrophic factors

Development of the vertebrate nervous system is characterized by an overproduction of neurons followed by naturally occurring, programmed cell death (apoptosis). During embryogenesis, neuronal differentiation and death of neurons are regulated by trophic factors supporting distinct neuronal populations (Hefti, 1994). The process is cell-type specific. For example, whereas embryogenic cell death of cranial and spinal motoneurons can be modified by muscle extract, this is not the case for sensory and sympathetic neurons (Seeburger and Springer, 1993). In the adult, neurotrophic factors play an important role in plasticity, structural integrity and repair subsequent to injury (DiStefano, 1993; Lindholm, 1994; Gao *et al.*, 1995; Ikeda *et al.*, 1995a). With maturation, there is some evidence suggesting that motoneuronal trophic dependence shifts from peripheral to centrally derived signals, implying there are trophic factors that also modulate the maintenance of corticomotoneuronal connections (Lindholm, 1994; Hefti, 1994). Large numbers of neurotrophic factors have been identified and unquestionably more will follow. There has been

Table 7.4. *Clinical trials using neurotrophic factors in ALS*

Growth factor	Current status	Comments
rhIGF-1 (insulin-like growth factor-1, myotrophin)	NDA to FDA	Phase III studies in 449 patients European and North American studies
GDNF (glial cell-derived neurotrophic factor)	Phase I	Intraventricular injection
BDNF (brain-derived neurotrophic factor)	Phase III	Negative; endpoints survival and FVC 283 patients
	Phase I	Intrathecal injection underway
rhCNTF (ciliary neurotrophic factor)	Phase III	Negative
Sanofi SR 57746A (orally active neurotrophic factor)	Phase III	Underway

NDA = new drug application; FDA = Food and Drug Administration.

a recent surge of clinical trials using a variety of trophic factors in ALS; they are summarized in Table 7.4.

Neurotrophins

Neurotrophins are a related family of neurotrophic peptides which includes nerve growth factor (NGF), BDNF and NT-3 and NT-4/5. They are expressed in a variety of adult brain regions and exert their actions by binding to cell surface receptors. BDNF promotes survival of developing motoneurons, inhibits the axotomy-induced cell death of motoneurons, and prevents glutamate-induced neuronal cell death (Lindholm, 1994). It also retards motor dysfunction in wobbler mice, a mouse model of PMA (Ikeda *et al.*, 1995a). BDNF has undergone phase III clinical trials involving 283 patients. The drug appears safe and was well tolerated. Initial studies were encouraging and appeared to induce significant improvement in FVC. However, final analysis of the trials with BDNF was negative (see Table 7.4).

Ciliary neurotrophic factor

Ciliary neurotrophic factor is a cytosolic molecule that is expressed post-natally in myelinating Schwann cells and in a subpopulation of astrocytes (Sendtner *et al.*, 1992). High levels of CNTF are detected in Schwann cells, where it may be released as a result of nerve injury and thereby reduce death of motoneurons. CNTF normally has a role in maintaining mature motoneurons and is protective against inherited lower motoneuron disease in the wobbler mouse, retarding disease progression and improving muscle strength (Mitsumoto *et al.*, 1994). Disruption of the mouse CNTF gene results in progressive muscle atrophy, reduction in muscle strength and loss of motoneurons in adult mice (Masu *et al.*, 1993). Compared to normal controls, CNTF-immunoreactivity is markedly decreased in the ventral horn of spinal cord from ALS patients but apparently not in the motor cortex (Anand *et al.*, 1994). These observations form the basis on which trials using CNTF in ALS were begun. Two recently completed multicentre, double-blind, placebo-controlled trials, each involving about 600 patients, were negative. The drug was administered subcutaneously, for six months in three dosage arms, randomized to 0.5, 2 or 5 μg/kg per day of recombinant CNTF (rhCNTF). The primary efficacy endpoint was the change from baseline to the last on-treatment value of a combination megascore for limb strength (maximum voluntary isometric contraction) and pulmonary function. The four treatment groups were similar at base-line with respect to age, sex, disease duration and muscle strength values. There was no beneficial effect with any of the doses tested and there was an increased number of deaths at the highest dose level (Miller *et al.*, 1996c).

The failure of rhCNTF to improve ALS is probably due to a combination of factors. Some of these are shared by other neurotrophic factors and include difficulty in delivery of the drug, short half-life of the drug as measured in the cerebrospinal fluid, and limited ability to target the drug to neurons that are specifically involved in ALS. The highest tolerable dose of rhCNTF that was administered (5 μg/kg) is probably far too small to have an effect. rhCNTF is not detected in cerebrospinal fluid even at doses of 20 μg/kg (Dittrich, Thoenen and Sendtner, 1994). Even if higher concentrations were achievable, the drug dissipates in a few minutes (Longo, 1994). Long-term therapy is likely to be associated with antibody formation and drug inactivation, but details about this are not known. Higher, effective, concentrations could be achieved using intrathecal injections and/or use of an infusion pump. A novel and possibly a more rewarding approach is the use of gene therapy (Aebischer and Kato, 1994). Polymer encapsulated cells genetically engineered to release a neurotrophic factor can be implanted subcutaneously or even intrathe-cally, permitting slow, continuous release of their active proteins. Rejec-tion of cells can be prevented or minimized by their isolation using a semipermeable membrane. This also removes the risk of tumour forma-tion. The polymer is readily removable in the event of a problem.

Insulin-like growth factors

Insulin-like growth factors IGF-1 and IGF-2 are structurally related but encoded by distinct genes. In brain cell cultures they promote neuronal survival and neurite outgrowth (Carson *et al.*, 1993), and IGF-1 can induce sprouting of spinal motoneurons. In ALS, spinal cord IGF-1 binding is increased (up-regulation) compared to controls. This occurs in a widespread fashion and is not restricted to the ventral grey matter of the spinal cord (Adem *et al.*, 1994; Gimenez-Gallego and Cuevas, 1994; Doré *et al.*, 1996). Recent North American and European placebo-controlled studies, using recombinant human IGF-1 (rhIGF-1, myotrophin) showed some efficacy in ALS (Murphy *et al.*, 1995; Lange *et al.*, 1996). Treatment of 449 patients with ALS was randomized to placebo or 0.05 or 0.10 mg/kg per day of subcutaneous myotrophin given over a period of nine months. Change in the Appel ALS (AALS) rating scale (which assesses swallowing, speech, respiratory and muscle function) was used as the primary endpoint. Patients receiving the 0.10 mg/kg dose showed approximately 35 per cent less deterioration in the AALS rating scale, as compared to the placebo group. The improvement occurred especially in relation to preservation of vital capacity and was matched by improvement in quality of life as measured by the SIP. Injections were well tolerated and there were no important adverse experiences that could be attributable to rhIGF-1. Survival was not a primary endpoint, but information regarding this variable was obtained during a subsequent period of open-label treatment. Analysis of all patients based on randomization showed a significant difference in survival, with survival time averaging 164 days longer in the 0.10 mg/kg per day treatment group.

Glial cell-derived neurotrophic factor

Glial cell-derived neurotrophic factor has been shown to produce significant protective and survival-promoting effects on motoneurons. When applied locally to the nerve, injected subcutaneously or administered directly into the cerebrospinal fluid, GDNF protects motoneurons from the effects of axotomy. A phase I study involving 24 patients in six centres and administering GDNF intraventricularly is presently underway. Endpoints include FVC, survival and isometric muscle strength testing. Preclinical studies have indicated that this method of administration is 100 times more potent than subcutaneous administration and that distribution to the upper motoneurons may be more effective with intraventricular administration than with intrathecal injection.

Fibroblast growth factors

Fibroblast growth factors include a family of nine members; six of which are biologically and structurally closely related. (For a recent review on FGFs, see Gimenez-Gallego and Cuevas, 1994.) FGFs induce a remarkably broad spectrum of biological activities, including mitogenesis in practically all mesoderm and neuroectoderm derived cells. In healthy animals, only two (acidic and basic FGFs) are detectable and are widely distributed. For example, acidic FGF is associated with neurons and basic FGF with astrocytes. FGFs are specifically abundant in neurons where mitogenesis is sparse. Up to the present time, there have been no trials in ALS using FGFs.

Sanofi-SR57746A

Sanofi-SR57746A is under development. It is a potent, orally active neurotrophic factor that also has neuroprotective properties (Fournier *et al.*, 1993). It penetrates the blood–brain barrier. The compound may mimic the activity of a number of endogenous neurotrophins, either acting directly on neurons as a neurotrophic factor or by activating the synthesis of neurotrophins. In vivo, SR57746A reduces histological, neurochemical and functional deficits produced in a variety of neuronal central and peripheral nerve models in rodents and primates. It is also a $5HT_{1A}$ receptor ligand and has anxiolytic and antidepressant effects in animal models. SR57746A in doses of 1–4 mg has been used in preliminary (phase II) studies in France involving 117 healthy volunteers and 110 patients with ALS. The ALS patients showed slower rates of decline in muscle strength testing, less decrease in vital capacity, and improved limb and bulbar functional scales, compared to non-treated patients after 32 weeks of treatment with 2 mg of SR57746A. A large (1000 patients) multi-national, multicentre, phase III trial of SR57746A is underway.

Therapy combining two or more neurotrophic factors

The original concept that trophic factors are strictly target-tissue derived needs revision. It has become apparent that several different factors may be compartmentalized within a 'functional system' (Nishi, 1994). For example, in the motor unit, acidic FGF is present in the anterior horn cell, basic FGF in the astrocyte, CNTF in the Schwann cell and BDNF and FGF-5 in the muscle fibres. It is possible that therapy with trophic factors may be more efficacious when two or more factors are used in combination. It might be anticipated that cocktails containing several growth factors would be considered in the future treatment of ALS. This statement is made in the knowledge that currently there is no evidence for defective neurotrophism in ALS. However, when mice were treated with both CNTF and BDNF, administered on alternate days, the combined therapy was able to arrest disease progression for one month (Mitsumoto *et al.*, 1994b). Either factor alone slows but does not arrest the disease process.

Calcium channel blockade

Glutamate-induced excitotoxicity is complex and multifactorial but a major component of the terminal events mediating neuronal injury and death involves excessive influx of calcium into neurons through ionic channels (Eisen, 1995). NMDA receptor activation and/or increased neuronal calcium activate a series of intracellular enzymes (e.g. protein kinase C, phospholipases, proteases, protein phosphatases and nitric oxide synthase). In theory, calcium channel blockers, which interrupt this final common process, should be of therapeutic value.

Verapamil, a derivative of papaverine, blocks calcium in neurons (as well as smooth and cardiac muscle fibres) (Greenberg, 1994). Verapamil was administered at a maximum dose of 240 mg/day by mouth to 72 ALS patients using a cross-over design. Two natural history periods of 1–3 months pretreatment and 10–12 months post-treatment were compared with a treatment period of 4–9 months. The endpoints measured were pulmonary function and limb megascores by TQNE. The medication was ineffective in slowing disease progression (Ziv *et al.*, 1994; Miller *et al.*, 1996d). Further, larger trials with calcium channel blockers are probably warranted.

Symptomatic measures in ALS

Respiratory care

Resistive inspiratory training and low doses of theophylline, which improves diaphragmatic contraction, can both help respiratory function.

However, the use of BIPAP, which actively assists the inspiratory phase of respiration, is rapidly becoming standard in North America (Hopkins *et al.*, 1996). Its use is more limited in Europe. Most patients learn to use the device confidently within a short time period, but in about 10 per cent of patients the nasal mask or nasal pillows employed to deliver pressure during inspiration cannot be tolerated. Little is known regarding the appropriate time to initiate BIPAP or the proper settings to use, and objective measures of efficacy need to be determined. Respiratory failure may be imminent when FVC falls below 50 per cent of age-predicted norms. This is frequently associated with paradoxical respiration, the inward abdominal movement on inspiration, as the paretic diaphragm is pulled up into the chest by the accessory muscles of respiration.

Despite these vagaries, it is already evident that BIPAP results in major symptomatic improvement: appetite returns and nutrition improves. Early morning headache, a common manifestation of hypoxia and carbon dioxide retention, is relieved and, with better sleep, daytime somnolence is reduced or abolished. We began instituting early BIPAP about two years ago and found it induces a significant increase in survival of patients with ALS (see Fig. 7.1). The Kaplan–Meier analysis for the patients who were looked after at the British Columbia ALS Clinic is compared with the survival curves of the worldwide riluzole 100 mg dose and the placebo arm of the trial. Many of the patients who had BIPAP were also on 100 mg of riluzole daily as part of an open-label extension study. We do not have comparative results regarding the time of instituting BIPAP, for how many hours it was used or clinical status of the patient. Nevertheless, the difference in survival is significant ($p < 0.01$) and underscores the impression of others that timely institution of BIPAP may be very important. It is also likely that timely institution of BIPAP may reduce the incidence of unexpected sudden death. This appears most frequently in patients who have upper motoneuron dysfunction and associated poor respiratory drive. Shortness of breath when supine and a FVC of $\leqslant 50$ per cent of the age–height-predicted value are both good indications to institute BIPAP (Renston, DiMarco and Supinski, 1994; Kramer *et al.*, 1995; Elliott and Simonds, 1995). We also now monitor diaphragmatic EMG routinely (see Chapter 4). If denervation is present, as indicated by moderate or profuse fibrillation potentials, we like to consider the use of BIPAP even if other measures (a significantly compromised FVC and clinical features of respiratory difficulty) are absent. There is probably a good correlation between FVC and diaphragmatic denervation, but statistical evidence for this needs to be determined.

Further studies are also required to determine how chest wall (intercostal) involvement versus diaphragmatic denervation influences outcome.

Ventilatory support using BIPAP eventually fails and then the issue of tracheotomy and long-term ventilation needs consideration. It raises many ethical dilemmas. Home ventilation, although available, is expensive and puts additional burden on the family and care-givers. The annual cost of home ventilation is about US$250 000, including rental, nursing care and maintenance. The annual cost of BIPAP is around US$5000. Modern ventilators are relatively small in size and weight and are quite mobile. They can be fitted with a Passy–Muir valve or similar adaptation that allows speech to be maintained. This encourages their use in a few patients. Steven Hawkins, the renowned physicist and mathematician, is a notable example of an ALS patient having led a useful and fulfilling life on a 'permanent' ventilator. However, in our experience, fewer than 5 per cent of patients elect to go this route. There are cultural differences; for example in Japan, use of tracheotomy in ALS is more frequent than elsewhere. In some respects the development of BIPAP has lessened the concern for tracheotomy ventilation. It is vital that the issue of permanent ventilation is discussed in a timely fashion with patients and their relatives: there have been too many instances of unwanted tracheotomy precipitated by an acute respiratory event. Nevertheless, the view that once instituted, long-term ventilation cannot be stopped is untrue in many countries. Legal authorities do not regard withdrawal of tracheotomy and ventilation as being assisted suicide. In Canada this view has been tested in the courts and the ruling was in favour of allowing discontinuation of permanent ventilation.

Nutritional care

Like BIPAP, enteral nutrition delivered via percutaneous endoscopically placed gastrostomy (PEG) is associated with a significant increase in survival of ALS patients (Kasarskis and Neville, 1996). In some patients, inserting the tube into the jejunum (J-tube) is preferred since it obviates the problem of gastric reflux which can occur with a PEG. Most patients with ALS have a decreased caloric intake. The events leading to this are complex and not fully understood. A lack of food intake is probably the major factor producing a negative caloric balance, but despite this an adequate protein consumption is often maintained. Energy demands are increased as respiratory function becomes compromised and this, even in the face of relative immobility, adds to the negative caloric balance. It is possible that the chronic deficit in caloric intake in ALS hastens muscle degradation over and above that resulting from loss of anterior horn cells. This scenario dictates timely, if not relatively early, institution of feeding via a PEG tube; a view more frequently held in North America than in Europe. Once patients understand the rationale behind employment of PEG, and the fact that it does not preclude taking food by mouth, they are much more likely to agree to have the procedure.

The beneficial effects of BIPAP and PEG are an important consideration in evaluating the outcome of new clinical trials. Their effects may mask those of drug efficacy, especially if drug effects are rather marginal.

Rehabilitative measures

Any improvement in muscle strength, albeit temporary, is appreciated by ALS patients. However, conventional physiotherapy cannot achieve much improvement in muscle strength in ALS. The effect of exercise has never been well studied in this disorder, but vigorous exercise and isometric weights are possibly counterproductive. Increasing release of acetylcholine at the neuromuscular junction may result in temporarily improved muscle function. Use of the slow potassium channel blocker 3,4-diaminopyridine (DAP), which enhances acetylcholine release from the nerve terminal, has been shown to be well tolerated and associated with a gain in muscle strength in ALS (Aisen *et al.*, 1995). Similarly, pyridostigmine (Mestinon) given in modest doses of 60 mg t.i.d. may also produce a temporary increase in muscle strength. However, the main aim should be directed to allowing patients to function as comfortably as possible given their neurological deficit. Table 7.5 lists some of the measures that can help with daily living.

Excessive salivation and thick mucus

Both are common problems in ALS. Several means can be used to tackle excessive salivation. We have found transdermal patches containing scopolamine applied twice weekly very helpful. A home suction machine is usually required in more advanced cases. We have recently started a trial of small-dose radiation to the submandibular glands. Of 12 ALS patients, five had more than three months of marked relief. Two others had no improvement in salivation, and the rest had modest but short-lasting relief. One patient developed a radiation rash that lasted a week but that responded to prednisone. Otherwise there were no side-effects. Thick

Table 7.5. *Some aids in daily living for patients with ALS*

Mobility
Neck support
Arm slings/wrist splints
Cane
Walker
Ankle foot orthotic
Electric wheelchair, scooter

Communication
Foam-padded pen
Magic pad/pen and paper
Computerized writing
Voice-activated computer

Disability clothing
Button hooks
Zipper pulls
Velcro shoe lacing and fastening

Home modifications
Wheelchair-accessible ramps
Grab bars
Adaptive utensils
Wheelchair-accessible kitchen and bathroom
Hoyer lift

mucus is a less frequent problem and can be managed by use of a mucolytic agent such as Mucomyst in a dose of 1–2 cc twice daily.

Future therapeutic directions

Despite the encouraging advances that have occurred in the treatment of ALS, the therapeutic effects of specific medications have been only modest or marginal. Nevertheless, when comparing Kaplan–Meier survival curves in our clinic between 1980–1987 and 1988–1996, the difference is very significant, with an increased survival of approximately 12 months. We suspect the same holds true for other large ALS clinics. There are at least three reasons for the longer survival in recent years: the earlier and more frequent implementation of gastrostomy, the institution of CPAP and BIPAP, and better monitoring of patients through better organized clinics. That these measures alone can add to survival so dramatically is encouraging, and predicts that, with the addition of other drug combinations, one can anticipate continued lengthening of survival for patients with ALS.

New drug delivery systems

The rationale that underscores some of the most promising medications (antioxidants, glutamate antagonists and growth factors) is well founded but largely limited by an inability to achieve high concentrations of drug at target neurons. Possible methods for better delivery include infusion pumps, liposomal packaging of drugs, delivery via a skin patch or inhalation. A phase II trial of the first intraventricular delivery in ALS using GDNF is presently underway.

Gene therapy

With ageing, genetic information becomes subject to random errors and damage to informational molecules. Eventually, the number of cells that can function normally is reduced to a critical level, which results in the failure of specific physiological functions. All diseases, to some degree, have a genetic component. Many genes are 'susceptibility' genes; that is, they do not cause the disease per se but render one susceptible when other events occur. Drugs can be targeted to counteract the effects of deleterious genes or to replace the malfunctioning or non-functioning proteins that result from gene mutations. Better still, mutant genes will soon be able to be replaced by normal genes through gene transfer. There are many technical problems to overcome before gene therapy becomes a reality, but this technique is no longer in the realms of science fiction. Many, probably 100 or more, disease genes that predispose to a variety of disorders will be identified in the future. Some genes degrade with ageing in association with oxidative stress, mitochondrial failure, excitotoxicity and other mechanisms yet to be clarified. It is these that are probably responsible for neurodegeneration and ALS. The total human genome is estimated to have 50 000 to 100 000 genes. It will become possible to perform genetic fingerprinting and determine the potential of future health and disease, and possibly predict those who are at risk for ALS. Neuroprotective therapy will then have a rational basis. The susceptibility genes, and there are likely to be several specific to ALS, need to be determined. Some possible candidate genes for sporadic ALS include the P2 blood group gene, the NF-H gene – although abnormalities of it in ALS have only rarely been described – and possibly the PV gene. The fact that even some of the Cu/Zn–SOD mutations, usually identified with familial ALS, have been described in some cases which appear to be sporadic ALS is commented on in Chapter 1. The susceptibility genes have very diverse functions, and a common thread, if there is one, is not apparent. However, they all lie in close contiguity to the terminal part of the long arm of the chromosome which they occupy. Telomerase is an enzyme that regulates the growth of the chromosome's terminal (the telomere) where there is a piece of DNA that is critical to ageing. Degradation of this may be responsible for the breakdown of genetic material in this region.

Summary

Survival of patients with ALS has improved considerably in recent years. This is mainly due to the more frequent and timely implementation of BIPAP and PEG. Drug trials have become large, multinational and expensive. However, their sophistication has led to the establishment of many ALS clinics with improved levels of care. An international consortium, under the auspices of the Research SubCommittee of the WFN on Motor Neuron Diseases, has been established for the design and performance of drug trials in ALS. It should help facilitate interactions between pharmaceutical companies and governmental regulatory agencies, which is essential for the development of combination therapies. It will also help establish the best endpoints to measure sample size and duration of trials. Currently, only riluzole (which inhibits glutamate release at synapses) has been approved for specific use in ALS. This medication confers modest benefit only, and this is likely to be the case for other drugs marketed for ALS. It can be anticipated that appropriate combination therapy, as has been utilized in cancer, will lengthen the survival of ALS patients. The efficacy of some of the medications that currently only induce modest benefit may be improved by better delivery systems, such as liposomal packaging, use of patch or inhalation and intraventricular pump reservoirs. Targeted therapy, using gene vectors, directed towards specific receptors will be important. However, at present, all medications in ALS have been directed towards tackling the final cascade of events or promoting sprouting of presumably sick neurons. The ultimate aim should be to develop a marker for the disease that will allow identification of people at risk so that early protective therapy can be instituted.

8

The overlap syndromes

As described in the previous chapters, the established view of ALS is that of a corticomotoneuronal system disease with involvement of bulbar and spinal motoneurons as well as corticospinal tracts and other descending pathways. The specific pattern of involvement makes the disease relatively unique. This particular selective vulnerability holds true for the majority of patients, but there are some who exhibit features of motoneuron destruction and loss of descending tracts with additional features indicative of involvement of structures outside the 'motor system'. For instance, some ALS patients have dementia, extrapyramidal features, sensory findings or autonomic involvement. How many such patients there are is difficult to determine. These cases are often identified in large ALS clinics where more vigorous case ascertainment is achieved. For example, overt clinical dementia occurs in fewer than 5 per cent of ALS patients (Strong et al., 1996). But, using formal psychometric testing, as many as 35 per cent of ALS patients show some evidence of cognitive impairment. PET has revealed abnormalities in dopamine metabolism in a number of ALS patients who do not have clinical evidence of PD. Also, functional MRI has demonstrated widespread abnormalities outside the primary motor cortex in many ALS patients with or without dementia or unusual clinical features. These variations of the typical presentation of ALS raise two important issues regarding the definition of the disease. First, to what extent are nervous system regions outside the 'motor system' involved in ALS? Secondly, to what degree is the pathogenesis of ALS shared by other neurodegenerative disorders which might account for the additional clinical features seen in otherwise typical ALS? Three important neurodegenerative disorders, AD, PD and ALS, share a number of characteristics. These are listed in Table 8.1. This chapter explores the boundaries of overlap between AD, PD and ALS. It is our contention that each of these

Table 8.1. *Epidemiological features of ALS, PD and AD*

	ALS	PD	AD
Mean age at onset (years)	59.3	61.9	71.9
Mean duration of disease (years)	2.4	10.5	7.3
Incidence/100 000	1.2	21	401
Prevalence/100 000	4.2	300	2155
Age of peak incidence	55–65	70–80	65–75
M : F ratio*	1.61:1	1.13:1	1.1:1
Familial occurrence (%)	< 10	< 10	< 10
Twin studies	Low concordance		

* Ratio reversed after age 75 years.
Adapted from Eisen and Calne (1992).

Table 8.2. *Atypical clinical presentations of ALS*

Dementia
Extrapyramidal features
Extraocular involvement
Sensory impairment
Autonomic disturbances

disorders is unique, but that the study of patients with overlapping features may give clues to the selective vulnerability of different anatomical regions.

Dementia and ALS

Dementia is but one of several atypical presenting clinical features of ALS (Table 8.2). All of the symptoms listed are, according to the El Escorial criteria for ALS, considered contrary to its diagnosis (Brooks, 1994).

Although dementia is regarded as an atypical feature of ALS, a number of reports have clearly demonstrated that dementia can occur in patients with sporadic and FALS. In an early epidemiological survey of this association, Jokelainen (1977) reported that 5 of 255 Finnish ALS patients had dementia, a prevalence of about 2 per cent. However, there were many more Finnish ALS patients with milder cognitive or behavioural abnormalities of uncertain significance (Jokelainen, 1977). In a large autopsy series, Brownell and her colleagues (1970) reported that dementia was present in one of their 36 cases. On the basis of these and other studies, the prevalence of dementia in sporadic ALS has been reported to range from 1 per cent to 5 per cent of patients (Hudson, 1981, 1991b; Strong *et al.*, 1996). A large-scale epidemiological survey of dementia in ALS needs to be performed to arrive at a more definitive prevalence figure (Strong *et al.*, 1996). The prevalence of dementia in ALS is likely to increase with better detection techniques and with the global increase in ALS incidence.

Over the last decade, increased attention has been paid to neuropsychological testing, imaging studies and neuropathological data. As a result, a clinical pattern is being delineated for ALS-associated dementia. Clinically, ALS associated with dementia has a presentation similar to that of typical ALS, but is accompanied by signs of cognitive impairment (Hudson, 1991b). The cognitive impairment may follow, but more usually precedes, the other features of ALS. These patients are often seen initially by a psychiatrist or in a dementia clinic and ALS is suspected only later because of fasciculations, weakness or amyotrophy. Conversely, electromyographers may initially make a diagnosis of typical ALS, only later to realize that cognition is impaired. Hudson (1981) claims that ALS patients present with either features of typical ALS or dementia, but that if dementia becomes apparent, it will do so within a year from the onset of the amyotrophy and weakness. In our own experience, the dementia usually preceded or accompanied the other features of ALS.

Formerly, in many circumstances, dementia with ALS was regarded as a form of Jakob–Creutzfeldt disease (CJD), AD or Pick's disease (Hudson, 1981; Strong *et al.*, 1996). However, the disorder had neither the characteristic EEG of CJD, nor could it be transmitted to a variety of animal species including non-human primates. No typical Alzheimer plaques, neurofibrillary tangles or Pick bodies were seen pathologically. The diagnoses in these cases were often unclear. More extensive study using psychometric testing has characterized the type of cognitive impairment in most cases of ALS–dementia as being 'frontal lobe' in type. Other designations include 'frontal lobe degeneration of non-Alzheimer type', 'dementia of frontal lobe type', 'frontal lobe dementia' and, more commonly, 'frontotemporal dementia' (Lund and Manchester Groups, 1994). Clinically, the dementia has relatively consistent behavioural and affective features sometimes associated with a speech disorder but with preserved spatial orientation and praxis until late in the disease. Memory is often surprisingly intact (see Case report 2.7, Chapter 2). The main behavioural abnormalities of ALS–dementia are summarized in Table 8.3.

Table 8.3. *Features of frontal lobe dementia*

Insidious onset with slow progression
Early loss of attention to personal hygiene and grooming
Loss of appropriate social behaviour with frequent misdemeanors
Erratic and unusual behaviour such as shop-lifting
Disinhibition with lack of sexual restraint, violent behaviour or restlessness
Perseveration and stereotyped behaviours with mannerisms or repeated actions and distractibility, impulsivity and impersistence
Prominent affective symptoms; e.g. depression, anxiety, hypochondria, emotional unconcern, lack of spontaneity
Speech disorders; e.g. progressive reduction in speech output, stereotyped speech with repetition of certain phrases or themes, echolalia and perseveration, late mutism

According to several recent classification schemes, this constellation of symptoms, which is typical of frontal lobe impairment, is particularly indicative of 'frontotemporal dementia'. Behavioural neurologists have defined several subtypes of frontotemporal dementia, and that associated with ALS represents one of these subtypes (Cummings and Benson,1992). The other major subtypes are Pick's disease and frontal lobe degeneration (Lund and Manchester Groups, 1994). A review of the literature suggests that frontotemporal dementia is the second most common cause of dementia after AD. The cases associated with ALS are infrequent compared to other subtypes of frontotemporal dementia, but have a number of features that strongly suggest ALS and are not found in other types of this dementia. These features include widespread fasciculations, upper limb atrophy, sialorrhoea and swallowing dysfunction (Lund and Manchester Groups, 1994). However, the specificity of these diagnostic criteria for the ALS-associated dementia has not been formally tested (Hooten and Lyketsos, 1996).

The neuropathological characteristics of the ALS-associated fronto-temporal dementia are also becoming clarified (Hudson, 1981; Rossi, 1994). In a review of 42 cases of sporadic ALS accompanied by dementia or Parkinsonism, Hudson (1981) reported that cerebral involvement almost universally affected frontal regions, with occasional loss of temporal structures. Involvement was also seen in several subcortical structures such as the globus pallidus, caudate nucleus, substantia nigra and, less frequently, the dentate nucleus of cerebellum and hippocampus. In addition to cell loss, status spongiosis was noted in some patients. The structures involved pathologically are consistent with clinical formulations of the topographic basis of the frontotemporal dementia in ALS. More recent neuropathological descriptions have confirmed and extended the older observations, including a more detailed definition of the neuronal loss, microvacuolation and gliosis, especially in superficial cortical layers of the frontotemporal regions (Rossi, 1994). A major characteristic is the presence of pale-staining cytoplasmic inclusions which are situated eccentric to the nucleus. They can be found in surviving neurons in all areas that demonstrate neuronal loss, including the anterior horn cells of spinal cord. The inclusions label strongly with antibodies directed against ubiquitin. The neuropathological description of the ALS-associated dementia is quite different from, and excludes, those cases having neuropathological features of other established causes of dementia such as AD and Pick's disease. An alternative interpretation for the cognitive changes seen in some cases of ALS is that it is a subcortical dementia, resulting from the widespread loss of subcortical tissue (Kushner *et al.*, 1991). This may be the case for some patients with ALS and dementia. However, a subcortical origin for the dementia in most patients is not supported by neuropathological evidence, since subcortical tissue loss in ALS is limited and appears overshadowed by the reduction in cortical tissue (see Chapter 2).

Recent advances in imaging techniques have extended our ability to evaluate morphological changes in the brains of ALS patients during life. For instance, CT scanning of demented ALS patients sometimes demonstrates cerebral atrophy with ventricular enlargement, which is most marked in the frontal lobes. Impaired frontal lobe function can also be inferred from reduced uptake of tracers using SPECT or PET. These topics are dealt with more extensively in Chapter 7. The prevalence of dementia in FALS is less well established than for sporadic ALS but has been estimated to be approximately 15 per cent (Hudson, 1981). If this figure is correct, it suggests that dementia in FALS is two to three times that of sporadic ALS. Although the number of descriptions is limited, the dementia usually appears to follow the amyotrophy and weakness, although it can sometimes precede or accompany these signs. The clinical and neuropathological findings are like those of sporadic ALS and are indicative of a frontotemporal type of dementia.

Case report 8.1: ALS-associated dementia

A 59-year-old man had a three-year history of increasing difficulty with behaviour and cognition. He was noted by his wife and his colleagues at work to be increasingly difficult to get along with. He had frequent outbursts of anger and would yell insults at people, especially on the golf course. He was thought to be uninhibited, impulsive and unpredictable. He complained of excess salivation. On examination, his memory was intact but he was noted to be distractable and would not complete tasks such as subtracting serial sevens from 100. Neurological examination was unremarkable. Over the following year his speech and swallowing deteriorated, especially over the last three months. On examination at that time he was found to have significant weight loss, with a low-amplitude, dysarthric voice. He had palatal weakness and tongue fasciculations as well as fasciculations in all limbs and diffuse atrophy. He died shortly after developing these neurological deficits from aspiration pneumonia. Autopsy revealed marked gyral atrophy, especially in the frontal region. No neurofibrillary tangles or senile plaques were found. Vacuolation of layer II of cortex was noted in frontal, temporal and parietal regions. Mild gliosis was seen in the subcortical white matter. No alteration of the substantia nigra was observed. Motoneuron loss was seen in the hypoglossal nucleus and spinal cord. Ubiquitin-immunoreactive neuronal cytoplasmic inclusions were observed in motoneurons and in neurons of the dentate gyrus granular layer.

Rapidly progressive dementia, CJD and ALS

Rapidly progressive dementia with features of motoneuron disease with or without myoclonus raises the possibility of CJD (Kirschbaum, 1968). Neuropathologically, CJD is associated with spongiform change in the cortex with reactive gliosis in the cortical and subcortical grey matter (Kretzschmar *et al.*, 1996). Diagnostic criteria for CJD are being established (Kretzschmar *et al.*, 1996). CJD is now known to be related to the presence of an abnormal isoform of a prion protein. These prion proteins are post-translationally modified glycoproteins that are anchored to the neuronal surface and are probably involved in normal synaptic transmission (Collinge *et al.*, 1994). Susceptibility to developing CJD and other prion diseases occurs in individuals with polymorphisms of the human prion protein and the majority of cases of CJD are seen in people who are homozygous for several specific alleles (Collinge, 1996). CJD has been reported to have a number of clinicopathologic subtypes, including those with presenile dementia and cortical blindness (Heidenhain type), an ataxic form, and others (Kirschbaum, 1968). Among the variants is a dementia with prominent amyotrophy. The description of this amyotrophic form of CJD has created confusion as to whether patients having prominent amyotrophy and dementia have ALS or CJD. The relation between amyotrophy, motoneuron loss and CJD is interesting, and the fundamentals of the association are unresolved. In the early studies on CJD, which were based largely on pathological findings, cases were recognized with bulbar motoneuron loss and degeneration of cortico-spinal tract pathways. In general, motoneuron loss was not prominent (Kirschbaum, 1968). Evidence for prominent amyotrophy was probably not reported before 1929, following a description by Meyer. Cases were then reported that were similar to those studied by Meyer, but whether they were actually CJD or ALS is debatable (Kirschbaum, 1968). A view of CJD at the beginning of the 1960s was typified by a neuropathologist who questioned 'whether the syndrome is more than a convenient dumping ground for otherwise unclassifiable dementias with interesting cross relations to certain systemic degenerations' (see Kirschbaum, 1968). Following observations on the transmissibility of CJD, the relation between amyotrophy and CJD was re-examined. In a review of 2000 patients who were suspected of having CJD based on clinical and pathological evidence, 231 cases could be identified with prominent lower motoneuron signs early in the disease, an incidence of about 12 per cent. Brain tissue from 33 of these 231 patients was inoculated into primates and the animals observed for features of a transmissible disease. Only two atypical cases of transmissible dementia occurred and 23 other cases were considered negative in terms of a transmissible disease. The other eight cases were indeterminant at the time of the study. It was concluded that when lower motoneuron signs do appear in CJD they develop late in the disease. That is, amyotrophy is present in the face of fulminant cerebral and cerebellar involvement (Salazar *et al.*, 1983). Based on neuropatholo-gical examinations, it was estimated that fewer than 1 per cent of cases, later shown to be CJD because of their transmissibility, would have motoneuron loss as a prominent clinical feature at the time of disease presentation (Salazar *et al.*, 1983). A further 11 per cent of patients would have neuropathological evidence of motoneuron loss during the course of their illness (Brown *et al.*, 1986). The current view is that it is likely that patients with dementia who have early amyotrophy have ALS and not the amyotrophic form of CJD. To add further complexity to the diagnostic problems associated with patients having amyotrophy and dementia, Connolly, Allen and Dermott (1988) reported a case of a patient who was initially believed to have the amyotrophic form of CJD. Brain tissue from this patient was inoculated into a monkey in 1971 which was still alive in 1983 and cited as negative for CJD by Salazar *et al.* (1983). However, the monkey died a year later and subsequent neuropathological examination revealed spongiform change compatible with CJD.

Thus, it appears likely that at least some of the cases of rapidly progressive dementia are amyotrophic CJD, although most are ALS. Unfortunately, until sensitive and specific diagnostic tests become available for the diagnosis of CJD, it will be unlikely that a satisfactory study can be undertaken to clarify this problem. A recent report has suggested that a specific, non-invasive test for CJD may soon become available (Hsich, Kenny and Gibbs, 1996).

Disinhibition–dementia–Parkinson–amyotrophy complex

Family studies of patients with ALS or ALS-like conditions have occasionally revealed a high incidence of associated disorders. One group of patients with amyotrophy resembling ALS had relatives with clinical features of psychotic disease. Further evaluation of these families suggested that many members had clinical evidence of behavioural 'disinhibition' as manifested by alcoholism, hyper-religiousity, aberrant sexual behaviour and bulimia. These psychological features were seen in more extreme degrees in several demented family members and attributed to a 'frontal-type' dementia. Parkinsonism was also present in some individuals. Neuropathological evaluation of affected members of one family demonstrated frontotemporal atrophy, spongiform change in the superficial cortex, as well as neuronal loss in cerebral cortex, amygdala and substantia nigra. Anterior horn cell loss was found in the two spinal cords which were examined. One family with this combination of clinical and pathological features has been recently evaluated using linkage analysis techniques. A locus for this disorder, named eponymically the 'disinhibition–dementia–Parkinson–amyotrophy complex' (DDPAC), has been mapped to a region on chromosome 17 (Wilhelmsen *et al.*, 1994). This locus is genetically distinct from other known loci for dementing illnesses. The locus is found in the vicinity of more than 100 identified genes but very few of the genes were thought by the authors to be related to DDPAC. Two genes of possible interest include the tau protein gene as well as the gene for the low-affinity NGF receptor. Although these genes may be of general relevance for neurodegenerative disorders, there is no specific information linking them to DDPAC. An important limitation of linkage studies on disorders such as DDPAC is that an initially positive linkage can be found to be spurious when more informative genetic markers become available. Furthermore, errors in linkage analysis can be made by assigning a normal status to 'at-risk' individuals, or by errors in the estimation of penetrance values. To substantiate the claims of linkage, distantly related members or other families with DDAPC would need to be identified. Nonetheless, linkage work on DDPAC is important as it supports and extends clinical observations that in some families amyotrophy resembling ALS, dementia and Parkinsonism could coexist, even in the same patient. It further serves to highlight the variability of clinical findings that can be seen even in a single family with a similar genetic defect. This phenotypic heterogeneity bears some similarity to the variety of presentations that can be seen in different transgenic mice having only minor changes in their pedigrees (see Chapter 3).

Other cognitive changes in ALS

A few case reports have described other cognitive changes occurring in ALS patients. These include:

1. Progressive aphasic dementia (Caselli *et al.*, 1993).
2. Thalamic dementia (Deymeer *et al.*, 1989).
3. Mild memory impairment with dementia.

The importance of these specific clinical presentations has yet to be determined.

In summary, dementia is clearly seen in a few patients with sporadic and familial ALS. The type of dementia is variable but the commonest form, frontotemporal dementia, has rather specific clinical, radiographic and pathological features. Evidence from these sources indicates that there is prominent involvement of frontotemporal cortical regions, as well as some subcortical structures. A few cases of amyotrophy resembling ALS, with dementia, turn out to have CJD. In these, amyotrophy is mild or modest whereas the dementia develops rapidly and is severe. Why so few patients with ALS manifest dementia and concomitant neuropathological abnormalities is entirely unknown. These patients may represent a different group of disorders with a specific phenotype, or the association could indicate a loss of the 'selective vulnerability' that normally restricts ALS to its conventional distribution. We know little, if anything, about the determinants of selective vulnerability. The clinical and pathological characteristics of most cases of ALS with dementia are quite unlike those of AD, so that the association is not merely an overlap syndrome of the two neurodegenerative disorders.

Subclinical Parkinsonism

Earlier neuropathological studies of patients with ALS reported neuron loss in the substantia nigra (see Hudson, 1981). However, these pathological changes were rarely accompanied by clinical features of Parkinsonism. When clinical Parkinsonism occurs in combination with ALS, it almost always does so in association with dementia (Hudson, 1981). As with ALS and dementia, Parkinsonian features may either precede or follow development of ALS. Several recent neuropathological studies have substantiated the earlier claims of involvement of substantia nigra in some cases of sporadic ALS. Burrow and Blumbergs (1992) examined the numbers of pigmented neurons in 14 patients with sporadic ALS without clinical Parkinsonism, compared to age-matched and sex-matched controls. No Lewy bodies or neurofibrillary tangles were observed in brain tissue from either group. However, the mean number of substantia nigra neurons was decreased in ALS cases compared to controls, although the ranges of surviving neurons in both groups were large and values overlapped considerably. The authors were not blinded to the clinical diagnoses. More recently, Kato, Oda and Tanabe (1993) evaluated the numbers of neurons at three levels of the substantia nigra in 15 patients with sporadic ALS and controls. The ALS patients had no clinical signs of Parkinsonism although three patients were demented, five had ophthalmoplegia and five had been on a respirator for one to eight years. Seven of the 15 ALS patients had significant reductions in the numbers of neurons in the substantia nigra. These reductions were seen especially in patients with dementia or ophthalmoplegia. There was no meaningful relationship between nigral neuron loss, the age of the patient, the duration of illness, or respirator use. No Lewy bodies or neurofibrillary tangles were seen in the autopsied tissues.

In a novel approach to the relationship between ALS and Parkinsonism, Takahashi and colleagues (1993) measured the striatal 6-fluorodopa (6-FD) uptake rate constants of 16 ALS patients without clinical Parkinsonism or dementia and 14 age-matched controls using PET scanning. From other work it is known that the 6-FD uptake rate constant is related to the number of dopaminergic neurons in the substantia nigra. The mean 6-FD uptake rate constants of the ALS patients and the controls were not significantly different in this study. Nonetheless, four ALS patients had rate constants which were substantially less than controls, raising the possibility that at least some of these ALS patients had significantly decreased numbers of nigral neurons. In general, ALS patients with lower numbers of substantia nigra neurons were those with longer duration disease, but the sample size was too small to infer much from this. There is an obvious difficulty in scanning severely affected ALS patients and this limitation would bias the sample to patients with less severe disease who have usually had symptoms for a shorter time.

Parkinsonism and ALS

A few reports have described the concurrence of symptomatic Parkinsonism and ALS. These reports can be subdivided, somewhat arbitrarily, into three groups: (i) sporadic or familial ALS presenting with Parkinsonian features, (ii) concurrent PD and ALS, and (iii) post-encephalitic ALS/PD. The association of Parkinsonism and FALS is infrequent and is almost invariably associated with dementia (Hudson, 1981). This topic is discussed below. A very limited number of studies have described patients with PD who later develop ALS (Eisen and Calne, 1992). The incidence of this association must be very low. In such cases, symptoms of PD nearly always precede ALS and the PD may respond to L-dopa. We are not aware of the presence of ALS in patients developing Parkinsonism following exposure to the neurotoxin N-methyl-4-phenyl-1,2,3,6-tetra-hydropyridine (MPTP).

A well-described Parkinsonian syndrome was seen following epidemics of encephalitis lethargica which occurred between 1915 and 1928. The nature of the virus responsible for this syndrome is unknown. Rarely, clinical features consistent with ALS were also seen after encephalitis lethargica. The amyotrophy invariably occurred after the Parkinsonian features had developed (Brait, Fahn and Schwarz, 1973; Hudson, 1981; Hudson and Rice, 1990). The course of the motoneuron dysfunction appeared to resemble closely typical sporadic ALS. In some cases, post-encephalitic PD–ALS progressed rather slowly and was accompanied by sensory symptoms (Brait *et al.*, 1973); dementia has not been reported in association with post-encephlitic ALS (Hudson, 1981). Neuropathologically, post-encephalitic ALS is characterized by prominent depigmentation of the substantia nigra, both the pars compacta and pars reticulata. Lewy bodies, typical of PD, are absent in post-encephalitic PD (Hudson and Rice, 1990). There is focal gliosis and severe neuron loss in the substantia nigra in the post-encephalitic syndrome. Neurofibrillary tangles are present in pigmented neurons but are also seen more generally throughout the cerebral cortex, basal ganglia, hypothalamus and tegmentum. Most neuropathologists regard post-encephalitic Parkinsonism as distinct from

PD, with a small region of unexplained overlap. The neurofibrillary changes, especially the neurofibrillary tangles, are reminiscent of Guamanian ALS, but occur without the presence of clinical dementia.

In summary, some ALS patients have a loss of neurons in the substantia nigra which is generally mild and may be more pronounced in patients with dementia or ophthalmoplegia, as occurs after long-term ventilatory support. Potentially, under some circumstances (e.g. rapidly progressive disease, long-duration disease), symptomatic Parkinsonism can result. This condition appears pathologically distinct from PD in that it invariably lacks Lewy bodies.

Dementia, Parkinsonism and ALS

The best-established descriptions of patients with ALS, Parkinsonism and dementia come from Guam and other regions in the western Pacific. Many aspects of this disease are discussed in Chapter 1. Recognition of overlap syndromes on Guam has served as an impetus for more recent epidemiological surveys of patients with sporadic ALS, FALS, and cases also having features of dementia and Parkinsonism. The features of ALS in the western Pacific are clinically indistinguishable from typical cases of sporadic ALS elsewhere and are characterized by muscle weakness and atrophy, spasticity and corticospinal tract involvement (Garruto and Yase, 1986; Rodgers-Johnson *et al.*, 1986). Extrapyramidal signs are clinically obvious in only 5 per cent of patients with Guamanian ALS and dementia in less (about 4 per cent) (Rodgers-Johnson *et al.*, 1986). Much more commonly, some members of a family have amyotrophy while others have Parkinsonism–dementia (Lavine *et al.*, 1991). True clinical overlap of amyotrophy, Parkinsonism and dementia in a single patient is therefore unusual, even in Guam, and its incidence is probably very close to that described in sporadic western ALS. This was appreciated in the 1800s by the native Chamorros, who coined the terms 'lytico' for the amyotrophy and 'bodig' for the Parkinsonism–dementia, recognizing that they seldom occurred together in the same person. When one of the authors (AE) visited Guam in 1989, more than 25 patients were seen with possible or probable ALS. None had clinical evidence of Parkinsonism or dementia. However, many reported these syndromes in one or several other family members.

Despite the lack of clinical overlap between ALS, Parkinsonism and dementia on Guam, neuropathological examination of these patients demonstrates neurofibrillary tangles and granulovacuolar change, both

Table 8.4. *Pathological features of Guamanian ALS and other disorders*

	Neuronal loss	Neurofibrillary tangles	Spheroids	Senile plaques	Granulovacuolar degeneration	Lewy bodies	Depigmentation of substantia nigra
Classical ALS							
Brain	+	−	−	−	−	−	−
Spinal cord	+ +	−	+ +	−	−	−	−
Guam ALS							
Brain	+ +	+ + +	+	−	+ +	−	+
Spinal cord	+ + +	+ + +	+ +	−	−	−	−
PD							
Brain	+	−	−	−	−	+ + +	+ + +
Spinal cord	−	−	−	−	−	−	−
Post-encephalitic PD/ALS							
Brain	+	+ + +	−	−	−	−	+ + +
Spinal cord	+	−	−	−	−	−	−
AD							
Brain	+ + +	+ + +	−	+ + +	+ + +	−	−
Spinal cord	−	−	−	−	−	−	−

Adapted from Garruto and Yase (1986). PD, Parkinson's disease; AD, Alzheimer's disease; − represents rarely present; + sometimes present; + + often present; + + + usually present.

in patients with ALS and in those with the ALS–Parkinsonism–dementia complex (Hirano *et al.*, 1966). The changes are widely distributed in the nervous system. The substantia nigra is involved in all ALS cases to varying degrees ranging from scattered neurofibrillary change in nigral neurons, to macroscopic atrophy (Hirano *et al.*, 1966). Of considerable interest is the observation that many asymptomatic, 'normal' Chamorros adults also had mild, but definite, histologic changes of the ALS–Parkinsonism–dementia syndrome (Hirano *et al.*, 1966). Pathological study of the spinal cords and medullas of unaffected family members did not reveal microscopic changes such as neuronal loss that would suggest ALS. A summary of some of these findings is shown in Table 8.4.

Two other western Pacific foci of ALS were described following the identification of Guamanian ALS and the ALS–Parkinsonism–dementia complex. One of these foci was in the Kii peninsula of Japan, on the main island of Honshu. A high incidence of ALS cases had been identified on this peninsula, possibly as early as 1911 (Shiraki and Yase, 1991). The highest concentration of ALS patients occurred in the districts of Hobara, which had an incidence of 15/100 000, and in Kozagawa, where there was an incidence of 55/100 000. These high incidences were sustained over a 20-year period but, like Guam, there has been a dramatic reduction in the incidence of ALS in Hobara and Kozagawa over the last decade or two. ALS has occasionally been seen with PD clinically, but there was no autopsy confirmation of such an association. The neuropathology of the Kii peninsula cases includes neurofibrillary tangles and appears similar to that of the Guamanian disease. A second focus of ALS was observed in western New Guinea among the native people of that region. Autopsies were not done, but in some cases with ALS there was an associated poliomyeloradiculitis (Shiraki and Yase, 1991). A few clusters of ALS outside the endemic regions of the western Pacific have been reported; these were unassociated with dementia or Parkinsonism (Kurtzke, 1991). The observations on the concurrence of ALS, Parkinsonism and dementia have played an important role in shaping the view that these disorders may have some fundamental similarities to the Guamanian disease. The implications of overlap between AD, PD and sporadic ALS or FALS are much less clear. These diseases are quite distinct from Guamanian ALS (Table 8.5). The current evidence dictates that they are related to Guamanian ALS only to the extent that both affect the same cell types and are progressive disorders. Overlap of syndromes in the Guamanian disease should not be construed as evidence that a similar association between AD, PD and sporadic ALS must be present.

Table 8.5. *Differences between Guamanian ALS and sporadic ALS*

Guamanian ALS	Sporadic ALS
High incidence in specific ethnic group	Uniform incidence in most ethnic groups
Young age of onset (approximately 45 years)	Older age of onset (approximately 60 years)
High incidence of dementia and Parkinsonism in family members	Incidence of dementia and Parkinsonism possibly increased in family members
Frequent neuronal loss in substantia nigra	Rare neuronal loss in substantia nigra
Frequent neurofibrillary degeneration	No neurofibrillary degeneration
Frequent granulovacuolar degeneration	No granulovacuolar degeneration
Normal glutamate contents in brain	Reduced glutamate contents in brain
Low taurine contents in brain	Elevated taurine contents in brain

Biochemical studies on patients with concurrent sporadic ALS, Parkinsonism and dementia are limited. In one study a single patient with dementia, Parkinsonism and fasciculations was evaluated postmortem (Gilbert, Kish and Chang, 1988). Neuropathologically, this patient had spongiform changes in cerebral cortex with mild gliosis, as well as neuron loss in substantia nigra and moderate anterior horn cell loss. The nucleus basalis was within normal limits. Neurochemically, choline acetyltransferase and γ-amino-butyric acid levels were unchanged compared to controls, but with reduced dopamine, homovanillic acid and serotonin in striatum (Gilbert *et al.*, 1988). These changes are dissimilar to those seen in Guamanian ALS (Perry *et al.*, 1990a).

Dementia and PD in family members of patients with ALS

Recent epidemiological studies have been used to determine the relative risk of dementia or Parkinsonism developing in family members or spouses of patients with ALS. Significant results in first-degree relatives would suggest a genetic defect that is common to ALS, PD and AD, and a significant outcome in a spousal study would point to an environmental factor(s) common to the household. Majoor-Krakaur and colleagues (1994) compared 150 newly diagnosed ALS patients, six of whom had FALS, and controls. Controls included patients undergoing neurological evaluation who did not have ALS, matched for age, gender and payment status. A Cox proportional hazard analysis was used to compute the relative rate for ALS, dementia and PD in the first-degree relatives of patients and controls. Patients with ALS and controls had similar participation rates, family sizes and sibships. The study was limited by recall bias, as subjects were asked to identify relatives who were demented on the basis of four specific questions. Support for a tentative diagnosis of dementia produced by the questionnaire could be obtained in only a small number of patients. No attempt was made to determine the nature of the dementia that was present. Relatives were characterized as having PD if a diagnosis of this disorder had been made by a physician. Dementia was reported to be present twice as frequently in relatives of ALS patients compared to relatives of controls. The increased dementia incidence in relatives of ALS patients was particularly associated with a greater cumulative incidence in parents and grandparents, but not in sibs. Although the risk of PD was twice as high in relatives of ALS patients as in controls, the difference was not statistically significant.

The low number of patients with FALS in this study (six patients) made the likelihood of finding a significant association in this group small (Majoor-Krakauer *et al.*, 1994). A case control study, in the Palermo region of Italy, was used to investigate the same issue (Savettieri *et al.*, 1991). Forty-six ALS patients and 92 matched controls, two for each patient, were subjected to a questionnaire. Matched triplet analysis was statistically evaluated using Mantel–Haenzsel estimate of the odds ratio. The relative risk for the presence of a neurological disease among first-degree relatives was higher for ALS patients than for controls, although this did not reach statistical significance. Several limitations of this study are evident. First was the small sample size (46 patients). Second, the presence of 'neurological disease' comprised a diverse group of neurological diseases, not just dementia or PD. Third, because of the small numbers of cases involved, a statistical analysis was not performed for individual neurological diseases such as dementia and PD.

In another case-control study examining possible associated factors in families of patients with ALS, Armon and colleagues (1991) administered questionnaires to 74 selected ALS patients, as well as to controls. No cases were selected with FALS. Among the possible factors that were examined was the hypothesis that patients with ALS were more likely to have relatives with neurodegenerative diseases than controls. Up to four controls were selected for each patient and comparison was made by rank-sum and chi-square tests. The proportion of relatives having neurodegenerative disease was higher for ALS patients than for controls, but this difference did not quite reach statistical significance. The percentage of ALS patients having a family member with a neurodegenerative disorder was also higher than for controls, but this also did not reach statistical significance. Several features of this study are relevant. First, the sample size was almost 50 per cent smaller than that of Majoor-Krakauer and colleagues (1994), making the statistical power smaller. Secondly, the patients and controls were also asked about maternal and paternal aunts and uncles, whereas studies such as that of Majoor-Krakauer *et al.* did not include data on second-degree relations. Possibly, this wider definition of family could lead to a 'dilution' of an association that might have been present in the first-order relatives. Thirdly, in the study of Armon *et al.* (1991) the percentage of ALS patients having a family member with a neurodegenerative disorder was close to statistical significance and it is possible that, with an increased sample size, a significant relationship would have been obtained.

Overlap of AD, PD and ALS in relation to neuronal ageing

Neurodegenerative disorders such as AD, PD and ALS do share the important feature of predominantly affecting older patients at a time when there might be normally occurring neuronal attrition. It has been proposed that AD, PD and ALS are due to an 'environmental insult' which affects neuronal populations specific for these disorders as individuals age, and that the neuronal damage remains subclinical for decades (Calne *et al.*, 1986). Clinical signs only become apparent when neuronal loss has reached a critical level, which transpires when 'physiological', age-related neuronal attrition is superimposed on the initial subclinical neuronal damage. To validate this hypothesis requires the ability to measure the size and decline of functioning neuronal populations over time. This has been achieved, in a limited fashion, for neurons of the substantia nigra using longitudinal PET studies with FD in normal, ageing individuals (Snow, 1994). These studies, which correlate well with post-mortem examinations, indicate that approximately 50 per cent of nigral neurons must be lost before clinical Parkinsonism develops. This implies that there is a reserve capacity of surviving substantia nigra neurons able to support compensatory mechanisms such as terminal sprouting and possibly vesicular storage. Also, FD PET studies in asymptomatic human subjects and primates exposed to the neurotoxin MPTP have demonstrated reduced striatal accumulation of FD, with a mean value falling between those for normal subjects and patients with

Parkinsonian symptoms. In some of these patients it was possible to predict that Parkinsonism would later develop.

It has been difficult to evaluate the extent of physiological (naturally occurring) neuronal loss. It has yet to be established whether an environmental insult leading to the development of neurodegeneration produces a change in the rate of naturally occurring cell death or an immediate decline in the neuronal population, which would subsequently be affected by physiological neuronal loss. The data regarding the attrition of cortical neurons as they relate to ALS and AD are very limited, and the extent to which specific areas of the cerebral cortex demonstrate age-related neuronal attrition is unknown. There is no specific information regarding a change in the number of human corticomotoneurons with ageing (Terry *et al.*, 1987; Mann, 1994). Pathological studies suggest an age-dependent reduction of pyramidal cells (but not specifically corticomotoneurons) ranging from 15 per cent to 40 per cent. Other studies conclude there is shrinkage of the perikaryon and dendritic arbor of cortical neurons, but with little, if any, loss of cells. Physiological studies using PSTHs do indicate that there is a linear decline in the number of corticomotoneurons with age (Eisen *et al.*, 1996). About one-third of the corticomotoneurons are lost between the ages of 35–40 and 60 years (see Chapter 4). If this can be confirmed, it indicates that demise of corticomotoneurons precedes that of anterior horn cells, which only starts after 60 years of age (W. F. Brown, 1994; McComas, 1994).

Neurodegenerative overlap syndrome

The identification of patients who might have symptoms or signs indicating features of ALS, Parkinsonism and dementia in various combination has been labelled by some authors as constituting a 'neurodegenerative overlap syndrome' (Eisen and Calne, 1992; Uitti *et al.*, 1995). Although the concept of this type of overlap is tantalizing, there is little evidence to support it. A further consideration is the possibility that age-related, 'naturally-occurring' neuronal attrition may result in mild distal atrophy or fasciculations and be of little clinical significance. The argument that 'overlap syndrome' patients represent 'forme frustes' of traditional diagnostic categories can be countered by evidence that many such patients have atypical forms of well-established neurodegenerative diseases, with or without changes that are often seen in similarly aged patients. Some aspects of neuronal ageing are reviewed below.

Naturally occurring neuronal death

Spinal motoneurons

Naturally occurring motoneuron death has been well described. It occurs late in embryogenesis and is possibly related to the development of voltage-dependent ionic channels, synaptic activity at the neuromuscular junction, as well as retrograde influences from muscle. It is thought that outside of this brief period of 'physiological' motoneuron death in embryogenesis, there is limited cell loss, at least in the early postnatal period (Lawson *et al.*, 1997). There is some evidence that motoneuron loss occurs later in life and that motoneurons demonstrate a number of age-related changes. These include an accumulation of lipofuscin (Mann and Yates, 1974), altered dendritic morphology, a reduction in neuron size and a decline in neuromuscular area (see Johnson, 1996). Biochemically, older motoneurons have a reduction in NADH-diaphorase and other enzymes. Axotomy has been used to model some of the effects of ALS on the motoneuron (Pullen, 1996). There are morphological and biochemical differences in axotomized motoneurons in young versus older rodents (Johnson, 1996). To explore further the hypothesis that ageing motoneurons are more vulnerable to injury than adult motoneurons, Johnson (1996) studied morphological changes in thoracic motoneurons subjected to nerve crush or nerve transection and ligation in adult and very old cats. He found that the effects of axotomy on Nissl body ultrastructure and calcitonin gene-related peptide (CGRP) immunoreactivity were similar, regardless of age. There was no more extensive axotomy-induced moto-neuronal degeneration in the older animals (Johnson, 1996). Johnson and colleagues conclude that at least for 'target-dependent' properties of motoneurons such as Nissl body ultrastructure and synaptic terminals, no major differences are apparent between younger and older animals in relation to axotomy.

Human studies are obviously more difficult, but a number of reports have addressed the changes which occur in normal spinal cord and motoneurons with advancing age. Summarizing these findings reveals: (i) that there is considerable variability in motoneuron counts between normal individuals, even at similar ages (Tsukagoshi *et al.*, 1979); (ii) that there is probably not much change in motoneuron number between young adulthood and the age of 60 (Tomlinson and Irving, 1977); (iii) that in adults at ages greater than 60 years, changes are seen in motoneuron counts revealing a diminished motoneuron population in which cell loss appears to be uniform throughout all segments and is unaccompanied by obvious morphological change; and (iv) that electrophysiological studies that have estimated motoneuron numbers and followed them longitudinally over time show there is little change until after age 60 years (W. F. Brown, 1994; McComas, 1994).

Motoneuron loss as a predisposition to developing ALS

Earlier, the hypothesis was raised that ALS is characterized by a toxic insult which produces subclinical damage to motoneurons and which only later becomes clinically manifest as motoneuron loss because of age-related motoneuron attrition. If this were true, it might be expected that any condition characterized by motoneuron destruction would later result in ALS. The best example is poliomyelitis. Even though there can be a large depletion of bulbar and spinal motoneurons in poliomyelitis, there has not been a convincing report of the subsequent development of ALS. Spinal cords from patients previously infected with polio contain the usual number of normal motoneurons and a higher number of abnormal, but surviving motoneurons (Dalakas, 1994). Under these conditions, ALS would be expected to develop more rapidly than usual. A syndrome known as post-polio progressive muscular atrophy (PPMA) has been defined as slowly progressive muscle weakness and atrophy which is generally painless and unaccompanied by sensory changes. These patients have objective evidence of motoneuron dysfunction including: (i) increasing weakness and atrophy, (ii) fatigue, (iii) myalgia, (iv) fasciculations, (v) bulbar muscle weakness, (vi) respiratory function compromise, and (vii) sleep apnoea (Dalakas, 1994). The PPMA syndrome begins about 30 years after the original attack of poliomyelitis. The progression of weakness is very slow and difficult to establish clinically (approximately 1 per cent per year). These data indicate that the tempo of progression of PPMA is very different from that in ALS. Furthermore, as indicated above, there is little evidence of 'physiological', age-dependent motoneuron attrition prior to 60 years. As many patients with ALS develop symptoms before 60 years of age, this also would cast doubt on the 'ageing hypothesis' of ALS. One might argue that the age-dependent motoneuron attrition in ALS may depend on the health of the motoneurons. Yet, even in polio, although many of the motoneurons surviving the initial episode of polio do not function normally, they still apear to be capable of maintaining function longer than is typically seen in ALS. This evidence argues against a model of ALS based on an interaction between ageing and the environment. This 'ageing' hypothesis appears to hold more strongly for PPMA than for ALS.

Summary

This chapter examines the shared aspects and possible overlap between AD, PD and ALS. The possibility of such an overlap developed largely from two independent observations. First, patients with the Guamanian form of ALS have a remarkably high coexistence of dementia, Parkinsonism and amyotrophy. Secondly, dementia is observed in between 1 per cent and 5 per cent of patients with sporadic ALS and in a slightly larger percentage of patients with FALS. The chapter also examines features of the Guamanian form of ALS. It concludes that it possesses features that are so distinct from those of sporadic ALS that it probably consitutes a separate disorder, although it may share some pathophysiological mechanisms with sporadic ALS.

Dementia associated with ALS is now a well-described entity and is unquestionably distinct from AD. It is characterized by extensive involvement of cerebral cortex, especially in frontotemporal regions. The contribution of subcortical white matter and deep nuclei to the dementia remains to be clarified. The identification of this ALS-associated dementia raises interesting questions about the nature of neuronal vulnerability in ALS. Could cerebral involvement reflect the wider limits of a selective vulnerability which exists for ALS? In this scheme, there is a high probability of motoneuron and corticospinal tract involvement in ALS, whereas the probability of sensory involvement is low. There is an intermediate probability of involvement of frontal cortex adjacent to motor cortex, which might relate to the presence or quantity of a cell surface epitope or enzyme.

In rapidly progressive dementia the presence of amyotrophy raises the possibility of CJD. The amyotrophy seen in CJD generally occurs late in the disease and is accompanied by fulminant cerebral and cerebellar involvement. Transmission studies suggest that early amyotrophy is rare in CJD. Possibly, new diagnostic tests for CJD will be helpful in clarifying whether this clinical profile is due to ALS or CJD. Neuropathological examination may be misleading in some cases as spongiform change in cortex is often observed in some non-transmissible cases of dementia attributable to ALS.

ALS can sometimes be seen with Parkinsonian signs. The prevalence of this association is unknown, and it sometimes occurs concurrently with dementia. The overlap between Parkinsonism and ALS appears to be the end of a spectrum in which reduced numbers of neurons are seen in substantia nigra even without Parkinsonian features. These patients having substantial involvement of substantia nigra, do not have Lewy bodies and may have a higher incidence of dementia and ophthalmoplegia. Although some authors have suggested that Parkinsonian features and dementia represent a neurodegenerative disease 'overlap syndrome', we suggest that this association depends critically on how these disorders are defined.

Although the connection between motoneuron loss that occurs in normal ageing and ALS is intriguing, there is no obvious causal relation between the two. In cases where there is a known disorder of motoneurons, such as poliomyelitis, age-related motoneuron attrition does not result in ALS. Instead, motoneuron loss occurs at a slow rate (the post-polio syndrome).

References

Abdel Hamid KM, Baimbridge KG. (1997). The effects of artificial calcium buffers on calcium responses and glutamate-mediated excitotoxicity in cultured hippocampal neurons. Neuroscience; 81:673–87.

Abe K, Fujimura H, Toyooka K, *et al.* (1993). Single-photon emission computed tomographic investigation of patients with motor neuron disease. Neurology; 43:1569–73.

Abe K, Fujimura H, Toyooka K, *et al.* (1997). Cognitive function in amyotrophic lateral sclerosis. J Neurol Sci; 148:95–100.

Abrahams S, Goldstein LH, Kew JJM, *et al.* (1996). Frontal lobe dysfunction in amyotrophic lateral sclerosis. A PET study. Brain; 119:2105–20.

Adem A, Ekblom J, Gillberg PG, *et al.* (1994). Insulin-like growth factor-1 receptors in human spinal cord: Changes in amyotrophic lateral sclerosis. J Neural Transm; 97:73–84.

Aebischer P, Kato AC. (1994). Treatment of amyotrophic lateral sclerosis using gene therapy approach. Europ Neurol; 35:65–8.

Aisen ML, Sevilla D, Gibson G, *et al.* (1995). 3,4-Diaminopyridine as a treatment for amyotrophic lateral sclerosis. J Neurol Sci; 129:21–4.

Al-Chalabi A, Powell JF, Leigh PN. (1995). Neurofilaments, free radicals, excitotoxins and amyotrophic lateral sclerosis. Muscle & Nerve; 18:540–5.

Alexianu ME, Ho B-K, Mohamed AH, *et al.* (1994). The role of calcium-binding proteins in selective motoneuron vulnerability in amyotrophic lateral sclerosis. Ann Neurol; 36:846–58.

Allaoua H, Chaudieu I, Krieger C, *et al.* (1992). Alterations in spinal cord excitatory amino acid receptors in amyotrophic lateral sclerosis patients. Brain Res; 579:169–72.

Amassian VE, Stewart M, Qirk GJ, Rosenthal JL. (1987). Physiological basis of motor effects of a transient stimulus to cerebral cortex. Neurosurgery; 20:74–93.

Anand P, Cedarbaum J, Lindsay RM, *et al.* (1994). Marked depletion of ciliary neurotrophic factor in ventral horn of spinal cord but not cerebral motor cortex in amyotrophic lateral sclerosis. Ann Neurol; 36:318p.

Andersen K, Launer LJ, Ott A, *et al.* (1995). Do nonsteroidal anti-inflammatory drugs decrease the risk for Alzheimer's disease? The Rotterdam Study. Neurology; 45:1441–5.

Andersen PM. (1997). Amyotrophic lateral sclerosis and CuZn-superoxide dismutase. UmU Tryckeri, Umea, Sweden, pp. 1–681.

Andersen PM, Forsgren L, Binzer M, *et al.* (1996). Autosomal recessive adult-onset amyotrophic lateral sclerosis associated with homozygosity for AsP90Ala CuZn-superoxide dismutase mutation: a clinical and genealogical study of 36 patients. Brain; 119:1153–72.

Andres PL, Finison L, Conlon T. (1988). Use of composite scores (megascores) to measure deficit in ALS. Neurology; 38:405–8.

Ang LC, Bhaumick B, Munoz DG, *et al.* (1992). Effects of astrocytes, insulin, insulin-like growth factor I on the survival of motoneurons in vitro. J Neurol Sci; 109:168–72.

Antel JP, Cashman NR. (1995). Immunological findings in amyotrophic lateral sclerosis. Springer Semin Immunopathol; 17:17–28.

Appel SH, Smith RG, Alexianu MF, *et al.* (1995). Autoimmunity as an etiological factor in sporadic amyotrophic lateral sclerosis. In: Pathogensesis and therapy of amyotrophic lateral sclerosis, Searratrice G, Munsat T, eds. Advances in Neurology, Vol. 68. Philadelphia: Lippincott-Raven Publishers, pp. 47–57.

Appel SH, Smith RG, Engelhardt JI, Stefani E. (1993). Evidence for autoimmunity in amyotrophic lateral sclerosis. J Neurol Sci; 118:169–74.

Appel V, Stewart SS, Smith G, Appel SH. (1987). A rating scale for amyotrophic lateral sclerosis: description and preliminary experience. Ann Neurol; 22:328–33.

Aquilonius SM, Jossan SS, Ekblom JG, *et al.* (1992). Increased binding of 3H-L-deprenyl in spinal cords from patients with amyotrophic lateral sclerosis. J Neural Transmission; 89:111–22.

Aran FA. (1850). Recherches sur une maladie non encore decrite du systeme musculaire (atrophie muculaire progressive). Arch Gen Med; 24:5, 172.

Armon C, Kurland LT, Daube JR, O'Brien P. (1991). Epidemiologic correlates of sporadic amyotrophic lateral sclerosis. Neurology; 41:1077–84.

Arsac C, Raymond C, Martin-Moutot N, *et al.* (1996). Immunoassays fail to detect antibodies against neuronal calcium channels in amyotrophic lateral sclerosis serum. Ann Neurol; 40:695–700.

Ashby P, Stalberg E, Winkler T, Hunter JP. (1987). Further observations of group Ia facilitation of motoneurons by vibration in man. Exp Brain Res; 69:1–6.

Ashby P, Zilm D. (1982a). Characteristics of postsynaptic potentials produced in single human motoneurons by homonymous group I volleys. Exp Brain Res; 47:41–8.

Ashby P, Zilm D. (1982b). Relationship between EPSP shape and cross-correlation profile explored by computer simulation studies on human motoneurons. Exp Brain Res; 47:33–40.

Asmark H, Aquilonius SM, Gillberg PG, *et al.* (1993). A pilot trial of dextromethorphan in amyotrophic lateral sclerosis. J Neurol Neurosurg Psychiatry; 56:197–200.

Averback P, Crocker P. (1982). Regular involvement of Clarke's nucleus in sporadic amyotrophic lateral sclerosis. Arch Neurol; 39:155–6.

Awiszus F, Feistner H. (1993). Abnormal EPSPs evoked by magnetic brain stimulation in hand muscle motoneurons of patients with amyotrophic lateral sclerosis. Electroenceph Clin Neurophysiol; 89:408–14.

Awiszus F, Feistner H. (1995). Comparison of single motor unit responses to transcranial magnetic and peroneal nerve stimulation in the tibialis anterior muscle of patients with amyotrophic lateral sclerosis. Electroenceph Clin Neurophysiol; 97:90–5.

Azulay J-Ph, Rihet P, Pouget J, *et al.* (1997). Long term follow up of multifocal motor neuropathy with conduction block under treatment. J Neurol Neurosurg Psychiatry; 62:391–4.

Baimbridge KG, Celio MR, Rogers JH. (1992). Calcium-binding proteins in the nervous system. Trends Neurosci; 15:259–64.

Barker AT, Freeston IL, Jalinous R, *et al.* (1985). Magnetic stimulation of the human brain. J Physiol; 369:3p.

Bawa P, Lemon RN. (1993). Recruitment of motor units in response to transcranial magnetic stimulation in man. J Physiol; 471:445–64.

Bazzoni F, Beutler B. (1996). The tumor necrosis factor ligand and receptor families. New Engl J Med; 334:1717–24.

Beal F. (1995). Aging, energy, and oxidative stress in neurodegenerative diseases. Ann Neurol; 38:357–66.

Beaulieu EE. (1991). Neurosteroids: a new function in the brain. Biol Cell; 71:3–10.

Beckman JS, Carson M, Smith CD, Koppenol WH. (1993). ALS, SOD and peroxynitrite. Nature; 364:584.

Beghi E, The Italian ALS Study Group. (1993). Branched-chain amino acids and amyotrophic lateral sclerosis: A treatment failure? Neurology; 43:2466–70.

Bell C. (1830). The nervous sytem of the human body. London: Longman.

Bellizzi MC, Franklin MF, Duthie GG, James WP. (1994). Vitamin E and coronary heart disease: the European paradox. Europ J Clin Nutrition; 48:822–31.

Ben Hamida M, Hentati F, Ben Hamida C. (1990). Hereditary motor system diseases (chronic juvenile amyotrophic lateral sclerosis): conditions combining a bilateral pyramidal syndrome with limb and bulbar amyotrophy. Brain; 113:347–63.

Bensimon G, Lacombiez L, Meininger V, The ALS/Riluzole Study Group. (1994). A controlled trial of riluzole in amyotrophic lateral sclerosis. N Engl J Med; 330:585–91.

Berger ML, Veitl M, Malessa S, *et al.* (1992). Cholinergic markers in ALS spinal cord. J Neurol Sci; 108:114–17.

Bergmann M, Volpel M, Kuchelmeister K. (1995). Onuf's nucleus is frequently involved in motor neuron disease/amyotrophic lateral sclerosis. J Neurol Sci; 129:141–6.

Beric A. (1993). Transcranial electrical and magnetic stimulation. In: Advances in neurology, Vol. 63. Electrical and magnetic stimulation of the brain and spinal cord, Devinsky O, Beric A, Dogali M, eds. New York: Raven Press, pp. 29–42.

Berry H, Kong K, Husdon AR, Moulton RJ. (1995). Isolated suprascapular nerve palsy: a review of nine cases. Can J Neurol Sci; 22:301–4.

Bird CE, Murphy J, Boroomand K, *et al.* (1978). Dehydroepiandrosterone: kinetics of metabolism in normal men and women. J Clin Endocrinol Metab; 47:818–22.

Birkenhager-Gillesse EG, Derksen J, Lagaay AM. (1994). Dehydroepiandrosterone sulphate (DHEAS) in the oldest old aged 85 and over. In: The aging clock: the pineal gland and other pacemakers in the progression of aging and carcinogenesis. Third Stromboli Conference on Aging and Cancer, Pierpaoli W, Regelson W, Fabris N, eds. Ann NY Acad Sci; 719:543–51.

Birnbaumer L, Campbell KP, Catterall WA, *et al.* (1994). The naming of calcium channels. Neuron; 13:505–6.

Blexrud MD, Windebank AJ, Daube JR. (1993). Long-term follow up of 121 patients with benign fascicualtions. Ann Neurol; 34:622–5.

Blin O, Samuel D, Nieoullon A, Serratrice G. (1994). Changes in CSF amino acid concentrations during the evolution of amyotrophic lateral sclerosis. J Neurol Neurosurg Psychiat; 57:119–21.

Blot S, Poirier C, Dreyfus PA. (1995). The mouse mutation muscle deficient (mdf) is characterized by a progressive motoneuron disease. J Neuropath Exp Neurol; 54:812–25.

Bolton CF, Grand'maison F, Parkes A, Shkrum M. (1992). Needle electromyography of the diaphragm. Muscle & Nerve; 15:678–81.

Boniface SJ, Mills KR, Schubert M. (1991). Responses of single motoneurons to magnetic brain stimulation in healthy subjects and patients with multiple sclerosis. Brain; 114:643–62.

Boniface SJ, Schubert M, Mills KR. (1994). Suppression and long latency excitation of single spinal motoneurons by transcranial magnetic stimulation in health, multiple sclerosis and stroke. Muscle & Nerve; 17:642–6.

Bouche P, Moulonguet A, Younes-Chennoufi AB, et al. (1995). Multifocal motor neuropathy with conduction block: a study of 24 patients. J Neurol Neurosurg Psychiatry; 59:38–44.

Bowling AC, Schulz JB, Brown RH Jr, Beal MF. (1993). Superoxide dismutase activity, oxidative damage, and mitochondrial energy metabolism in familial and sporadic amyotrophic lateral sclerosis. J Neurochem; 61:2322–5.

Bradley WG, Good P, Rassool CG, Adelman LS. (1984) Morphometric and biochemical studies of peripheral nerves in amyotrophic lateral sclerosis. Ann Neurol; 14:267–77.

Brain WR, Croft PB, Wilkinson M. (1965). Motor neurone disease as a manifestation of neoplasm (with a note on the course of classical motor neurone disease). Brain; 88:479–500.

Brait K, Fahn S, Schwarz GA. (1973). Sporadic and familial parkinsonism and motor neuron disease. Neurology; 23:990–1002.

Bredesen DE. (1995). Neural apoptosis. Ann Neurol; 38:839–51.

Bredesen DE, Wiedau-Pazos M, Goto JJ, et al. (1996). Cell death mechanisms in ALS. Neurology; 47(Suppl. 2):S36–S39.

Breitner JC, Gau BA, Welsh KA, et al. (1994). Inverse association of anti-inflammatory treatments and Alzheimer's disease: initial results of a co-twin control study. Neurology; 44:227–32.

Bremnar FD, Baker JR, Stephens JA. (1991). Variation in the degree of synchronization exhibited by motor units lying in different finger muscles in man. J Physiol; 432:381–99.

Briani C, Marcon M, Dam M, et al. (1996). Motor neuron disease in the Padua district of Italy. Neuroepidemiology; 15:173–9.

Brodie MJ. (1992). Lamotrigine. Lancet; 339:1397–400.

Bromberg MB. (1993). Motor unit estimation: reproducibility of the spike-triggered averaging technique in normal and ALS subjects. Muscle & Nerve; 16:466–71.

Bromberg MB, Abrams JL. (1995). Sources of error in the spike-triggered averaging method of motor unit number estimation (MUNE). Muscle & Nerve; 18:1139–46.

Brooks BR. (1994). World Federation of Neurology Sub Committee on Neuromuscular Diseases. El Escorial criteria for the diagnosis of amyotrophic lateral sclerosis. J Neurol Sci; 124(Suppl.):96–107.

Brooks BR, Lewis D, Rawling J, et al. (1994). The natural history of amyotrophic lateral sclerosis. In: Motor neuron disease, Williams AC, ed. London: Chapman & Hall, pp. 131–69.

Brooks BR. (1996). Clinical epidemiology of amyotrophic lateral sclerosis. Neurologic Clin; 14:399–421.

Brouwer B, Ashby P. (1990). Corticospinal projections to upper and lower limb spinal motoneurons in man. Electroenceph Clin Neurophysiol; 76:509–19.

Brown P, Cathala F, Castaigne P, Gajdusek DC. (1986). Creutzfeldt–Jakob disease: Clinical analysis of a consecutive series of 230 neuropathologically verified cases. Ann Neurol; 20:597–602.

Brown P. (1994). Transmissible human spongiform encephalopathy (infectious cerebral amyloidosis): Creutzfeld–Jakob disease, Gerstmann–Straussler–Scheinker syndrome, and Kuru. In: Neurodegenerative diseases, Calne DB, ed. Philadelphia: WB Saunders, pp. 839–76.

Brown RH Jr. (1995). Amyotrophic lateral sclerosis: recent insights from genetics and transgenic mice. Cell; 80:687–92.

Brown RH Jr. (1996). Superoxide dismutase and familial amyotrophic lateral sclerosis: New insights into mechanisms and treatments. Ann Neurol; 39:145–6.

Brown WF. (1994). Neurophysiological changes in aging. AAEM Plenary Session 1: Aging: Neuromuscular function and disease. Rochester, Mn: Johnson Printing Co, pp. 17–23.

Brown WF, Strong MJ, Snow R. (1988). Methods for estimating numbers of motor units in biceps-brachialis muscles and losses of motor units with aging. Muscle & Nerve; 11:423–32.

Brownell B, Oppenheimer DR, Hughes T. (1970). The central nervous system in motor neurone disease. J Neurol Neurosurg Psychiatry; 33:338–57.

Bruijn LI, Cleveland DW. (1996). Mechanisms of selective motor neuron death in ALS: insight from transgenic mouse models of motor neuron disease. Neuropathol Appl Neurobiol; 22:373–87.

Bruyn RP, Koelman JH, Troost D, de Jong JM. (1995). Amyotrophic lateral sclerosis arising from longstanding primary lateral sclerosis. J Neurol Neurosurg Psychiatry; 58:742–4.

Brzustowicz LM, Lehner T, Castilla H, *et al.* (1990). Genetic mapping of chronic childhood-onset spinal muscular atrophy to chromosome 5q11.2–13.3. Nature; 344:540–1.

Burrow JNC, Blumbergs PC. (1992). Substantia nigra degeneration in motor neuron disease: a quantitative study. Aust NZ J Med; 22:469–72.

Calne DB, Eisen A, McGeer E, Spencer P. (1986). Alzheimer's disease, Parkinson's disease and motoneurone disease: abiotropic interaction between aging and environment? Lancet; 2:1067–70.

Cambier J, Serratrice J. (1995). Clues to the diagnosis of amyotrophic lateral sclerosis. In: Pathogenesis and therapy of amyotrophic lateral sclerosis, Serratrice G, Munsat T, eds. Advances in neurology, Vol. 68. Philadelphia: Lippincott-Raven, pp. 161–2.

Campbell MJ, McComas AJ, Petito F. (1973). Physiological changes in aging muscle. J Neurol Neurosurg Psychiatry; 36:174–82.

Camu W, Billiard M, Baldy-Moulinier M. (1993). Fasting plasma and CSF amino acid levels in amyotrophic lateral sclerosis: a subtype analysis. Acta Neurol Scand; 88:51–5.

Cantello R, Gianelli M, Cirardi C, Mutani R. (1990). Magnetic brain stimulation: The silent period after the motor evoked potential. Neurology; 42:1951–9.

Caramia MD, Cicinelli P, Paradiso C, *et al.* (1991). Excitability changes of muscular responses to magnetic brain stimulation in patients with central motor disorders. Electroenceph Clin Neurophysiol; 81:243–50.

Cardoso F, Jankovic J. (1994). Progressive supranuclear palsy. In: Neurodegenerative diseases, Calne DB, ed. Philadelphia: WB Saunders, pp. 769–86.

Carpenter S. (1968). Proximal axonal enlargement in motor neuron disease. Neurology; 18:841–51.

Carson MJ, Behringer RR, Brinster RL, *et al.* (1993). Insulin-like growth factor 1 increases brain growth and central nervous system myelination in transgenic mice. Neuron; 10:729–40.

Carter JE, Gallo JM, Anderson VER, *et al.* (1996). Aggregation of neurofilaments in NF-L transfected neuronal cells: Regeneration of the filamentous network by a protein kinase C inhibitor. J Neurochem; 57 (5):1997–2004.

Carvalho M, Schwartz MS, Swash M. (1995). Involvement of the external anal sphincter in amyotrophic lateral sclerosis. Muscle & Nerve; 18:843–53.

Caselli RJ, Windebank AJ, Petersen RC, *et al.* (1993). Rapidly progressive aphasic dementia and motor neuron disease. Ann Neurol; 33:200–7.

Celio MR. (1990). Calbindin D-28K and parvalbumin in rat nervous system. Neuroscience; 35:375–475.

Cha CH, Patten BM. (1989). Amyotrophic lateral sclerosis: abnormalities of the tongue on magnetic resonance imaging. Ann Neurol; 25:468–72.

Chancellor AM, Hendry A, Caird FI, Warlow CP, Weir AI. (1993a). Motor neuron disease: a disease of old age. Scottish Med J; 38:178–82.

Chancellor AM, Swingler RJ, Fraser H, *et al.* (1993b). Utility of Scottish morbidity and mortality data for epidemiological studies of motor neuron disease. J Epidemiol Comm Health; 47:116–20.

Chancellor AM, Warlow CP. (1992). Adult onset motor neuron disease: worldwide mortality, incidence and distribution since 1950. J Neurol Neurosurg Psychiatry; 55:1106–15.

Charcot JM. (1865). Sclerose des cordons lateraux de la moelle epinere chez femme hysterique atteinte de contracture permanente des quatre membres. Bull Soc Med Hop Paris; 2(Suppl. 2):24–42.

Charcot JM. (1874). De la sclerose laterale amyotrophique. Proges Med; 2:325, 341, 453.

Charcot JM, Joffroy A. (1869). Deux cas d'atrophie musculaire progressive avec lesions de la substance grise et des faisceaux anteriolateraux de la moelle epiniere. Arch Physiol Norm Pathol; 2:354–67, 629–49, 744–60.

Chaudhuri KR, Crump S, Al-Sarraj S, *et al.* (1995). The validation of El Escorial criteria for the diagnosis of amyotrophic lateral sclerosis: a clinicopathological study. J Neurol Sci; 129(Suppl.):11–12.

Chen KM. (1995). Disappearance of ALS from Guam: implications for exogenous causes. Rinsho Shinkeigaku – Clin Neurol; 35:1549–53.

Chen R, Grand'Maison F, Brown JD, Bolton CF. (1997). Motor neuron disease presenting as acute respiratory failure: electrophysiological studies. Muscle & Nerve; 20:517–19.

Chen R, Grand'Maison F, Strong MJ, *et al.* (1996). Motor neuron disease presenting as acute respiratory failure: clinical and pathological study. J Neurol Neurosurg Psychiatry; 60:455–8.

Cheung G, Gawel MJ, Cooper PW, Farb RI, Ang LC. (1995). Amyotrophic lateral sclerosis: correlation of clinical and MRI imaging findings. Radiology; 194:263–70.

Choi DW. (1988). Glutamate neurotoxicity and diseases of the nervous system. Neuron; 1:623–34.

Choi DW, Peters S, Viseskul V. (1987). Dextrorphan and levorphanol selectively block N-methyl-D-aspartate receptor mediated neurotoxicity on cortical neurons. J Pharmacol Exp Ther; 242:713–20.

Chokroverty S, Chokroverty M. (1992). Magnetic stimulation of the spinal roots. In: Clinical applications of magnetic transcranial stimulation, Lissen MA, ed. Leuven, Belgium: University Press; pp. 107–25.

Chou SM. (1994). Pathology of motor system disorder. In: Motor neuron disease, Leigh PN, Swash M, eds. London: Springer-Verlag, pp. 53–92.

Chou SM, Norris FH. (1993). Amyotrophic lateral sclerosis: lower motor neuron disease spreading to upper motor neurons. Muscle & Nerve; 16:864–9.

Chou SM, Wang HS, Komai K. (1996). Colocalization of NOS and SOD1 in neurofilament accumulation within the motor neurons of amyotrophic lateral sclerosis: an immunohistochemical study. J Chem Neuroanat; 10:249–58.

Christensen PB, Hojer-Pedersen E, Jensen NB. (1990). Survival of patients with amyotrophic lateral sclerosis in 2 Danish counties. Neurology; 40:600–4.

Church J, Lodge D, Berry SC. (1985). Differential effects of dextrorphan and levorphan on the excitation of rat spinal neurons by amino acids. Eur J Pharmacol; 111:185–90.

Clough JFM, Kernell D, Phillips CG. (1968). The distribution of monosynaptic excitation from the pyramidal tract and from primary spindle afferents to motoneurons of the baboon's hand and forearm. J Physiol; 195:145–66.

Cohen G, Werner P. (1994). Free radicals, oxidative stress, and neurodegeneration. In: Neurodegenerative diseaese, Calne DB, ed. Philadelphia: WB Saunders, pp. 139–61.

Colebatch JG, Rothwell JC, Day BL, Thompson PD, Marsden CD. (1990). Cortical outflow to proximal arm muscles in man. Brain; 113:1843–56.

Collard JF, Côté F, Julien JP. (1995). Defective axonal transport in a transgenic mouse model of amyotrophic lateral sclerosis. Nature; 375:61–4.

Collinge J. (1996). New diagnostic tests for prion diseases. N Engl J Med; 335:963–65.

Collinge J, Whittington MA, Sidle KC, et al. (1994). Prion protein is necessary for normal synaptic function. Nature; 370:295–7.

Colton CA, Pagan F, Snell J, et al. (1995). Protection from oxidation enhances the survival of cultured mesencephalic neurons. Exp Neurol; 132:54–61.

Conde F, Lund JS, Jacobowitz DM, Baimbridge KG, Lewis DA. (1994). Local circuit neurons immunoreact for calretinin, calbindin D-28k or parvalbumin in monkey prefrontal cortex: Distribution and morphology. J Comp Neurol; 341:95–116.

Connolly JH, Allen IV, Dermott E. (1988). Transmissible agent in the amyotrophic form of Creutzfeldt–Jakob disease. J Neurol Neurosurg Psychiatr; 51:1459–60.

Conradi S, Grimby L, Lundemo G. (1982). Pathophysiology of fasciculations in ALS as studied by electromyography of single motor units. Muscle & Nerve; 5:202–8.

Cope TC, Fetz EE, Matsumura M. (1987). Cross-correlation assessment of synaptic strength of single Ia fibre connections with triceps surae motor neurons in cats. J Physiol; 390:161–88.

Côté F, Collard JF, Julien JP. (1993). Progressive neuronopathy in transgenic mice expressing the human neurofilament heavy gene: a mouse model of amyotrophic lateral sclerosis. Cell; 73:35–46.

Cottell E, Hutchinson M, Simon J, Harrington MG. (1990). Plasma glutamate levels in normal subjects and in patients with amyotrophic lateral sclerosis. Biochem Soc Trans; 18:283.

Coulpier M, Junier M-P, Peschanski M, Dreyfus PA. (1996). Bcl-2 sensitivity differentiates two pathways for motoneuronal death in the wobbler mutant mouse. J. Neurosci; 16:5897–904.

Couratier P, Hugon J, Sindou P, et al. (1993). Cell culture evidence for neuronal degeneration in amyotrophic lateral sclerosis being linked to glutamate AMPA/kainate receptors. Lancet; 341:265–8.

Coyle JT, Puttfarken P. (1993). Oxidative stress, glutamate, and neurodegenerative disorders. Science; 262:689–95.

Cummings JL, Benson DF. (1992). Dementia, a clinical approach. Boston: Butterworths.

Cwik VA, Hanstock CC, Boyd C, et al. (1997). Regional neuronal dysfunction in amyotrophic lateral sclerosis (ALS): In vivo measurement with proton magnetic resonance spectroscopy (MRS). Neurology; 48(Suppl):A216.

Czeh G, Gallego R, Kudo N, Kuno M. (1978). Evidence for the maintenance of motoneuron properties by muscle activity. J Physiol; 281:239–52.

Dalakas MC. (1994). Post-polio motor neurone disease. In: Motor neurone disease, Williams AC, ed. London: Chapman & Hall, pp. 83–108.

Dalakas MC, Hatazawa J, Brooks RA, Di Chiro G. (1987). Lowered cerebral glucose utilization in amyotrophic lateral sclerosis. Ann Neurol; 22:580–6.

Dal Canto MC, Gurney ME. (1994). Development of central nervous system pathology in a murine transgenic model of human amyotrophic lateral sclerosis. Am J Pathol; 145:1271–9.

Dantes M, McComas AJ. (1991). The extent and time-course of motoneuron involvement in amyotrophic lateral sclerosis. Muscle & Nerve; 14:416–21.

Date ES, Mar EY, Bugola MR, Teraoka JK. (1996). The prevalence of lumbar paraspinal spontaneous activity in asymptomatic subjects. Muscle & Nerve; 19:350–4.

Datta AK, Farmer SF, Stephens JA. (1991). Central nervous pathways underlying synchronization of human motor unit firing studied during voluntary contractions. J Physiol; 432:401–25.

Daube JR. (1985). Electrophysiological studies in the diagnosis and prognosis of motor neuron diseases. Neurol Clin; 3:477–93.

Daube JR. (1997). Motor unit estimates in ALS. In: Physiology of ALS and related diseases, Kimura J, Kaji R, eds. Amsterdam: Elsevier Science, pp. 203–16.

Davenport RJ, Swingler RJ, Chancellor AM, Warlow CP. (1996). Avoiding false positive diagnosis of motor neuron disease: lessons from the Scottish Motor Neuron Disease Register. J Neurol Neurosurg Psychiatry; 60:147–51.

Day BL, Dressler D, Maertens de Noordhout A, et al. (1989). Electrical and magnetic stimulation of human motor cortex: surface EMG and single unit responses. J Physiol; 412:449–73.

Day BL, Rothwell JC, Thompson PD, et al. (1987). Motor cortex stimulation in intact man: II Multiple descending volleys. Brain; 110:1191–209.

de Belleroche J, Recordati A, Rose FC. (1984). Elevated levels of amino acids in the CSF of motor neurone disease patients. Neurochem Pathol; 2:1–6.

DeFelipe J, Hendry SH, Jones EG. (1989). Synapses of double-bouquet cells in monkey cerebral cortex visualized by calbindin immunoreactivity. Brain Res; 503:49–54.

DeFelipe J, Jones EG. (1992). High-resolution light and electron microscopic immunohistochemistry of colocalized GABA and calbindin D-28k in somata and double bouquet cell axons of monkey somatosensory cortex. Euo J Neurosci; 4:46–60.

Deibel MA, Ehmann WD, Candy JM, et al. (1997). Aluminum in motor neuron disease spinal cord. Trace Elements in Medicine; 14:51–4.

Delbono O, Garcia J, Appel SH, Stefani E. (1991). Calcium current and charge movement of mammalian muscle: action of amyotrophic lateral sclerosis immunoglobulins. J Physiol; 444:723–42.

Delisle MB, Carpenter S. (1984). Neurofibrillary axonal swellings in amyotrophic lateral sclerosis. J Neurol Sci; 63:241–50.

Deng HX, Hentati A, Tainer JA, et al. (1993). Amyotrophic lateral sclerosis and structural defects in Cu,Zn superoxide dismutase. Science; 261:1047–51.

Dengler R, Konstanzer A, Kuther G, et al. (1990). Amyotrophic lateral sclerosis: macro EMG and twitch forces of single motor units. Muscle & Nerve; 13:545–50.

Desiato MT, Caramia MD. (1997). Towards a neurophysiological marker of amyotrophic lateral sclerosis as revealed by changes in cortical excitability. Electroencephalogr Clin Neurophysiol; 105:1–7.

Devaney KO, Johnson HA. (1980). Neuron loss in the aging visual cortex of man. J Gerontol; 35:836–41.

Deymeer F, Smith TW, DeGirolami U, Drachman DA. (1989). Thalamic dementia and motor neuron disease. Neurology; 39:58–61.

Dietl MM, Sanchez M, Probst A, Palacios JM. (1989). Substance P receptors in the human spinal cord: decrease in amyotrophic lateral sclerosis. Brain Research; 483:39–49.

DiMuzio A, Delli Pizzi C, Lugaresi A, et al. (1994). Benign monomelic amyotrophy of lower limb: a rare entity with characteristic muscular CT. J Neurol Sci; 126:153–61.

DiStefano PS. (1993). Neurotrophic factors in the treatment of motor neuron disease and trauma. Expt Neurol; 124:56–9.

Dittrich F, Thoenen H, Sendtner M. (1994). Ciliary neurotrophic factor: pharmacokinetics and acute phase response in rat. Ann Neurol; 35:151–63.

Doherty TJ, Brown WF. (1993). The estimated numbers and relative sizes of thenar motor units as selected by multiple point stimulation in young and older adults. Muscle & Nerve; 16:355–66.

Doherty TJ, Simmons Z, O'Connell B, et al. (1995). Methods for estimating the numbers of motor units in human muscles. J Clin Neurophysiol; 12:565–84.

Donaghy M, Duchen LW. (1986). Sera from patients with motor neurone disease and associated paraproteinemia fail to inhibit experimentally induced sprouting of motor nerve terminals. J Neurol Neurosurg Psychiatr; 49:817–19.

Doré S, Krieger C, Kar S, Quirion R. (1996). Distribution and levels of insulin-like growth factor (IGF-I and IGF-II) and insulin receptor binding sites in the spinal cords of amyotrophic lateral sclerosis (ALS) patients. Mol Brain Res; 41:128–33.

Doroudchi MM, Durham HD. (1996). Activation of protein kinase C induces neurofilament fragmentation, hyperphosphorylation of perikaryal neurofilaments and proximal dendritic swellings in cultured motor neurons. J Neuropathol Exp Neurol; 55:246–56.

Drachman DB, Chaudhry V, Cornblath D, *et al.* (1994). Trial of immunosuppression in amyotrophic lateral sclerosis using total lymphoid irradiation. Ann Neurol; 35:142–50.

Drachman DB, Fishman PS, Rothstein JD, *et al.* (1995). Amyotrophic lateral sclerosis: An autoimmune disease? In: Pathogensesis and therapy of amyotrophic lateral sclerosis, Serratrice G, Munsat T, eds, Advances in Neurology, Vol. 68. Philadelphia: Lippincott-Raven Publishers, pp. 59–65.

Duberley RM, Johnson IP, Anand P, *et al.* (1997). Neurotrophin-3-like immunoreactivity and Trk C expression in human spinal motoneurons in amyotrophic lateral sclerosis. J Neurol Sci; 148:33–40.

Duchenne G. (1853). Étude comparee des lesions anatomiques dans l'atrophie musculaire progressive et dans paralysie generale. L'Union Med; 7:202.

Duncan MW, Kopin IJ, Lavine L, *et al.* (1988). The putative neurotoxin BMAA in cycad-derived foods is an unlikely cause of ALS-PD. Lancet; ii:631–2.

Duval C, Poelman MC. (1995). Scavenger effect of vitamin E and derivatives on free radicals generated by photoirradiated pheomelamin. J Pharm Sci; 84:107–10.

Ebeling P, Koivisto VA. (1994). Physiological importance of dehydroepiandrosterone. Lancet; 343:1479–81.

Edgley SA, Eyre JA, Lemon RN, Miller S. (1990). Excitation of the corticospinal tract by electromagnetic and electrical stimulation of the scalp in the macaque monkey. J Physiol; 425:301–20.

Eisen A. (1992). Cortical and peripheral nerve magnetic stimulation. Methods in Clin Neurophysiol; 4:65–84.

Eisen A. (1994). Clinical electrophysiology of amyotrophic lateral sclerosis. In: Neurodegenerative diseases, Calne DB, ed. Philadelphia: W.B. Saunders, pp. 489–505.

Eisen A. (1995). Amyotrophic lateral sclerosis is a multifactorial disease. Muscle & Nerve; 18:741–52.

Eisen A, Bertrand G. (1972). Isolated accessory nerve palsy of spontaneous origin: A clinical and electromyographic study. Arch Neurol; 27:496–502.

Eisen A, Calne D. (1992). Amyotrophic lateral sclerosis, Parkinson's disease and Alzheimer's disease: phylogenetic disorders of the human neocortex sharing many characteristics. Can J Neurol Sci; 19(Suppl.):117–20.

Eisen A, Entezari-Taher M, Stewart H. (1996). Estimating the size of the cortico-motoneuronal core: Changes with aging and amyotrophic lateral sclerosis. Neurology; 46:1396–404.

Eisen A, Kim S, Pant B. (1992). Amyotrophic lateral sclerosis (ALS): a phylogenetic disease of the corticomotoneuron? Muscle & Nerve; 15:219–28.

Eisen A, Krieger C. (1993). Pathogenic mechanisms in amyotrophic lateral sclerosis. Can J Neurol Sci; 20:286–96.

Eisen A, McComas AJ. (1993). Motor neuron disorders. In: Clinical electromyography, 2nd ed., Brown WF, Bolton CF, eds. Stoneham, Mass.: Butterworth–Heinemann, pp. 427–50.

Eisen A, Nakajima M, Enterzari-Taher M, Stewart H. (1997). The corticomotoneuron: aging sporadic amyotrophic lateral sclerosis (ALS) and first degree relatives. In: Physiology of ALS and related diseases, Kimura J, Kaji R, eds. Amsterdam: Elsevier Science, pp. 155–75.

Eisen A, Pant B, Stewart H. (1993a). Cortical excitability in amyotrophic lateral sclerosis: a clue to pathogenesis. Can J Neurol Sci; 20:11–16.

Eisen A, Pearmain J, Stewart H. (1995). Dehydroepiandrosterone sulphate

(DHEAS) concentrations and amyotrophic lateral sclerosis. Muscle & Nerve; 18:1481–83.

Eisen A, Schulzer M, MacNeil M, Pant B, Mak E. (1993b). Duration of amyotrophic lateral sclerosis is age dependent. Muscle & Nerve; 16:27–32.

Eisen A, Shytbel W, Murphy K, Hoirch M. (1990). Cortical magnetic stimulation in amyotrophic lateral sclerosis. Muscle & Nerve; 13:146–51.

Eisen A, Stewart H, Cameron D, Schulzer M. (1993c). Anti-glutamate therapy in amyotrophic lateral sclerosis using Lamotrigine. Can J Neurol Sci; 20:297–301.

Ellaway PH. (1978). Cumulative sum technique and its application to the analysis of peri-stimulus time histograms. Electroencephalogr Clin Neurophysiol; 34:302–4.

Elliott MW, Simonds AK. (1995). Nocturnal assisted ventilation using bilevel positive airway pressure: the effect of expiratory positive airway pressure. Europ Respiratory J; 8:436–40.

Elliott JL, Snider WD. (1996). Motor neuron growth factors. Neurology; 47(Suppl. 2):S47–S53.

Enterzari-Taher M, Eisen A, Stewart H, Nakajima M. (1997). Abnormalities of cortical inhibitory neurons in amyotrophic lateral sclerosis. Muscle & Nerve; 20:65–71.

Erecinska M, Nelson D. (1990). Activation of glutamate dehydrogenase by leucine and its non-metabolized analogue in rat brain synaptosomes. J Neurochem; 65:59–67.

Eyer J, Peterson A. (1994). Neurofilament-deficient axons and perikaryal aggregates in viable transgenic mice expressing a neurofilament-beta-galactosidase fusion protein. Neuron; 12:389–405.

Eyre JA, Miller S, Ramesh V. (1991). Constancy of central conduction delays during development in man: investigation of motor and somatosenory pathways. J Physiol; 434:441–52.

Fahr P, Agostino R, Hallett M. (1991). Spinal motor neuron excitability during the silent period after cortical stimulation. Electroenceph Clin Neurophysiol; 81:257–62.

Ferrante MA, Wilbourn AJ. (1997). The characteristic electrodiagnostic features of Kennedy's disease. Muscle & Nerve; 20:323–9.

Fetz EE, Cheney PD. (1980). Post-spike facilitation of forelimb muscle activity by primate corticomotoneuronal cells. J Neurophysiol; 44:751–72.

Fetz EE, Gustafsson B. (1983). Relation between shapes of postsynaptic potentials and changes in the firing probability of cat motoneurons. J Physiol; 341:387–410.

Figlewicz DA, Krizus A, Martinoli MG, et al. (1994). Variants of the heavy neurofilament subunit are associated with development of amyotrophic lateral sclerosis. Hum Mol Genet; 3:1757–61.

Flament D, Goldsmith P, Buckley JC, Lemon RN. (1993). Task-dependence of responses in first dorsal interosseus muscle to magnetic brain stimulation in man. J Physiol; 464:361–78.

Flood JF, Smith GE, Roberts E. (1988). Dehydroepiandrosterone and its sulfate enhance memory retention in mice. Brain Res; 447:269–78.

Forster FM, Alpers BJ. (1946). Effects of denervation on fasciculations in human muscle. Arch Neurol Psychiat; 56:276–82.

Forsyth PA, Dalmau J, Graus F, et al. (1997). Motor neuron syndromes in cancer patients. Ann Neurol; 41:722–30.

Friedman DP, Tartaglino LM. (1993). Amyotrophic lateral sclerosis:

Hyperintensity of the corticospinal tracts on MR images of the spinal cord. Am J Roentgenol; 160:604–6.

Friess E, Trachsel L, Guldner J, *et al.* (1995). DHEA administration increases rapid eye movement sleep and EEG power in the sigma frequency range. Amer J Physiol; 268(1):E107–E113.

Fournier J, Steinberg R, Gauthier T, *et al.* (1993). Neuroprotective effects of SR57746A in central and peripheral models in rodents and primates. Neurosci; 55:629–41.

Gallassi R, Montagna P, Morreale A, *et al.* (1989). Neuropsychological, electroencephalogram and brain computed tomography findings in motor neurone disease. Eur Neurol; 29:115–20.

Gandevia SC, Rothwell JC. (1980). Activation of the human diaphragm from the motor cortex. J Physiol; 303:351–64.

Gandevia SC, Plassman BL. (1988). Responses in human intercostal and truncal muscles to motor cortical and spinal stimulation. Resp and Physiol; 73:325–38.

Gao W-Q, Dybdal N, Shinsky N, *et al.* (1995). Neurotrophin-3 reverses experimental cisplatin-induced peripheral sensory neuropathy. Ann Neurol; 38:30–7.

Garruto RM, Yase Y. (1986). Neurodegenerative disorders of the Western Pacific: the search for mechanisms of pathogenesis. Trends Neurosci; 9:368–75.

Garruto RM. (1987). Neurotoxicity of trace and essential elements: factors provoking the high incidence of motor neuron disease, Parkinsonism and dementia in the Western Pacific. In: Motor neuron disease: global clinical patterns and interational research, Gouri-Devi M, ed. New Delhi: Oxford and IBH Publishing Co, pp. 73–82.

Garruto RM, Yanagihara R. (1991). Amyotrophic lateral sclerosis in the Mariana Islands. Handbook of Clinical Neurology; 15(59):253–71.

Ghez C, Hening W, Gordon J. (1991). Organization of voluntary movement. Curr Opin Neurobiol; 1:664–71.

Gibbs CJ, Gajdusek DC. (1982). An update on long-term in vivo and in vitro studies designed to identify a virus as the cause of amyotrophic lateral sclerosis, Parkinsonism dementia, and Parkinson's disease. Adv. Neurol; 36:343–53.

Gilbert JJ, Kish SJ, Chang LJ. (1988). Dementia, parkinsonism, and motor neuron disease: neurochemical and neuropathological correlates. Ann Neurol; 24:688–91.

Gillberg PG, Aquilonius SM. (1985). Cholinergic, opioid and glycine receptor binding sites localized in human spinal cord by in vitro autoradiography: changes in amyotrophic lateral sclerosis. Acta Neurol Scand; 72:299–306.

Gilliatt RW, Willison RG, Dietz V, Williams IR. (1978). Peripheral nerve conduction in patients with cervical rib and band. Ann Neurol; 4:124–9.

Gimenez-Gallego G, Cuevas P. (1994). Fibroblast growth factors, proteins with a broad spectrum of biological activities. Neurol Res; 16:212–316.

Goodkin DS, Rowley HA, Olney RK. (1988). Magnetic resonance imaging in amyotrophic lateral sclerosis. Ann Neurol; 23:418–20.

Goodridge AE, Feasby TE, Ebers GC, Brown WF, Rice GP. (1987). Hand wasting due to mid-cervical spinal cord compression. Can J Neurol Sci; 14:309–11.

Gorell JM, Johnson CC, Rybicki BA, *et al.* (1997). Occupational exposures to metals as risk factors for Parkinson's disease. Neurology; 48:650–8.

Gouin A, Bloch-Gallego E, Tanaka H, Henderson CE. (1996). Transforming growth factor $\beta3$, glial cell line-derived neurotrophic factor and fibroblast growth factor-2 act in different manners to promote motoneuron survival in vitro. J Neurosci Res; 43:454–64.

Gredal O, Moller SE. (1995). Effect of branched-chain amino acids on glutamate metabolism in amyotrophic lateral sclerosis. J Neurol Sci; 129:40–3.

Gredal O, Rosenbaum S, Topp S, *et al.* (1997). Quantification of brain metabolites in amyotrophic lateral sclerosis by localized proton magnetic resonance spectroscopy. Neurology; 48:878–81.

Greenberg DA. (1994). Calcium channels and neuromuscular disease. Ann Neurol; 35:131–2.

Gubbay SS, Kahana E, Ziber N, *et al.* (1985). Amyotrophic lateral sclerosis – a study of its presentation and prognosis. J Neurol; 232:295–300.

Guiloff RJ, Modarres-Sadeghi H. (1992). Voluntary activation and fiber density of fasciculations in motor neuron disease. Ann Neurol; 31:416–24.

Gunnarsson LG, Lygner PE, Veiga-Cabo J, de Pedro-Cuesto J. (1996). An epidemic-like cluster of motor neuron disease in a Swedish county during the period 1973–1984. Neuroepidemiol; 15:142–52.

Gurney ME, Belton AC, Cashman N, Antel JP. (1984). Inhibition of terminal sprouting by serum from patients with amyotrophic lateral sclerosis. N Engl J Med; 311:933–9.

Gurney ME, Pu H, Chiu AY, *et al.* (1994). Motor neuron degeneration in mice that express a human Cu,Zn superoxide dismutase mutation. Science; 164:1772–5.

Gurney ME, Yamamoto H, Kwon Y. (1992). Induction of motor neuron sprouting in vivo by ciliary neurotrophic factor and basic fibroblast growth factor. J Neurosci; 12:3241–7.

Haase G, Kennel P, Pettman B, *et al.* (1997). Gene therapy of a murine motor neuron disease using adenoviral vectors for neurotrophic factors. Nature Med; 3:429–36.

Hammer Jr RP, Tomiyasu U, Scheibel AB. (1979). Degeneration of the human Betz cell due to amyotrophic lateral sclerosis. Exp Neurol; 63:336–46.

Harding AE, Thomas PK, Baraitser M, *et al.* (1982). X-linked recessive bulbospinal neuronopathy: A report of ten cases. J Neurol Neurosurg Psychiatry; 45:1012–19.

Hasham MI, Pelech SL, Koide HB, Krieger C. (1997). Activation of protein kinase C by intracellular calcium in the motoneuron cell line NSC-19. Biochim Biophys Acta; 1360:177–91.

Hastings KEM. (1992). Gene expression in motor neurons. In: Handbook of amyotrophic lateral sclerosis, Smith RA, ed. New York: Marcel Dekker, pp. 709–37.

Haub O, Goldfarb M. (1991). Expression of the fibroblast growth factor-5 gene in the mouse embryo. Development; 112:397–406.

Haug BA, Schönle PW, Knoblock C, Köhne M. (1992). Silent period measurement revived as a valuable diagnostic tool with transcranial magnetic stimulation. Electroenceph Clin Neurophysiol; 85:158–60.

Hausmanowa-Petrusewicz I. (1991). Spinal muscular atrophies: How many types? In: Advances in neurology, Vol. 56: Amyotrophic lateral sclerosis and other motor neuron diseases, Rowland LP, ed. New York: Raven Press, pp. 157–67.

Hebert T, Drapeau P, Pradier L, Dunn RJ. (1994). Block of the rat brain IIA sodium channel alpha subunit by the neuroprotective drug riluzole. Mol Pharmacol; 45:1055–60.

Hefti F. (1994). Neurotrophic factor therapy for nervous system degenerative diseases. J Neurobiol; 25:1418–35.

Henderson CE, Camu W, Mettling C, *et al.* (1993). Neurotrophins promote motor neuron survival and are present in embryonic limb bud. Nature; 363:266–70.

Henderson CE, Phillips HS, Pollock RA, Davies AM, *et al.* (1994). GDNF: A potent survival factor for motoneurons present in peripheral nerve and muscle. Science; 266:1062–4.

Henderson G, Tomlinson BE, Gibson P. (1980). Cell counts in human cerebral cortex in normal adults throughout life using an image analysing computer. J Neurol Sci; 46:113–36.

Henderson JT, Javaheri M, Kopko S, Roder JC. (1996). Reduction of lower motor neuron degeneration in wobbler mice by N-acetyl-cysteine. J Neurosci; 16:7574–82.

Henneman E, Somjen G, Carpenter DO. (1965). Functional significance of cell size in spinal motoneurons. J Neurophysiol; 28:560–80.

Hess CW, Mills KR, Murray NMF. (1987). Responses in small hand muscles from magnetic stimulation of the human brain. J Physiol; 388:397–419.

Hideo T, Takashi A, Mika S, *et al.* (1996). A-tocopherol quinone level is remarkably low in the cerebrospinal fluid of patients with sporadic amyotrophic lateral sclerosis. Neurosci Lett; 207:5–8.

Hill R, Martin J, Hakim A. (1983). Acute respiratory failure in motor neuron disease. Arch Neurol; 40:30–2.

Hirano A. (1996). Neuropathology of ALS: An overview. Neurology; 47(Suppl. 2):S63–S66.

Hirano A, Iwata M. (1979). Pathology of motor neurons with special reference to amyotrophic lateral sclerosis and related diseases. In: Amyotrophic lateral sclerosis, Tsubaki T, Toyokura Y, eds. Baltimore: University Park Press, pp. 107–34.

Hirano A, Malamud N, Elizan T, Kurland LT. (1966). Amyotrophic lateral sclerosis and Parkinsonism–dementia complex on Guam. Arch Neurol; 15:35–51.

Hirayama K. (1991). Non-progressive juvenile spinal muscular atrophy of the distal upper limb (Hirayama's disease). Handbook of clinical neurology 15 (59): Diseases of the motor system, d Jong JMBV, ed. Amsterdam: Elsevier Science Publishers, pp. 107–20.

Hirayama K, Toyokura Y, Tsubaki T. (1959). Juvenile muscular atrophy of unilateral upper extremity – a new clinical entitiy. Psychiatr Neurol Jpn; 61:2190–7.

Hirokawa N. (1991). Molecular architecture and dynamics of the neuronal cytoskeleton. In: The neuronal cytoskeleton, Burgoyne RD, ed. New York: Wiley-Liss, pp. 5–74.

Hjorth RJ, Walsh JC, Willison RG. (1973). The distribution and frequency of spontaneous fasciculations in motor neurone disease. J Neurol Sci; 18:469–74.

Ho B-K, Alexianu ME, Colom LV, *et al.* (1996). Expression of calbindin-D28k in motoneuron hybrid cells after retroviral infection with calbindin-D28k cDNA prevents amyotrophic lateral sclerosis IgG-mediated cytotoxicity. Proc Natl Acad Sci USA; 93:6796–801.

Hochberg F, Miller G, Valenzuela R, *et al.* (1997). Occupational exposures to metals as risk factors for Parkinson's diseases. Neurology; 48:650–7.

Hollander D, Pradas J, Kaplan R, *et al.* (1994). High-dose dextromethorphan in amyotrophic lateral sclerosis: Phase 1 safety and pharmacokinetic studies. Ann Neurol; 36:920–4.

Holmgren H, Larson LE, Pedersen S. (1990). Late muscular responses to transcranial cortical stimulation in man. Electroenceph Clin Neurophysiol; 75:161–72.

Hooten WM, Lyketsos CG. (1996). Frontotemporal dementia: A clinicopathological review of four postmortem studies. J Neuropsychiat Clin Neurosci; 8:10–19.

Hopkins LC, Tatarian GT, Pianta TF. (1996). Management of ALS: Respiratory care. Neurology; 47(Suppl. 2):S123–S125.

Houenou LJ, Turner PL, Li L, *et al.* (1995). A serine protease inhibitor, protease nexin-1, rescues motoneurons from naturally occurring and axotomy-induced cell death. Proc Natl Acad Sci USA; 92:895–9.

Howard RS, Murray NM. (1992). Surface EMG in the recording of fasciculations. Muscle & Nerve; 15:1240–5.

Howlett WP, Brubaker GR, Milingi GR, Rosling H. (1990). Konzo, an epidemic upper motor neuron disease studied in Tanzania. Brain; 113:223–35.

Hsich G, Kenny K, Gibbs CJ. (1996). The 14–3–3 brain protein in cerebrospinal fluid as a marker for transmissible spongiform encephalopathies. New Engl J Med; 335:924–30.

Hubert JP, Delumeau JC, Glowiniski J, *et al.* (1994). Antagonism by riluzole of entry of calcium evoked by NMDA and veratridine in rat cultured granule cells: evidence for dual mechanism of action. Br J Pharmacol; 113:261–7.

Hudson AJ. (1981). Amyotrophic lateral sclerosis and its association with dementia, Parkinsonism and other neurological disorders: A review. Brain; 104:217–47.

Hudson AJ. (1991a). Amyotrophic lateral sclerosis/Parkinsonism/dementia: Clinico-pathological correlations relevant to Guamanian ALS/PD. Can J Neurol Sci; 18:387–9.

Hudson AJ. (1991b). Dementia and parkinsonism in amyotrophic lateral sclerosis. Handbook of Clinical Neurology; 15(59):231–40.

Hudson AJ, Rice GPA. (1990). Similarities of Guamanian ALS/PD to postencephalitic parkinsonism/ALS: possible viral cause. Can J Neurol Sci; 17:427–33.

Hufnagel A, Elger CE, Marx W, Ising A. (1990). Magnetic stimulation motor-evoked potentials in epilepsy: effects of the disease and anticonvulsant medications. Ann Neurol; 28:680–6.

Hugon J, Lubeau M, Tabarard F, Chazot F, Vallat JM, Dumas M. (1987). Central motor conduction in motor neuron disease. Ann Neurol; 22:544–6.

Hugon J, Vallat JM, Spencer PS, *et al.* (1989). Kainic acid induces early and delayed degenerative neuronal changes in rat spinal cord. Neurosci Lett; 104:258–62.

Humphrey DR. (1986). Representation of movements and muscles within the primate precentral motor cortex: historical and current perspectives. Fed Proc; 45:2687–99.

Ikeda K, Kinoshita M, Iwasaki Y, *et al.* (1995a). Lecithinized superoxide dismutase retards wobbler mouse motoneuron disease. Neuromusc Disord; 5:383–90.

Ikeda K, Klinkosz B, Greene T, *et al.* (1995b). Effects of brain-derived neurotrophic factor on motor dysfunction in wobbler mouse motor neuron disease. Ann Neurol; 37:505–11.

Ikonomidou C, Qin YQ, Labruyere J, Olney JW. (1996). Motor neuron degeneration induced by excitotoxin agonists has features in common with those seen in the SOD-1 transgenic mouse model of amyotrophic lateral sclerosis. J Neuropath Exp Neurol; 55:211–24.

Ince P, Stout N, Shaw P, *et al.* (1993). Parvalbumin and calbindin D-28k in the human motor system in motor neuron disease. Neuropath & Appl Neurobiol; 19:291–9.

Ingram DA, Swash M. (1987). Central motor conduction is abnormal in motor neuron disease. J Neurol Neurosurg Psychiatry; 50:159–66.

Irani K, Xia Y, Zweier JL, *et al.* (1997). Mitogenic signalling mediated by oxidants in Ras-transformed fibroblasts. Science; 275:1649–52.

Ishikawa K, Nagura H, Yokota T, Yamanouchi H. (1993). Signal loss in the motor cortex on magnetic resonance images in amyotrophic lateral sclerosis. Ann Neurol; 33:218–21.

Iwasaki Y, Ikeda K, Kinoshita M. (1992a). MRI lesions in motor neuron disease. J Neurol; 239:112–13.

Iwasaki Y, Ikeda K, Kinoshita M. (1992b). Plasma amino acid levels in patients with amyotrophic lateral sclerosis. J Neurol Sci; 107:219–22.

Iwasaki Y, Ikeda K, Shiojima T, *et al.* (1994a). Clinical significance of hypointensity in the motor cortex on T2-weighted images. Neurology; 44:1181.

Iwasaki Y, Ikeda K, Shiojima T, *et al.* (1994b). Deprenyl enhances neurite outgrowth in cultured rat spinal ventral horn neurons. J Neurol Sci; 125:11–13.

Iwatsubo T, Kuzuhara S, Kanemitsu B, *et al.* (1990). Corticofugal projections to the motor nuclei of the brainstem and spinal cord in humans. Neurology; 40:309–12.

Jablecki CK, Berry C, Leach J. (1989). Survival prediction in amyotrophic lateral sclerois. Muscle & Nerve; 12:833–41.

Jankowska E, Patel Y, Tanaka R. (1975). Projections of pyramidal tract cells to a-motoneurones innervating hind-limb muscles in monkey. J Physiol; 249:637–67.

Jansen PHP, Joosten EMG, Jaspar HHJ, Vingerhoets HM. (1986). A rapidly progressive autosomal dominant scapulohumeral form of spinal muscular atrophy. Ann Neurol; 20:538–40.

Johnson IP. (1996). Target dependence of motoneurons. In: The neurobiology of disease, Bostock H, Kirkwood PA, Pullen AH, eds. Cambridge: Cambridge University Press, pp. 379–94.

Jokelainen M. (1977). Amyotrophic lateral sclerosis in Finland. Acta Neurol Scand; 56:194–201.

Jones AP, Gunawardena WJ, Coutinho CMA, *et al.* (1995). Preliminary results of proton magnetic resonance spectroscopy in motor neuron disease (amyotrophic lateral sclerosis). J Neurol Sci; 129(Suppl.):85–9.

Jones KR, Farinas I, Backus C, Reichardt LF. (1994). Targetted disruption of the BDNF gene perturbs brain and sensory nerve development but not motor neuron development. Cell; 76:989–99.

Josson SS, Ekblom J, Aquilonius SM, Oreland L. (1994a). Monoamine oxidase-B in motor cortex and spinal cord in amyotrophic lateral sclerosis studied by quantitative autoradiography. J Neural Transm; 41(Suppl.):243–8.

Josson SS, Ekblom J, Gudjonsson O, Hagbarth KE, Aquilonius SW. (1994b).
    Double blind cross-over trial with deprenyl in amyotrophic lateral sclerosis.
    J Neural Transm; 41:237–41.
Julien JP. (1995). A role for neurofilaments in the pathogenesis of amyotrophic
    lateral sclerosis. Biochem Cell Biol; 73:593–7.
Julien JP. (1997). Neurofilaments and motor neuron disease. Trends Cell Biol;
    7:243–9.
Juneja T, Pericak-Vance A, Laing NG, *et al.* (1997). Prognosis and survival in
    familial amyotrophic lateral sclerosis: Progression and survival in patients
    with glu100gly and ala4val mutations in Cu,Zn superoxide dismutase.
    Neurology; 48:55–7.
Kaji R. (1997). Physiological and technical basis of peripheral nerve and
    motoneuron testing. In: Physiology of ALS and related diseases, Kimura J,
    Kaji R, eds. Amsterdam: Elsevier Science, pp. 15–41.
Kalimi M, Regelson W, eds. (1990). The biological role of
    dehydroepiandrosterone (DHEA). New York: Walter de Gruyter.
Kandel ER, Schwartz JH. (1991). Directly gated transmission at central synapses.
    In: Principles of neural science, 3rd ed., Kandel ER, Schwartz JH, Jessell
    TM, eds. New York: Elsevier, pp. 153–72.
Kaplan JC, Fontaine B. (1996). Neuromuscular disorders: gene location.
    Neuromusc Disord; 6:I–IX.
Kasarskis EJ, Neville HE. (1996). Management of ALS: Nutritional care.
    Neurology; 47(Suppl. 2):S118–S120.
Kato S, Oda M, Tanabe H. (1993). Diminution of dopaminergic neurons in the
    substantia nigra of sporadic amyotrophic lateral sclerosis. Neuropathol
    Appl Neurobiol; 19:300–4.
Kato S, Oda M, Hayashi H, *et al.* (1994). Participation of the limbic system and
    its associated areas in the dementia of amyotrophic lateral sclerosis. J Neurol
    Sci; 126:62–9.
Kawamura Y, Dyck PJ, Shimono M, *et al.* (1981). Morphometric comparison of
    vulnerability of peripheral motor and sensory neurons in amyotrophic
    lateral sclerosis. J Neuropathol Exp Neurol; 40:667–75.
Kennedy WR, Alter M, Sung JH. (1968). Progressive proximal spinal and bulbar
    muscular atrophy of late onset: a sex-linked recessive trait. Neurology;
    18:671–80.
Kernell D, Wu CP. (1967). Responses of pyramidal tract to stimulation of the
    baboon's motor cortex. J Physiol (Lond.); 191:653–72.
Kew JJ, Brooks DJ, Passingham RE, *et al.* (1994). Cortical function in
    progressive lower motor neuron disorders and amyotrophic lateral sclerosis:
    a comparative PET study. Neurology; 44:1101–10.
Kew JJM, Goldstein LH, Leigh PN, *et al.* (1993). The relationship between
    abnormalities of cognitive function and cerebral activation in amyotrophic
    lateral sclerosis. A neuropsychological and positron emission tomography
    study. Brain; 116:1399–423.
Khawli FA, Reid MB. (1994). N-acetylcysteine depresses contractile function and
    inhibits fatigue of diaphragm in vitro. J Applied Physiol; 77:317–24.
Kiernan JA, Hudson AJ. (1991). Changes in sizes of cortical and lower motor
    neurons in amyotrophic lateral sclerosis. Brain; 114:843–53.
Kiernan JA, Hudson AJ. (1993). Anti-neurone antibodies are not characteristic
    of ALS. Neuroreport; 4:427–30.
Kiernan JA, Hudson AJ. (1994). Frontal lobe atrophy in motor neuron diseases.
    Brain; 117:747–57.

Kimura J. (1997). Multifocal motor neuropathy and conduction block. In: Physiology of ALS and related diseases, Kimura J, Kaji R, eds. Amsterdam: Elsevier Science, pp. 57–72.

Kirschbaum W. (1968). Jakob–Creutzfeldt disease. New York: Elsevier.

Kisby GE, Ross SM, Spencer PS, *et al.* (1992). Candidate neurotoxins for western Pacific amyotrophic lateral sclerosis/Parkinsonism–dementia complex. Neurodegeneration; 1:73–82.

Kishimoto T, Taga T, Akira S. (1994). Cytokine signal transduction. Cell; 76:253–62.

Kitani K, Kanai S, Carrillo MC, Ivy GO. (1994). (-)Deprenyl increases the life span as well as activities of superoxide dismutase and catalase but not of glutathione peroxidase in selelctive brain regions in Fischer rats. Ann NY Acad Sci; 717:60–71.

Knight JM, Jones AP, Redmond JP, Shaw IC. (1996). Identification of brain metabolites by magnetic resonance spectroscopy in MND/ALS. J Neurol Sci; 139(Suppl.):104–9.

Kohara N, Kaji R, Kojima Y, *et al.* (1996). Abnormal excitability of the corticospinal pathway in patients with amyotrophic lateral sclerosis: a single motor unit study using transcranial magnetic stimulation. Electroencephalogr Clin Neurophysiol; 101:32–41.

Kornberg AJ, Pestronk A. (1995). Chronic motor neuropathies. In: Pathogenesis and therapy of amyotrophic lateral sclerosis, Serratrice G, Munsat T, eds. Advances in Neurology, Vol. 68. Philadelphia: Lippincott-Raven Publishers, 113–19.

Kozlowski MA, Williams C, Hinton DR, Miller CA. (1989). Heterotopic neurons in spinal cord of patients with ALS. Neurology; 39:644–8.

Kramer N, Meyer TJ, Meharg J, Cece RD, Hill NS. (1995). Randomized, prospective trial of noninvasive positive pressure ventilation in acute respiratory failure. Amer J Respiratory & Critical Care Medicine; 151:1799–806.

Kretzschmar HA, Ironside JW, DeArmond SJ, Tateishi J. (1996). Diagnostic criteria for sporadic Creutzfeldt–Jakob disease. Arch Neurol; 53:913–20.

Krieger C, Hansen S, Heyes MP. (1993a). Amyotrophic lateral sclerosis: Quinolinic acid levels in cerebrospinal fluid and spinal cord. Neurodegeneration; 2:237–41.

Krieger C, Lai R, Mitsumoto H, Shaw C. (1993b). The wobbler mouse: quantitative autoradiography of glutamatergic ligand binding sites in spinal cord. Neurodegeneration; 2:9–17.

Krieger C, Lanius RA, Pelech SL, Shaw CA. (1996a). Amyotrophic lateral sclerosis: the involvement of intracellular Ca^{2+} and protein kinase C. Trends Pharmacol Sci; 17:114–20.

Krieger C, Mezei M, Hasham MI, Lanius RA. (1996b). Neurotransmitter receptor modification in neurological disease. In: Receptor dynamics in neural development, CA Shaw, ed. Boca Raton: CRC Press, pp. 321–36.

Krieger C, Wagey R, Lanius RA, Shaw CA. (1993c). Activation of PKC reverses apparent NMDA receptor reduction in ALS. NeuroReport; 4:931–4.

Krieger C, Wagey R, Shaw CA. (1993d). Amyotrophic lateral sclerosis: quantitative autoradiography of [^{3}H]MK-801/NMDA binding sites in spinal cord. Neurosci Lett; 159:191–4.

Kurland LT, Choi NW, Sayre GP. (1969). Implications of incidence and geographic patterns on the classification of amyotrophic lateral sclerosis. In:

Motor neuron diseases: Research on amyotrophic lateral sclerosis and related disorders, Norris FH, Kurland LT, eds. New York: Grune and Stratton, pp. 28–50.

Kurland LT, Molgaard CA. (1982). Guamanian ALS: hereditary or acquired? In: Human motor neuron diseases, Rowland LP, ed. New York: Raven Press, pp. 165–71.

Kurtzke JF. (1991). Risk factors in amyotrophic lateral sclerosis. In: Ayotrophic lateral sclerosis and other motor neuron diseases, Rowland LP, ed. Advances in Neurology, Vol. 56. New York: Raven Press, 245–70.

Kushner PD, Stephenson DT, Wright S. (1991). Reactive astrogliosis is widespread in the subcortical white matter of amyotrophic lateral sclerosis brain. J Neuropathol Exp Neurol; 50:263–77.

Kuwabara S, Nakajima M, Matsuda S, Hattori T. (1997). Magnetic resonance imaging at the demyelinating foci in chronic inflammatory demyelinating polyneuropathy. Neurology; 48:874–7.

Lacomblez L, Bensimon G, Leigh PN, Guillet P, Meininger V, The ALS/ Riluzole Study Group-II. (1996). A dose-ranging study of riluzole in amyotrophic lateral sclerosis. Lancet; 347:1425–31.

Lambert EH. (1969). Electromyography in amyotrophic lateral sclerosis. In: Motor neuron disease: Research on amyotrophic lateral sclerosis and related disorders, Norris FN Jr, Kurland LT, eds. New York: Grune & Stratton, pp. 135–53.

Lane RJM, Bandopadhyay R, de Belleroche J. (1993). Abnormal glycine metabolism in motor neurone disease: Studies on plasma and cerebrospinal fluid. J Roy Soc Med; 86:501–5.

Lange DJ, Felice KJ, Festoff BW, et al. (1996). Recombinant human insulin-like growth factor-1 in ALS. Description of a double-blind, placebo-controlled study. Neurology; 47(Suppl. 2):S93–S95.

Lanius RA, Krieger C, Wagey R, Shaw CA. (1993). Increased [^{35}S]glutathione binding sites in spinal cords from patients with sporadic amyotrophic lateral sclerosis. Neurosci Lett; 163:89–92.

Lanius RA, Paddon HB, Mezei M, et al. (1995). A role for amplified protein kinase C activity in the pathogenesis of amyotrophic lateral sclerosis. J Neurochem; 65:927–30.

Lanius RA, Shaw CA, Wagey R, Krieger C. (1994). Characterization, distribution and protein kinase C-mediated regulation of [^{35}S]glutathione binding sites in spinal cords. J Neurochem; 63:155–60.

Lanthier A, Patwardhan VV. (1986). Sex steroids and 5-en-3b-hydroxysteroids in specific regions of the human brain and cranial nerves. J Steroid Biochem; 25:445–9.

Lavine L, Steele JC, Wolfe N, et al. (1991). Amyotrophic lateral sclerosis/ Parkinsonism/dementia complex in Southern Guam: Is it disappearing? Adv Neurol; 56:271–85.

Lawson SJ, Davies HJ, Bennett JP, Lowrie MB. (1997). Evidence that spinal interneurons undergo programmed cell death postnatally in the rat. Eur J Neurosci; 9:101–6.

Layzer RB. (1982). Diagnostic implications of clinical fasciculations and cramps. Adv Neurol; 36:23–7.

Layzer RB. (1994). The origin of muscle fasciculations and cramps. Muscle & Nerve; 17:1243–9.

Lee JRJ, Annegers JF, Appel SH. (1995). Prognosis of amyotrophic lateral sclerosis and the effect of referral selection. J Neurol Sci, 132:207–15.

Lee MK, Marszalek JR, Cleveland DW. (1994). A mutant neurofilament subunit causes massive, selective motor neuron death: implications for the pathogenesis of human motor neuron disease. Neuron; 13:975–88.

Leigh PN. (1994). Pathogenic mechanisms in amyotrophic lateral sclerosis and other motor neuron disorders. In: Neurodegenerative diseases, Calne DB, ed. Philadelphia: WB Saunders, pp. 473–88.

Leigh PN, Swash M. (1991). Cytoskeletal pathology in motor neuron diseases. In: Amyotrophic lateral sclerosis and other motor neuron diseases. Rowland LP, ed. Advances in Neurology, Vol. 56. New York: Raven Press, pp. 115–24.

Leigh PN, Whitwell H, Garofalo O. (1991). Ubiquitin-immunoreactive intraneuronal inclusions in amyotrophic lateral sclerosis. Brain; 114:775–88.

Lemon RN. (1993). The G.L. Brown prize lecture: Cortical control of the primate hand. Exp Physiol; 78:263–301.

Lennon VA, Kryzer TJ, Griesmann GE, et al. (1995). Calcium-channel antibodies in the Lambert–Eaton syndrome and other paraneoplastic syndromes. N Engl J Med; 332:1467–74.

Leveugle B, Spik G, Perl DP, et al. (1994). The iron-binding protein lactotransferrin is present in pathological lesions in a variety of neurodegenerative disorders: A comparative immunohistochemical analysis. Brain Res; 650:320–31.

Lewis ME, Neff NT, Contreras PC, et al. (1993). Insulin-like growth factor 1: potential for treatment of motor neuronal disorders. Exp Neurol; 124:73–88.

Li M, Sobue G, Doyu M, et al. (1995). Primary sensory neurons in X-linked recessive bulbospinal neuronopathy: Histopathology and androgen receptor gene expression. Muscle & Nerve; 18:301–8.

Lillienfeld DE, Chan E, Ehland J, et al. (1989). Rising mortality from motoneuron disease in the USA, 1982–84. Lancet; 1:710–12.

Lindholm D. (1994). Role of neurotrophins in preventing glutamate induced neuronal cell death. J Neurol; 242(Suppl. 1):16–18.

Lipton SA, Rosenberg PA. (1994). Excitatory amino acids as a final common pathway for neurologic disorders. N Engl J Med; 330:613–22.

Llinas R, Sugimori M, Cherksey BD, et al. (1993). IgG from amyotrophic lateral sclerosis patients increases current through P-type calcium channels in mammalian cerebellar Purkinje cells and in isolated channel protein in lipid bilayer. Proc Natl Acad Sci USA; 90:11743–7.

Longo FM. (1994). Will ciliary neurotrophic factor slow progression of motor neuron disease? Ann Neurol; 36:125–7.

Louis ED, Hanley AE, Brannagan TH, Sherman W, et al. (1996). Motor neuron disease, lymphoproliferative disease and bone marrow biopsy. Muscle & Nerve; 19:1334–7.

Louwerse ES, Weverling GJ, Bossuyt PMM, et al. (1995). Randomized, double-blind, controlled trial of acetylcysteine in amyotrophic lateral sclerosis. Arch Neurol; 52:559–64.

Lowe J. (1994). New pathological findings in amyotrophic lateral sclerosis. J Neurol Sci; 124:38–51.

Ludolph AC, Elger CE, Bottger IW, et al. (1989). N-Isopropyl-p-^{123}I-amphetamine single photon emission computer tomography with motor neuron disese. Eur Neurol; 29:255–60.

Ludolph AC, Langen KJ, Regard M, et al. (1992). Frontal lobe function in amyotrophic lateral sclerosis: a neuropsychological and positron emission tomography study. Acta Neurol Scand; 85:81–9.

Lund and Manchester Groups. (1994). Clinical and neuropathological criteria for frontotemporal dementia. J Neurol Neurosurg and Psychiat; 57:416–19.

Mailis A, Ashby P. (1990). Alterations in group Ia projections to motoneurons following spinal lesions in humans. J Neurophysiol; 64:637–47.

Majoor-Krakaur D, Ottman R, Johnson WG, Rowland LP. (1994). Familial aggregation of amyotrophic lateral sclerosis, dementia, and Parkinson's disease. Neurology; 44:1872–7.

Manaker S, Caine SB, Winokur A. (1988). Alterations in receptors for thyrotropin-releasing hormone, serotonin and acetylcholine in amyotrophic lateral sclerosis. Neurology; 38:1464–74.

Manaker S, Shulman LH, Winokur A, Rainbow TC. (1985). Autoradiographic localization of thyrotropin-releasing hormone receptors in amyotrophic lateral sclerosis spinal cord. Neurology; 35:1650–3.

Mann DM. (1994). Vulnerability of specific neurons to aging. In: Neurodegenerative diseases, Calne DB, ed. Philadelphia: WB Saunders, pp. 15–31.

Mann DM, Yates PO. (1974). Lipoprotein pigments: Their relationship to aging in the human nervous system. Brain; 97:481–8.

Mannen T, Iwata M, Toyokura Y, Nagashima K. (1977). Preservation of a certain motoneurone group of the sacral cord in amyotrophic lateral sclerosis: its clinical significance. J Neurol Neurosurg Psychiatr; 40:464–9.

Mantz J, Laudmbach V, Lecharny JB, et al. (1994). Riluzole, a novel antiglutamate, blocks GABA uptake by striatal synaptosomes. Eur J Pharmacol (Netherlands); 257:R7–8.

Mao CC, Ashby P, Wang M, McCrae D. (1984). Synaptic connections from large muscle afferents to the motoneurons of leg muscles in man. Exp Brain Res; 56:341–50.

Markesbury WR, Ehmann WD, Candy JM, et al. (1995). Neutron activation analysis of trace elements in motor neuron disease spinal cord. Neurodegeneration; 4:383–90.

Marti-Fabregas J, Pujol J. (1990). Selective involvement of the pyramidal tract on magnetic resonance imaging in primary lateral sclerosis. Neurology; 40:1799–800.

Martin D, Thompson MA, Nadler JV. (1993). The neuroprotective agent riluzole inhibits release of glutamate and aspartate from slices of hippocampal area CA1. Eur J Pharmacol; 250:473–6.

Martin JE, Mather K, Swash M. (1993). Heterotopic neurons in amyotrophic lateral sclerosis. Neurology; 43:1420–2.

Masu Y, Wolf E, Holtman B, et al. (1993). Disruption of the CNTF gene results in motor neuron degeneration. Nature; 365:27–32.

Mathias CJ, Williams AC. (1994). The Shy–Drager syndrome (and multiple system atrophy). In: Neurodegenerative diseases, Calne DB, ed. Philadelphia: WB Saunders, pp. 743–67.

Mathur C, Prasad VVK, Raju VS, et al. (1993). Steroids and their conjugates in the mammalian brain. Biochemistry; 90:85–8.

Mattman A, Feldman H, Forster B, et al. (1997). Regional HmPAO SPECT and CT measurements in the diagnosis of Alzheimer's disease. Can J Neurol Sci; 24:22–8.

Mayo W, Dellu F, Robel P, et al. (1993). Infusion of neurosteroids into nucleus basalis magnocellularis affects cognitive processes in the rat. Brain Res; 607:324–8.

McComas AJ. (1977). Neuromuscular function and disorders. London: Butterworths, pp. 101–8.

McComas AJ. (1987). Motor neuron disorders. In: Clinical electromyography, Brown WF, Bolton CF, eds. Boston: Butterworths, pp. 431–51.

McComas AJ. (1991). Invited review: motor unit estimation: methods, results and present status. Muscle & Nerve; 14:585–97.

McComas AJ. (1994). Motor unit estimation: Anxieties and achievements. Nineteenth annual Edward H Lambert Lecture of the AAEM. Rochester, Minn., Johnson Printing Co Inc., pp. 39–48.

McComas AJ, Fawcett PRW, Campbell MJ, Sica REP. (1971). Electrophysiological estimation of the number of motor units within a human muscle. J Neurol Neurosurg Psychiatry; 34:121–31

McCormick DA. (1992). Neurotransmitter actions in the thalamus and cerebral cortex. J Clin Neurophysiol; 9:212–23.

McCormick DA, Wang Z, Huguenard J. (1993). Neurotransmitter control of neocortical neuronal activity and excitability. Cerebral Cortex; 3:387–98.

McGeer EG, McGeer PL. (1994). Neurodegeneration and the immune system. In: Neurodegenerative diseases, Calne DB, ed. Philadelphia: WB Saunders, pp. 277–99.

McGeer PL, Rogers J, McGeer EG. (1994). Neuroimmune mechanisms in Alzheimer's disease pathogenesis. Alzheimer's Disease & Associated Disorders; 8:149–58.

McGuire V, Longstreth WT, Koepsell TD, van Belle G. (1996). Incidence of amyotrophic lateral sclerosis in three counties in western Washington state. Neurology; 47:571–3.

McHolm GB, Aguilar MJ, Norris FH. (1984). Lipofuscin in amyotrophic lateral sclerosis. Arch Neurol; 41:1187–8.

McLarnon JG. (1995). Potassium currents in motoneurons. Prog Neurobiol; 47:513–31.

Meier DH, Schott KJ. (1988). Free amino acid pattern of cerebrospinal fluid in amyotrophic lateral sclerosis. Acta Neurol Scand; 77:50–3.

Melki J, Abdelhak S, Sheth P, et al. (1990). Gene for chronic proximal spinal muscular atrophies maps to chromosome 5q. Nature; 344:767–8.

Merton PA, Morton HB. (1980). Stimulation of cerebral cortex in intact human subject. Nature; 285;227–8.

Migheli A, Cavalla P, Piva R, Giordana MT, et al. (1994). bcl-2 protein expression in aged brain and neurodegenerative diseases. NeuroReport; 5:1906–8.

Miles TS, Turker KS, Le TH. (1989). Ia reflexes and EPSPs in human soleus motor neurons. Exp Brain Res; 77:628–36.

Miller RG, Bouchard JP, Duquette P, et al. (1996a). Clinical trials of riluzole in patients with ALS. Neurology; 47(Suppl. 2):S86–S92.

Miller RG, Gelinas D, Moore M, et al. (1996b). A placebo-controlled trial of gabapentin in amyotrophic lateral sclerosis. Neurology; 46(Suppl. 2):A469.

Miller RG, Petajan JH, Bryan WW. (1996c). A placebo-controlled trial of recombinant human ciliary neurotrophic (rh CNTF) factor in amyotrophic lateral sclerosis. Ann Neurol; 39:256–60.

Miller RG, Smith SA, Murphy JR, et al. (1996d). A clinical trial of verapamil in amyotrophic lateral sclerosis. Muscle & Nerve; 19:511–15.

Mills KR. (1995). Motor neuron disease: Studies of the corticospinal excitation of single motor neurons by magnetic brain stimulation. Brain; 118:971–82.

Mills KR, Kohara N. (1997). Magnetic brain stimulation in ALS: Single motor unit studies. In: Physiology of ALS and related diseases, Kimura J, Kaji R, eds. Amsterdam: Elsevier Science, pp. 177–92.

Mirowitz S, Sartor K, Gado M, Torack R. (1989). Focal signal-intensity variations in the posterior internal capsule: normal MR findings and distinction from pathologic findings. Radiology; 172:535–9.

Mitchell JD. (1997). Disorders of anterior horn cell. In: Spinal cord disease: Basic science, diagnosis and management, Crtitchley E, Eisen A, eds. London: Springer-Verlag, pp. 347–65.

Mitsumoto H, Pioro EP. (1995). Animal models of amyotrophic lateral sclerosis. Adv Neurol; 68:73–91.

Moriwaka F, Okumura H, Tashiro K, *et al.* (1993). Motor neuron disease and past poliomyelitis. Geographic study in Hokkaido, the northern-most island of Japan. ALS Study Group. J Neurol; 240:13–16.

Morrison KE. (1996). Advances in SMA research: review of gene deletions. Neuromusc Disord; 6:397–408.

Munoz DG, Greene C, Perl DP, Selkoe DJ. (1988). Accumulation of phosphorylated neurofilaments in anterior horn motoneurons of amyotrophic lateral sclerosis patients. J Neuropath Exp Neurol; 47:9–18.

Munsat TL. (1995). Issues in amyotrophic lateral sclerosis clinical trial design. In: Pathogenesis and therapy of amyotrophic lateral sclerosis, Searratrice G, Munsat T, eds. Advances in Neurology, Vol. 68. Philadelphia: Lippincott-Raven Publishers, pp. 209–18.

Munsat TL. (1996). Issues in clinical trial design 1: Use of natural history controls. A protagonist view. Neurology; 47(Suppl.):S96–S97.

Munsat TL, Andres PL, Finison L, *et al.* (1988). The natural history of motoneuron loss in amyotrophic lateral sclerosis. Neurology; 38:409–13.

Murphy MF, Felice K, Gawel M, *et al.* (1995). A double-blind, placebo-controlled study of myotrophin (CEP-151) in the treatment of amyotrophic lateral sclerosis. Ann Neurol; 38:335.

Murray NMF. (1993). Motor evoked potentials. In: Electrodiagnosis in clinical neurology, 2nd ed., Aminoff MJ, ed. New York: Churchill Livingstone, pp. 605–26.

Nag S, Riopelle RJ. (1990). Spinal neuronal pathology associated with continuous intrathecal infusion of N-methyl-D-aspartate in the rat. Acta Neuropath; 81:7–13.

Nakajima M, Eisen A, McCarthy R, *et al.* (1996). Reduced corticomotoneuronal excitatory postsynaptic potentials (EPSPs) with normal Ia afferent EPSPs in amyotrophic lateral sclerosis. Neurology; 47:1555–65.

Nakamura R, Kamakura K, Kwak S. (1994). Late onset selective damage in the rat spinal cord induced by continuous intrathecal administration of AMPA. Brain Res; 654:279–85.

Nakano I, Hirayama K, Terao K. (1987). Hepatic ultrastructural changes and liver dysfunction in amyotrophic lateral sclerosis. Arch Neurol; 44:103–6.

Nasman B, Olsson T, Backstrom T, *et al.* (1991). Serum dehydroepiandrosterone sulphate in Alzeimer's disease and multi-infarct dementia. Biol Psychiatry; 30:684–90.

Neilson S, Robinson I, Clifford Rose F, Hunter M. (1993). Rising mortality from motor neuron disease: an explanation. Acta Neurol Scand; 87:184–91.

Nelson LM. (1996). Epidemiology of ALS. Clin Neurosci; 3:327–31.

Nihei K, Kowall NW, McKee AC. (1992). Degeneration of non-pyramidal local circuit neurons in the motor cortex of amyotrophic lateral sclerosis patients (abstract). J Neuropathol Exp Neurol; 51:322.

Nihei K, McKee AC, Kowall NW. (1993). Patterns of neuronal degeneration in the motor cortex of amyotrophic lateral sclerosis patients. Acta Neuropathol; 86:55–64.

Nishi R. (1994). Neurotrophic factors: two are better than one. Science; 265:1052–3.

Nixon RA, Sihag RK. (1991). Neurofilament phosphorylation: a new look at regulation and function. Trends Neurosci; 14:501–6.

Nobile-Orazio E. (1996). Editorial: Multifocal motor neuropathy. J Neurol Neurosurg Psychiatry; 60:599–603.

Norris FH Jr. (1965). Synchronous fasciculations in motor neuron disease. Arch Neurol; 13:495–500.

Norris FH Jr. (1992). Amyotrophic lateral sclerosis: The clinical disorder. In: Handbook of amyotrophic lateral sclerosis, Smith RA, ed. New York: Marcel Dekker, pp. 3–38.

Norris FH, Engle WK. (1965). Carcinomatous amyotrophic lateral sclerosis. In: The remote effects of cancer on the nervous system, Brain WR, Norris FH, eds. New York: Grune & Stratton, pp. 24–34.

Nyormoi O. (1996). Proteolytic activity in amyotrophic lateral sclerosis preparations. Ann Neurol; 40:701–6.

Oba H, Araki T, Monzawa S, et al. (1992). MR imaging of amyotrophic lateral sclerosis. Nippon Acta Radiol; 52:427–35.

O'Doherty DS. (1961). The amyotrophic lateral sclerosis syndrome. Dis Nerv Syst; 22:305–12.

O'Gara RW, Brown JM, Whiting MG. (1964). Induction of hepatic and renal tumours by topical application of aqueous extract of the cycad nut to artificial skin ulcers in mice. Third Conference on Toxicity of Cycads. Fed Proc; 23:1383

Olanow CW. (1993). A rationale for monoamine oxidase inhibition as neuroprotective therapy for Parkinson's disease. Movement Disorders; 8(Suppl. 1):1–7.

Olanow CW, Arendash GW. (1994). Metals and free radicals in neurodegeneration. Current Opinion in Neurol; 7:548–58.

Ono S, Yamauchi M. (1992). Collagen cross-linking of skin in patients with amyotrophic lateral sclerosis. Ann Neurol; 31:305–10.

Ono S, Yamauchi M. (1994) Elastin cross-linking in the skin from patients with amyotrophic lateral sclerosis. J Neurol Neurosurg Psychiat; 57:94–6.

Oppenheim RW. (1991). Cell death during development of the nervous system. Annu Rev Neurosci; 14:453–501.

Oppenheim RW, Houenou LJ, Johnson JE, Lin L-FH, et al. (1995). Developing motor neurons rescued from programmed and axotomy-induced cell death by GDNF. Nature; 373:344–6.

Oppenheim RW, Qin-Wei Y, Prevette D, Yan Q. (1992). Brain-derived neurotrophic factor rescues developing avian motoneurons from cell death. Nature; 360:755–7.

O'Reilly SA, Roedica J, Nagy D, et al. (1995). Motor neuron–astrocyte interactions and levels of Cu,Zn superoxide dismutase in sporadic amyotrophic lateral sclerosis. Exp Neurol; 131:203–10.

Palmer E, Ashby P. (1992a). Corticospinal projections to upper limb motoneurons in humans. J Physiol; 448:397–411.

Palmer E, Ashby P. (1992b). The transcortical nature of the late reflex responses in human small hand muscle to digital nerve stimulation. Exp Brain Res; 91:320–6.

Palmer SS, Fetz EE. (1985). Effects of single intracortical microstimuli in motor cortex on activity of identified forearm motor units in behaving monkeys. J Neurophysiol; 54:1194–212.

Pamphlett R, Kril J, Hng TM. (1995). Motor neuron disease: A primary disorder of corticomotoneuron? Muscle & Nerve; 18:314–18.

Pant B, Eisen A, Stewart H. (1992). Some fasciculations in ALS result from corticomotoneuronal drive. Neurology; 42(Suppl. 3):468.

Pardo, CA, Xu Z, Borchelt DR, et al. (1995). Superoxide dismutase is an abundant component in cell bodies, dendrites, and axons of motor neurons and in a subset of other neurons. Proc Natl Acad Sci USA; 92:954–8.

Parry GJ. (1996). AAEM Case report No. 30: multifocal motor neuropathy. Muscle & Nerve; 19:269–76.

Parry GJ, Sumner AJ. (1992). Multifocal motor neuropathy. Neurologic Clinics; 10:671–84.

Patten BM, Harati Y, Acosta L, et al. (1978). Free amino acid levels in amyotrophic lateral sclerosis. Ann Neurol; 3:305–9.

Paty DW, Moore GRW. (1998). Magnetic resonance imaging changes as living pathology in multiple sclerosis. In: Multiple sclerosis, Paty DW, Ebers G, eds. Philadelphia: F.A. Davis, pp. 328–60.

Perl DP, Gajdusek DC, Garruto RM, et al. (1982). Intraneuronal aluminum accumulation in amyotrophic lateral sclerosis and Parkinsonism–dementia of Guam. Science; 217:1053–5.

Perry TL, Bergeron C, Steele JC, et al. (1990a). Brain amino acid contents are dissimilar in sporadic and Guamanian amyotrophic lateral sclerosis. J Neurol Sci; 99:3–8.

Perry TL, Hansen S. (1990). What excitotoxin kills striatal neurons in Huntington's disease? Clues from neurochemical studies. Neurology; 40:20–4.

Perry TL, Hansen S, Jones K. (1987). Brain glutamate deficiency in amyotrophic lateral sclerosis. Neurology; 37:1845–8.

Perry TL, Krieger C, Hansen S, Eisen A. (1990b). Amyotrophic lateral sclerosis: amino acid levels in plasma and cerebrospinal fluid. Ann Neurol; 28:12–17.

Perry TL, Krieger C, Hansen S, Tabatabaei A. (1991). Amyotrophic lateral sclerosis: fasting plasma levels of cysteine and inorganic sulfate are normal, as are brain contents of cysteine. Neurology; 41:487–90.

Pestronk A, Choksi R, Blume G, Lopate G. (1997). Multifocal motor neuropathy: serum IgM binding to a GM1 ganglioside-containing lipid mixture but not to GM1 alone. Neurology; 48:1104–6.

Phillips CG. (1975). Laying the ghost of 'muscles versus movements'. Can J Neurol Sci; 2:209–18.

Pioro EP, Antel JP, Cashman NR, Arnold DL. (1994). Detection of cortical neuron loss in motor neuron disease by proton magnetic resonance spectroscopy imaging in vivo. Neurology; 44:1933–8.

Plaitakis A. (1990). Glutamate dysfunction and selective motor neuron degeneration in amyotrophic lateral sclerosis: a hypothesis. Ann Neurol; 28:3–8.

Plaitakis A, Caroscio JT. (1987). Abnormal glutamate metabolism in amyotrophic lateral sclerosis. Ann Neurol; 22:575–9.

Plaitakis A, Constantakakis E. (1993). Altered metabolism of excitatory amino acids, N-acetyl-aspartate and N-acetyl-aspartyl-glutamate in amyotrophic lateral sclerosis. Brain Res Bull; 30:381–6.

Plaitakis A, Constantakakis E, Smith J. (1988a). The neuroexcitotoxic amino acids glutamate and aspartate are altered in the spinal cord and brain in amyotrophic lateral sclerosis. Ann Neurol; 24:446–9.

Plaitakas A, Fesdjian CO, Shashidharan P. (1996). Glutamate antagonists in amyotrophic lateral sclerosis: A review of their therapeutic potential. CNS Drugs; 5:437–56.

Plaitakis A, Mandeli J, Fesdjian C, Swak MA. (1991). Dysregulation of glutamate metabolism in ALS: correlation with gender and disease type. Neurology; 41(Suppl.):392.

Plaitakis A, Sivak M, Fesdjian CO, Mandeli J. (1992). Treatment of amyotrophic lateral sclerosis with branched chain amino acids (BCAA): Results of a second trial. Neurology; 42(Suppl. 3):454.

Plaitakis A, Smith J, Mandeli J, Yahr MD. (1988b). Pilot trial of branched-chain amino acids in amyotrophic lateral sclerosis. Lancet; 1:1015–18.

Porter R, Lemon R. (1993). Corticospinal function and voluntary movement. Monographs of the Physiological Society No.45. Oxford: Clarendon Press, pp. 1–421.

Pouget J, Schmied A, Morin D, *et al.* (1994). Comparison of single motor units electrical and mechanical properties in amyotrophic lateral sclerosis. J Neurol; 241(Suppl.):S15.

Pringle CE, Hudson AJ, Munoz DG, *et al.* (1992). Primary lateral sclerosis. Clinical features, neuropathology and diagnostic criteria. Brain; 115:495–520.

Prout AJ, Eisen A. (1994). The cortical silent period and amyotrophic lateral sclerosis. Muscle & Nerve; 17:217–23.

Przedborski S, Dhawan V, Donaldson DM, *et al.* (1996). Nigrostriatal dopaminergic function in familial amyotrophic lateral sclerosis patients with and without copper/zinc superoxide dismutase mutations. Neurology; 47:1546–51.

Pullen AH. (1996). Selective neuronal vulnerability in motor neurone diseases with reference to sparing of Onuf's nucleus, In: The neurobiology of disease, Bostock H, Kirkwood PA, Pullen AH, eds. Cambridge: Cambridge University Press, pp. 411–26.

Rabizadeh S, Gralla EB, Borchelt DR, *et al.* (1995). Mutations associated with amyotrophic lateral sclerosis convert superoxide dismutase from an antiapoptotic gene to a proapoptotic gene: studies in yeast and neural cells. Proc Natl Acad Sci USA; 92:3024–8.

Radunovic A, Leigh PN. (1996). Cu/Zn superoxide dismutase gene mutations in amyotrophic lateral sclerosis: correlation between genotype and clinical features. J Neurol Neurosurg Psychiatry; 61:565–72.

Reed DM, Kurland LT. (1963). Muscle fasciculation in a healthy population. Arch Neurol; 9:363.

Regelson W, Kalimi M. (1994). Dehydroepiandrosterone (DHEA) – the multifunctional steroid. In: The aging clock: The pineal gland and other pacemakers in the progression of aging and carcinogenesis. Third Stromboli Conference on Aging and Cancer. Pierpaoli W, Regelson W, Fabris N, eds. Ann NY Acad Sci; 719:564–72.

Regelson W, Kalimi M, Loria R. (1990). DHEA: some thoughts as to its biological and clinical action. In: Biological role of dehydroepiandrosterone (DHEA), Kalimi M, Regelson W, eds. New York: Walter de Gruyter, pp. 405–45.

Reid MB, Stokic DS, Koch SM, Khawli FA, Leis AA. (1994). N-acetylcysteine inhibits muscle fatigue in humans. J Clin Invest; 94:2468–74.

Reider CR, Paulson GW. (1997). Lou Gehrig and amyotrophic lateral sclerosis. Is Vitamin E to be revisited? Arch Neurol; 54:527–8.

Reiner A, Medina L, Figuerdo-Cardenas G, Anfinson S. (1995). Brainstem motoneuron pools that are selectively resistant in amyotrophic lateral sclerosis are preferentially enriched in parvalbumin: Evidence from monkey brainstem for a calcium-mediated mechanism in sporadic ALS. Exp Neurol; 131:239–50.

Renston JP, DiMarco AF, Supinski GS. (1994). Respiratory muscle rest using nasal BiPAP ventilation in patients with stable severe COPD. Chest; 105:1053–60.

Rich JB, Rasmusson DX, Carson KA, et al. (1995). Nonsteroidal anti-inflammatory drugs in Alzheimer's disease. Neurology; 45:51–5.

Riggs JE. (1993). Antecedent trauma and amyotrophic lateral sclerosis in young adult men. Military Med; 158:55–7.

Riggs JE. (1995). Trauma, axonal injury, and amyotrophic lateral sclerosis: a clinical correlate of a neuropharmacologic model. Clin Neuropharmacol; 18:273–6.

Riggs JE. (1996). Amyotrophic lateral sclerosis, heterogeneous susceptibility, trauma, and epidemiology. Arch Neurol; 53:225–7.

Ripps ME, Huntley CW, Hof PR, et al. (1995). Transgenic mice expressing an altered murine superoxide dismutase gene provide an animal model of amyotrophic lateral sclerosis. Proc Natl Acad Sci USA; 92:689–93.

Robberecht W, Sapp P, Kristina M, et al. (1994). Cu/Zn superoxide dismutase activity in familialand sporadic amyotrophic lateral sclerosis. J Neurochem; 62:384–7.

Rodgers-Johnson P, Garruto RM, Yanagihara R, et al. (1986). Amyotrophic lateral sclerosis and Parkinsonism–dementia on Guam: a 30-year evaluation of clinical and neuropathologic trends. Neurology; 36:7–13.

Rogers J, Kirby LC, Hempe SR, et al. (1993). Clinical trial of indomethacin in Alzheimer's disease. Neurology; 43:1609–11.

Roman GC. (1996). Neuroepidemiology of amyotrophic lateral sclerosis: clues to aetiology and pathogenesis. J Neurol Neurosurg Psychiatry; 61:131–7.

Rosen DR, Siddique T, Patterson D, et al. (1993). Mutations in Cu/Zn superoxide dismutase gene are associated with familial amyotrophic lateral sclerosis. Nature; 362:59–62.

Rosenfeld MR, Posner JB. (1991). Paraneoplastic motor neuron disease. In: Amyotrophic lateral sclerosis and other motor neuron diseases, Rowland LP, ed. Advances in Neurology, Vol. 56. New York: Raven Press, pp. 455–62.

Rosling H. (1986). Cassava, cyanide, and epidemic spastic paraparesis. A study in Mozambique on dietary cyanide exposure. Acta Univ Upsal; 19:1–52.

Rossi M. (1994). Classical pathology. In: Motor neuron disease, Williams AC, ed. London: Chapman & Hall, pp. 307–41.

Roth G. (1984). Fasciculations and their F-response – localization of their axonal origin. J Neurol Sci; 63:299–306.

Rothman SM. (1992). Excitotoxins: possible mechanisms of action. NY Acad Sci; 648:132–8.

Rothstein JD. (1996a). Excitotoxicity hypothesis. Neurology; 47(Suppl. 2):S19–S26.

Rothstein JD. (1996b). Excitotoxic mechanisms in the pathogenesis of amyotrophic lateral sclerosis. In: Pathogenesis and therapy of amyotrophic lateral sclerosis, Serratrice G, Munsat T, eds. Philadelphia: Lippincott-Raven Publishers, pp. 7–27.

Rothstein JD, Bristol LA, Hosler B, Brown RH Jr, *et al.* (1994). Chronic inhibition of superoxide dismutase produces apoptotic death in spinal neurons. Proc Natl Acad Sci; 91:4155–9.

Rothstein JD, Jin L, Dykes-Hoberg M, Kuncl RW. (1993). Chronic glutamate uptake inhibition produces a model of slow neurotoxicity. Proc Natl Acad Sci USA; 90:6591–5.

Rothstein JD, Kuncl R, Chaudhry V, *et al.* (1991). Excitatory amino acids in amyotrophic lateral sclerosis: An update. Ann Neurol; 30:224–5.

Rothstein JD, Martin L, Dykes-Hoberg M, *et al.* (1995). Selective loss of glial glutamate transporter GLT-1 in amyotrophic lateral sclerosis. Ann Neurol; 38:73–84.

Rothstein, JD, Martin LJ, Kuncl RW. (1992). Decreased glutamate transport by the brain and spinal cord in amyotrophic lateral sclerosis. New Engl J Med; 326:1464–8.

Rouleau GA, Clark AW, Rooke K, *et al.* (1996). SOD 1 mutation is associated with accumulation of neurofilaments in amyotrophic lateral sclerosis. Ann Neurol; 39:128–31.

Rowland LP. (1994a). Natural history and clinical features of amyotrophic lateral sclerosis and related motor neuron diseases. In: Neurodegenerative diseases, Calne DB, ed. Philadelphia: WB Saunders, pp. 507–21.

Rowland LP. (1994b). Riluzole for the treatment of amyotrophic lateral sclerosis: too soon to tell? N Engl J Med; 330:636–7.

Rowland LP. (1995). Amyotrophic lateral sclerosis with paraproteins and autoantibodies. In: Pathogenesis and therapy of amyotrophic lateral sclerosis, Serratrice G, Munsat T, eds. Advances in Neurology, Vol. 68. Philadelphia: Lippincott-Raven Publishers, pp. 93–105.

Rowland LP. (1997). Muscular atrophies, motor neuropathies, amyotrophic lateral sclerosis and immunology. In: Physiology of ALS and related diseases, Kimura J, Kaji R, eds. Amsterdam: Elsevier Science, pp. 3–11.

Rowland LP, Louis E, Youner DS, *et al.* (1994). Lymphoproliferative diseases and motor neuron diseases. In: ALS – From Charcot to the present and into the future, Rose FC, ed. London: Smith Gordon, pp. 113–16.

Roy DN, Spencer PS, Nunn PB. (1986). Toxic components of Lathyrus. In: Lathyrus and lathyrism, Kaul AK, Combes D, eds. New York: TWMRF Press, pp. 287–96.

Roy N, Mahadevan MS, McLean M, *et al.* (1995). The gene for neuronal apoptosis inhibitory protein is partially deleted in individuals with spinal muscular atrophy. Cell; 80:167–78.

Salazar AM, Masters CL, Gajdusek DC, Gibbs CJ Jr. (1983). Syndromes of amyotrophic lateral sclerosis and dementia: relation to transmissible Creutzfeldt–Jakob disease. Ann Neurol; 14:17–26.

Salemi G, Fierro B, Arcara A, *et al.* (1989). Amyotrophic lateral sclerosis in Palermo, Italy: an epidemiological study. Ital J Neurol Sci; 10:505–9.

Sales Luís ML, Hormigo A, Mauricio C, *et al.* (1990). Magnetic resonance imaging in motor neuron disease. J Neurol; 237:471–4.

Sardesai VM. (1995). Role of antioxidants in health maintenance. Nutrition in Clinical Practice; 10:19–25.

Savettieri G, Salemi G, Arcara A, *et al.* (1991). A case-control study of amyotrophic lateral sclerosis. Neuroepidemiol; 10:242–5.

Schmalbruch H, Jensen H-JS, Bjaerg M, *et al.* (1991). A new mouse mutant with progressive motor neuropathy. J Neuropathol Exp Neurol; 50:192–204.

Schriefer TN, Hess CW, Mills KR, Murray NM. (1989). Central motor conduction studies in motor neurone disease using magnetic brain stimulation. Electroencephal Clin Neurophysiol; 74:431–7.

Seeburger JL, Springer JE. (1993). Experimental rationale for the therapeutic use of neurotrophins in amyotrophic lateral sclerosis. Expt Neurol; 124:64–72.

Sendtner M, Holtmann B, Kolbeck R, *et al.* (1992). Brain-derived neurotrophic factor prevents the death of motoneurons in newborn rats after nerve section. Nature; 360:757–9.

Shaw PJ. (1993). Excitatory amino acid receptors, excitotoxicity, and the human nervous system. Curr Opin Neurol Neurosurg; 6:414–22.

Shaw PJ, Chinnery RM, Ince PG. (1994a). [3H]D-Aspartate binding sites in the normal human spinal cord and changes in motor neuron disease: a quantitative autoradiographic study. Brain Res; 655:195–201.

Shaw PJ, Chinnery RM, Ince PG. (1994b). Non-NMDA receptors in motor neuron disease (MND): a quantitative autoradiographic study in spinal cord and motor cortex using [3H]CNQX and [3H]kainate. Brain Res; 655:186–94.

Shaw PJ, Forrest V, Ince PG, *et al.* (1995). CSF and plasma amino acid levels in motor neuron disease: elevation of csf glutamate in a subset of patients. Neurodegeneration; 4:209–16.

Shibasaki H. (1997). Physiological abnormalities of motor cortex in motor neuron diseases studied by neuroimaging. In: Physiology of ALS and related diseases, Kimura J, Kaji R, eds. Amsterdam: Elsevier Science, pp. 193–200.

Shibata N, Hirano A, Kobayashi M, *et al.* (1993). Immunohistochemical demonstration of Cu/Zn superoxide dismutase in the spinal cord of patients with familial amyotrophic lateral sclerosis. Acta Histochem Cytochem; 26:619–22.

Shiraki H, Yase Y. (1991). Amyotrophic lateral sclerosis and Parkinsonism-dementia in the Kii Peninsula: comparison with the same disorders in Guam and with Alzheimer's disease. Handbook of Clinical Neurology; 15(59):273–300.

Shuldiner AR. (1996). Transgenic animals. N Engl J Med; 334:653–5.

Siddique T, Figlewicz DA, Percak-Vance MA, *et al.* (1991). Linkage of a gene causing familial amyotrophic lateral sclerosis to chromosome 21 and evidence of genetic-locus heterogeneity. N Engl J Med; 324:1381–4.

Siddique T, Nijhawan D, Hentati A. (1996). Molecular genetic basis of familial ALS. Neurology; 47(Suppl.):S27–S35.

Siklos L, Engelhardt J, Harati Y, Smith RG. (1996). Ultrastructural evidence for altered calcium in motor nerve terminals in amyotrophic lateral sclerosis. Ann Neurol; 39:203–16.

Sillevis Smitt PAE, de Jong JMBV. (1989). Animal models of amyotrophic lateral sclerosis and the spinal muscular atrophies. J Neurol Sci; 91:231–58.

Singh RB, Niaz MA, Bishnoi I, *et al.* (1994). Diet, antioxidant vitamins, oxidative stress and risk of coronary artery disease: the Peerzada Prospective Study. Acta Cardiologica; 49:453–67.

Slawnych MP, Laszlo CA, Hershler C. (1996). Motor unit estimates obtained using the new 'MUESA' method. Muscle & Nerve; 19:626–36.

Smith RG, Alexianu M, Crawford G, *et al.* (1994). Cytotoxicity of immunoglobulins from amyotrophic lateral sclerosis patients on a hybrid motoneuron cell line. Proc Natl Acad Sci USA; 91:3393–7.

Smith RG, Engelhardt JL, Tajti J, Appel SH. (1993). Experimental immune-mediated motor neuron disease: models for human ALS. Brain Res Bull; 30:373–80.

Smith RG, Hamilton S, Hofmann F, *et al.* (1992). Serum antibodies to L-type calcium channels in patients with amyotrophic lateral sclerosis. N Engl J Med; 327:1721–8.

Snider WD. (1995). Parvalbumin is a marker of ALS-resistant motor neurons. Neuroreport; 6:449–52.

Snow B. (1994). Positron emission tomography. In: Neurodegenerative diseases, Calne DB, ed. Philadelphia: W.B. Saunders, pp. 427–44.

Sohal RS, Kua HH, Agarwal S, Forster Mj, Lal H. (1994). Oxidative damage, mitochondrial oxidant generation and antioxidant defenses: during aging and in response to food restriction in the mouse. Mech Aging Devel; 74:121–33.

Spencer PS, Allen CN, Kisby GE, *et al.* (1991). Lathyrism and western Pacific amyotrophic lateral sclerosis: etiology of short and long latency motor system disorders. In: Amyotrophic lateral sclerosis and other motor neuron diseases, Rowland LP, ed. Advances in Neurology, Vol. 56. New York: Raven Press, pp. 287–310.

Spencer PS, Kisby GE, Ross SM, *et al.* (1993). Guam ALS-PDC: possible causes. Science; 262:825–6.

Spencer PS, Nunn PB, Hugon J, *et al.* (1987). Guam amyotrophic lateral sclerosis–Parkinsonism–dementia linked to a plant excitant neurotoxin. Science; 237:517–22.

Stålberg E. (1986). Single fiber EMG, Macro EMG, and scanning EMG, new ways of looking at the motor unit. Crc Crit Rev Clin Neurobiol; 2:125–67.

Stålberg E. (1990). Macro EMG. Methods in Clin Neurophysiol; 1:1–14.

Stålberg E, Sanders DB. (1984). The motor unit in ALS studied with different neurophysiological techniques. In: Progress in motor neurone disease, Rose CF, ed. London: Pitman Books, pp. 105–22.

Steiner T, *et al.* (1994). Multinational trial of branched-chain amino acids in amyotrophic lateral sclerosis. Muscle & Nerve; Suppl. 1:S66.

Stewart GR, Olney JW, Pathikonda M, Snider WD. (1991). Excitotoxicity in the embryonic chick spinal cord. Ann Neurol; 30:758–66.

Strickland D, Smith SA, Dolliff G, *et al.* (1996). Amyotrophic lateral sclerosis and occupational history. A pilot case-control study. Arch Neurol; 53:730–3.

Strong M. (1994). Aluminum neurotoxicity: an experimental approach to the induction of neurofilamentous inclusions. J Neurol Sci; 124:20–6.

Strong MJ, Grace GM, Orange JB, Leeper HA. (1996). Cognition, language and speech in amyotrophic lateral sclerosis: a review. J Clin Exp Neuropsychol; 18:291–303.

Strong MJ, Hudson AJ, Alvord WG. (1991). Familial amyotrophic lateral sclerosis, 1850–1989: a statistical analysis of the world literature. Can J Neurol Sci; 13:317–19.

Swash M. (1995). The diagnosis of amyotrophic lateral sclerosis: A discussion. In: Pathogenesis and therapy of amyotrophic lateral sclerosis, Serratrice G, Munsat T, eds. Advances in Neurology, Vol. 68. Philadelphia: Lippincott-Raven Publishers, pp. 157–60.

Swash M, Leader M, Brown A, Swettenham KW. (1986). Focal loss of anterior horn cells in the cervical cord in motor neuron disease. Brain; 109:939–52.

Swash M, Schwartz MS. (1992). What do we really know about amyotrophic lateral sclerosis. J Neurol Sci; 113:4–16.

Swingler RJ, Fraser H, Warlow CP. (1992). Motor neuron disease and polio in Scotland. J Neurol Neurosurg Psychiatry; 55:1116–20.

Tahmoush AJ, Alonso RJ, Tahmoush GP, Heiman-Patterson TD. (1991). Cramp–fasciculation syndrome: a treatable hyperexcitable peripheral nerve disorder. Neurology; 41:1021–4.

Takahashi H, Snow BJ, Bhatt MH, *et al.* (1993). Evidence for a dopaminergic deficit in sporadic amyotrophic lateral sclerosis. Lancet; 342:1016–18.

Tanaka M, Kondo S, Hirai S, *et al.* (1993). Cerebral blood flow and oxygen metabolism in progressive dementia associated with amyotrophic lateral sclerosis. J Neuro Sci; 120:22–8.

Tandan R, Bromberg MB, Forshew D, *et al.* (1996). A controlled trial of amino acid therapy in amyotrophic lateral sclerosis: I. Clinical, functional, and maximum isometric torque data. Neurology; 47:1220–6.

Taylor CP. (1994). Emerging perspectives on the mechanism of action of gabapentin. Neurology; 44(Suppl. 5):S10–S16.

Teitlebaum JS, Zatorre RJ, Carpenter S, *et al.* (1990). Neurologic sequelae of domoic acid intoxication due to the ingestion of contaminated mussels. N Engl J Med; 322:1781–7.

Terao S-i, Sobue G, Yasuda T, *et al.* (1995). Magnetic resonance imaging of the corticospinal tracts in amyotrophic lateral sclerosis. J Neurol Sci; 133:66–72.

Terry RD, De Teresa R, Hansen LA. (1987). Neocortical cell counts in normal human adult aging. Ann Neurol; 21:530–9.

Testa D, Caraceni T, Fetoni V. (1989). Branched-chain amino acids in the treatment of amyotrophic lateral sclerosis. J Neurol; 236:445–7.

Thorpe JW, Moseley IF, Hawkes CH, *et al.* (1996). Brain and spinal cord MRI in motor neuron disease. J Neurol Neurosurg Psychiatry; 61:314–17.

Toma S, Shiozawa Z. (1995). Amyotrophic cervical myelopathy in adolescence. J Neurol Neurosurg Psychiatry; 58:56–64.

Tomlinson BE, Irving D. (1977). The number of limb motor neurons in the human lumbosacral cord throughout life. J Neurol Sci; 34:213–25.

Tomohiko M, Aki M, Shiozawa R, *et al.* (1990). Development of ophthalmoplegia in amyotrophic lateral sclerosis during long-term use of respirators. J Neurol Sci; 99:311–19.

Tonstad S. (1995). Antiksidanter og hjerte-og karsykdom – epidemiologiske aspekter. Bor tilskudd anbefales for hoyrisikopasienter? Tidsskrift for Den Norske Laegeforening; 115:227–9.

Triggs WJ, Macdonell RAL, Cros D, Chiappa KH, Shahani BT, Day BJ. (1992). Motor inhibition and excitation are independent effects of magnetic cortical stimulation. Ann Neurol; 32:345–51.

Trojaborg W, Buchthal F. (1965). Malignant and benign fasciculations. Acta Neurol Scand; 41(Suppl. 13):251–4.

Trojaborg W, Hays AP, Van Den Berg L, Younger DS, Latov N. (1995). Motor conduction parameters in neuropathies associated with anti-MAG antibodies and other types of demyelinating and axonal neuropathies. Muscle & Nerve; 18:730–5.

Troost D, Aten J, Morsink F, de Jong JMBV. (1995). Apoptosis in ALS is not restricted to motoneurons. J Neurol Sci; 129(Suppl.):79–80.

Tsai GC, Stauch-Slusher B, Sim L, *et al.* (1991). Reduction in acidic amino and N-acetylaspartylglutamate in amyotrophic lateral sclerosis CNS. Brain Res; 556:151–6.

Tsujihata M, Hazama R, Yoshimura T, *et al.* (1984). The motor endplate fine structure and ultrastructural localization of acetylcholine receptors in amyotrophic lateral sclerosis. Muscle Nerve; 7:243–9.

Tsukagoshi H, Yanigisawa N, Oguchi K, *et al.* (1979). Morphometric quantification of the cervical limb motor cells in controls and in amyotrophic lateral sclerosis. J Neurol Sci; 41:287–97.

Tu PH, Raju P, Robinson KA, *et al.* (1996). Transgenic mice carrying a human mutant superoxide dismutase transgene develop neuronal cytoskeletal pathology resembling human amyotrophic lateral sclerosis lesions. Proc Natl Acad Sci USA; 93:3155–60.

Tylleskar T, Banea M, Bikangi N, *et al.* (1992). Cassava cyanogens and konzo, an upper motor neuron disease found in Africa. Lancet; 339:208–11.

Tysnes OB, Vollset SE, Aarli JA. (1991). Epidemiology of amyotrophic lateral sclerosis in Hordaland county, western Norway. Acta Neurol Scand; 83:280–5.

Uchitel OD, Appel SH, Crawford F, Sczcupak L. (1988). Immunoglobulins from amyotrophic lateral sclerosis patients enhance spontaneous transmitter release from motor nerve terminals. Proc Natl Acad Sci USA; 85:7371–4.

Udaka F, Sawada H, Seriu N, *et al.* (1992). MRI and SPECT findings in amyotrophic lateral sclerosis. Neuroradiology; 34:389–93.

Uitti RJ, Berry K, Yasuhara O, *et al.* (1995). Neurodegenerative 'overlap' syndrome: clinical and pathological features of Parkinson's disease, motor neuron disease, and Alzheimer's disease. Parkin Rel Disord; 1:21–34.

Uozumi T, Tsuji S, Murai Y. (1991). Motor potentials evoked by magnetic stimulation of the motor cortex in normal subjects and patients with motor disorders. Electroenceph Clin Neurophysiol; 81:251–6.

Urca G, Urca R. (1990). Neurotoxic effects of excitatory amino acids in the mouse spinal cord: quisqualate and kainate but not N-methyl-D-aspartate induce permanent neural damage. Brain Res; 529:7–15.

Van Es HW, Van den Berg LH, Franssen H, *et al.* (1997). Magnetic resonance imaging of the brachial plexus in patients with multifocal motor neuropathy. Neurology; 48:1218–24.

Vatassery GT. (1992). Vitamin E. Neurochemistry and implications for neurodegeneration in Parkinson's disease. Ann NY Acad Sci; 669:97–109.

Veugelers B, Theys P, Lamme M, Van Hees JR. (1996). Pathological findings in a patient with amyotrophic lateral sclerosis and multifocal motorneuropathy with conduction block. J Neurol Sci; 136:64–71.

Vincent A, Drachman DB. (1996). Amyotrophic lateral sclerosis and antibodies to voltage-gated calcium channels – new doubts. Ann Neurol; 40:691–3.

Vinceti M, Guidetti D, Pinotti M, *et al.* (1996). Amyotrophic lateral sclerosis after long-term exposure to drinking water with high selenium content. Epidemiology; 7:529–32.

Wagey R, Krieger C, Shaw CA. (1997). Abnormal dephosphorylation effect on NMDA receptor regulation in ALS spinal cord. Neurobiol Dis; 4:350–5.

Wagey R, Lanius R, Charlton L, *et al.* (1996). Increased PI-3-kinase activity in ALS. Neurosci Abstr; 22:2143.

Wakayama I, Nerurkar VR, Strong MJ, Garruto RM. (1996). Comparative study of chronic aluminum-induced neurofilamentous aggregates with intracytoplasmic inclusions of amyotrophic lateral sclerosis. Acta Neuropath; 92:545–54.

Wang FC, Delwaide PJ. (1995). Number and relative size of thenar motor units estimated by an adapted multiple point stimulation method. Muscle & Nerve; 18:969–79.

Whitehouse PJ, Walmsley JK, Zarbin MA, *et al.* (1983). Amyotrophic lateral sclerosis: Alterations in neurotransmitter receptors. Ann Neurol; 14:8–16.

Wiedau-Pazos M, Goto JJ, Rabizadeh S, *et al.* (1996). Altered reactivity of superoxide dismutase in familial amyotrophic lateral sclerosis. Science; 271:515–17.

Wilhelmsen KC, Lynch T, Pavlou E, *et al.* (1994). Localization of disinhibition–dementia–Parkinsonism–amyotrophy complex to 17q21–22. Am J Hum Genet; 55:1159–65.

Williams DB. (1991). Familial amyotrophic lateral sclerosis. Handbook of Clinical Neurology; 59:241–51.

Wohlfart G. (1957). Collateral regeneration from residual motor nerve fibers in amyotrophic lateral sclerosis. Neurology; 7:124–34.

Wong PC, Pardo CA, Borchelt DR, *et al.* (1995). An adverse property of a familial ALS-linked SOD1 mutation causes motor neuron disease characterized by vacuolar degeneration of mitochondria. Neuron; 14:1105–16.

World Federation of Neurology Research Group on Neuromuscular Diseases Subcommittee on Motor Neuron Disease. (1995). Airlie House Guidelines: Therapeutic trials in amyotrophic lateral sclerosis. J Neurol Sci; 129(Suppl.):1–10.

Wu RM, Mohanakumar KP, Murphy DL, Chiueh CC. (1994). Antioxidant mechanism and protection of nigral neurons against MPP + toxicity by Deprenyl (selegiline) Ann NY Acad Sci; 738:214–21.

Xu Z, Cork LC, Griffin JW, Cleveland DW. (1993). Increased expression of neurofilament subunit NF-L produces morphological alterations that resemble the pathology of human motor neuron disease. Cell; 73:23–33.

Yamauchi H, Fukuyama H, Ouchi Y, *et al.* (1995). Corpus callosum atrophy in amyotrophic lateral sclerosis. J Neurol Sci; 134:189–96.

Yan Q, Matheson C, Lopez OT. (1995). In vivo neurotrophic effects of GDNF on neonatal and adult facial motor neurons. Nature; 373:341–4.

Yasui M, Yase Y, Ota K. (1991). Distribution of calcium in central nervous system tissue. J. Neurol Sci; 105:206.

Yielding KL, Tomkins GM. (1961). An effect of L-leucine and other essential amino acids on the structure and activity of glutamic dehydrogenase. Proc Natl Acad Sci USA; 47:983–9.

Yokota T, Yoshino A, Saito Y. (1996). Double cortical stimulation in amyotrophic lateral sclerosis. J Neurol Neurosurg Psychiatry; 61:596–600.

Younger DS, Rowland LP, Latov N, *et al.* (1990). Motor neuron disease and amyotrophic lateral sclerosis: relation of high CSF protein to paraproteinemia and clinical syndromes. Neurology; 40:595–9.

Younger DS, Rowland LP, Latov N, *et al.* (1991). Lymphoma, motor neuron diseases, and amyotrophic lateral sclerosis. Ann Neurol; 29:78–96.

Yuen EC, Mobley WC. (1996). Therapeutic potential of neurotrophic factors for neurological disorders. Ann Neurol; 40:346–54.

Zhainazarov AB, Annunziata P, Toneatto S, *et al.* (1994). Serum fractions from amyotrophic lateral sclerosis patients depress voltage-activated Ca^{2+} currents of rat cerebellar granule cells in culture. Neurosci Lett; 172:111–14.

Zhang ZX, Anderson DW, Mantel N, Roman GC. (1995). Motor neuron disease on Guam. Temporal occurrence, 1941–85. Acta Neurol Scand; 92:299–307.

Zhang ZX, Anderson DW, Mantel N, Roman GC. (1996). Motor neuron disease on Guam: geographic and and familial occurrence, 1956–85. Acta Neurol Scand; 94:1–9.

Zech VL, Telford IR. (1943). Negative therapeutic effect of massive doses of vitamin E on amyotrophic lateral sclerosis. Arch Neurol Psychiatry; 50:190–2.

Zeman S, Lloyd C, Meldrum B, Leigh PN. (1994). Excitatory amino acids, free radicals and the pathogenesis of motor neuron disease. Neuropath Appl Neurobiol; 20:219–31.

Ziv I, Achiron A, Djaldetti R, *et al.* (1994). Can nimodipine affect progression of motor neuron disease? A double blind study. Clin Neuropharmacol; 17:423–8.

Index

294

Printed in the United States
75647LV00001B/184-195